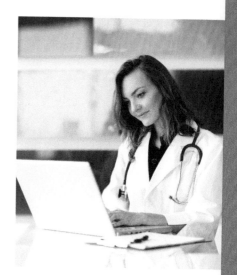

Cystic Fibrosis

Editor

JONATHAN L. KOFF

CLINICS IN CHEST MEDICINE

www.chestmed.theclinics.com

March 2016 • Volume 37 • Number 1

ELSEVIER

1600 John F. Kennedy Boulevard • Suite 1800 • Philadelphia, Pennsylvania, 19103-2899

http://www.theclinics.com

CLINICS IN CHEST MEDICINE Volume 37, Number 1
March 2016 ISSN 0272-5231, ISBN-13: 978-0-323-41641-2

Editor: Patrick Manley
Developmental Editor: Casey Jackson

Clinics in Chest Medicine (ISSN 0272-5231) is published quarterly by Elsevier Inc., 360 Park Avenue South, New York, NY 10010-1710. Months of issue are March, June, September, and December. Periodicals postage paid at New York, NY and additional mailing offices. Subscription prices are $345.00 per year (domestic individuals), $621.00 per year (domestic institutions), $100.00 per year (domestic students/residents), $380.00 per year (Canadian individuals), $771.00 per year (Canadian institutions), $470.00 per year (international individuals), $771.00 per year (international institutions), and $230.00 per year (international and Canadian students/residents). International air speed delivery is included in all Clinics subscription prices. All prices are subject to change without notice. **POSTMASTER:** Send address changes to Clinics in Chest Medicine, Elsevier Health Sciences Division, Subscription Customer Service, 3251 Riverport Lane, Maryland Heights, MO 63043. **Customer Service: Telephone: 1-800-654-2452** (U.S. and Canada); **1-314-447-8871** (outside U.S. and Canada). **Fax: 1-314-447-8029. E-mail: journalscustomerservice-usa@elsevier.com (for print support); journalsonlinesupport-usa@elsevier.com (for online support).**

Reprints. For copies of 100 or more of articles in this publication, please contact the Commercial Reprints Department, Elsevier Inc., 360 Park Avenue South, New York, NY 10010-1710. Tel.: 212-633-3874; Fax: 212-633-3820; E-mail: reprints@elsevier.com.

Clinics in Chest Medicine is covered in *MEDLINE/PubMed (Index Medicus), Current Contents/Clinical Medicine, EMBASE/Excerpta Medica, Science Citation Index,* and *ISI/BIOMED.*

Contributors

EDITOR

JONATHAN L. KOFF, MD
Director, Adult Cystic Fibrosis Program;
Associate Professor, Department of Medicine,
Yale University, New Haven, Connecticut

AUTHORS

DAVID N. ASSIS, MD
Assistant Professor of Medicine, Section of
Digestive Diseases, Yale School of Medicine,
New Haven, Connecticut

TRACEY L. BONFIELD, PhD, D(ABMLI)
Associate Professor, Division of Pulmonology,
Allergy and Immunology, Department of
Pediatrics, Case Western Reserve University
School of Medicine, Cleveland, Ohio

MOLLY BOZIC, MD
Assistant Professor of Clinical Pediatrics,
Pediatric Gastroenterology, Hepatology &
Nutrition, Riley Hospital for Children,
Indianapolis, Indiana

JOHN BREWINGTON, MD
Clinical Fellow, Division of Pulmonary Medicine,
Department of Pediatrics, Cincinnati Children's
Hospital Medical Center, Cincinnati, Ohio

EMANUELA M. BRUSCIA, PhD
Assistant Professor, Section of Respiratory
Medicine, Department of Pediatrics, Yale
University School of Medicine, New Haven,
Connecticut

J.P. CLANCY, MD
Professor, Division of Pulmonary Medicine,
Department of Pediatrics, Cincinnati Children's
Hospital Medical Center, Cincinnati, Ohio

DOUGLAS J. CONRAD, MD
Professor of Medicine, Division of Pulmonary,
Critical Care and Sleep Medicine, University of
California, San Diego, San Diego, California

CHARLES L. DALEY, MD
Professor, Department of Medicine, National
Jewish Health, Denver, Colorado; Department
of Medicine, University of Colorado Anschutz
Medical Campus, Aurora, Colorado

PAMELA B. DAVIS, MD, PhD
Dean and Senior Vice President for Medical
Affairs, Arline and Curtis Garvin Research
Professor of Pediatrics, Case Western Reserve
University School of Medicine, Cleveland, Ohio

MARK T. DRANSFIELD, MD
Department of Medicine, The UAB Lung Health
Center, University of Alabama at Birmingham,
Birmingham, Alabama

MARIE E. EGAN, MD
Professor, Departments of Pediatrics and
Cellular and Molecular Physiology, Yale School
of Medicine, New Haven, Connecticut

WAEL ELMARAACHLI, MD
Assistant Professor, Division of Pulmonary,
Critical Care and Sleep Medicine, University of
California, San Diego, San Diego, California

STEVEN D. FREEDMAN, MD, PhD
Professor of Medicine, Harvard Medical School
and Beth Israel Deaconess Medical Center,
Boston, Massachusetts

YVONNE J. HUANG, MD
Assistant Professor of Internal Medicine,
Division of Pulmonary/Critical Care Medicine,
University of Michigan Medical School, Ann
Arbor, Michigan

MARY ELLEN KLEINHENZ, MD
Director, UCSF Faculty Chest Practice and
Adult CF Program; Professor of Medicine;
Division of Pulmonary, Critical Care, Allergy
and Sleep Medicine, Department of Internal
Medicine, University of California, San
Francisco, San Francisco, California

JOHN J. LIPUMA, MD
Professor of Pediatrics, Department of
Pediatrics and Communicable Diseases,
University of Michigan Medical School, Ann
Arbor, Michigan

STACEY L. MARTINIANO, MD
Assistant Professor of Pediatrics,
Department of Pediatrics, Children's
Hospital Colorado, University of Colorado
Denver School of Medicine, Aurora,
Colorado

MARIA R. MASCARENHAS, MBBS
Section Chief, Nutrition; Director, Nutrition
Support Service; Medical Director, Clinical
Nutrition, The Children's Hospital of
Philadelphia; Associate Professor of
Pediatrics, Perelman School of Medicine,
University of Pennsylvania, Philadelphia,
Pennyslvania

MATTHEW R. MORRELL, MD
Medical Director, Lung Transplant
Program, University of Pittsburgh Medical
Center; Assistant Professor of Medicine,
University of Pittsburgh, Pittsburgh,
Pennsylvania

THOMAS S. MURRAY, MD, PhD
Associate Professor, Department of
Medical Sciences, Frank H Netter MD
School of Medicine, Quinnipiac University,
Hamden, Connecticut; Attending Physician,
Division of Infectious Diseases and
Immunology, Connecticut Children's
Medical Center, Hartford, Connecticut

DAVID P. NICHOLS, MD
Department of Medicine, University of
Colorado Denver School of Medicine, Aurora,
Colorado; Department of Pediatrics, National
Jewish Health, Denver, Colorado

JERRY A. NICK, MD
Professor, Department of Medicine,
National Jewish Health, Denver, Colorado;
Department of Medicine, University of
Colorado Denver School of Medicine,
Aurora, Colorado

MEGUMI J. OKUMURA, MD, MAS
Assistant Professor, Division of General
Pediatrics; Division of General Internal
Medicine; Philip R. Lee Institute for Health
Policy Studies, University of California,
San Francisco, San Francisco, California

JOSEPH M. PILEWSKI, MD
Co-Director, Adult Cystic Fibrosis Program,
Children's Hospital of Pittsburgh of UPMC;
Associate Chief for Clinical Affairs, Division of
Pulmonary, Allergy, and Critical Care Medicine,
University of Pittsburgh Medical Center;
Associate Professor of Medicine, Pediatrics,
and Cell Biology, University of Pittsburgh,
Pittsburgh, Pennsylvania

S. VAMSEE RAJU, BPharm, PhD
Department of Medicine and Cell
Developmental and Integrative Biology,
Gregory Fleming James Cystic Fibrosis
Research Center, University of Alabama at
Birmingham, Birmingham, Alabama

STEVEN M. ROWE, MD, MSPH
Departments of Medicine, Pediatrics, and Cell
Developmental and Integrative Biology,
Gregory Fleming James Cystic Fibrosis
Research Center, University of Alabama at
Birmingham, Birmingham, Alabama

GEORGE M. SOLOMON, MD
Department of Medicine, Gregory Fleming
James Cystic Fibrosis Research Center,
University of Alabama at Birmingham,
Birmingham, Alabama

MISSALE SOLOMON, MD
Assistant Professor of Medicine;
Director, Nutrition Services, Division
of Gastroenterology; Attending
Gastroenterologist, Drexel Adult Cystic
Fibrosis Center, Drexel University
College of Medicine, Philadelphia,
Pennsylvania

KIMBERLY A. SPOONHOWER, MD
Department of Pediatrics (retired), Case Western Reserve University School of Medicine, Cleveland, Ohio

JAIDEEP S. TALWALKAR, MD
Associate Director, Yale Adult Cystic Fibrosis Program; Assistant Professor, Departments of Internal Medicine and Pediatrics, Yale School of Medicine, New Haven, Connecticut

ANGELA C.C. WANG, MD
Staff Physician, Division of Chest and Critical Care Medicine, Scripps Clinic, San Diego, California

Contents

Improved quality of care and rapidly emerging therapeutic strategies to restore chloride transport profoundly impact the epidemiology and pathobiology of cystic fibrosis (CF) in the twenty-first century. CF now serves as a model for chronic illness management, continuous quality improvement via registry data, and a seamless link between basic science research, translational studies, clinical trials, and outcomes research to enable rapid expansion of treatment options.

Cystic fibrosis (CF) is a common life-shortening autosomal recessive genetic disorder caused by mutations in the gene that encodes for the cystic fibrosis transmembrane conductance regulator protein (CFTR). Almost 2000 variants in the CFTR gene have been identified. The mutational classes are based on the functional consequences on CFTR. New therapies are being developed to target mutant CFTR and restore CFTR function. Understanding specific CF genotypes is essential for providing state-of-the art care to patients. In addition to the variation in CFTR genotype, there are several modifier genes that contribute to the respiratory phenotype.

Cystic fibrosis (CF) lung disease is characterized by persistent and unresolved inflammation, with elevated proinflammatory and decreased anti-inflammatory cytokines, and greater numbers of immune cells. Hyperinflammation is recognized as a leading cause of lung tissue destruction in CF. Hyper-inflammation is not solely observed in the lungs of CF patients, since it may contribute to destruction of exocrine pancreas and, likely, to defects in gastrointestinal tract tissue integrity. Paradoxically, despite the robust inflammatory response, and elevated number of immune cells (such as neutrophils and macrophages), CF lungs fail to clear bacteria and are more susceptible to infections. Here, we have summarized the current understanding of immune dysregulation in CF, which may drive hyperinflammation and impaired host defense.

Cystic Fibrosis (CF) is a rare, multisystem disease leading to significant morbidity and mortality. CF is caused by defects in the cystic fibrosis transmembrane conductance regulator protein (CFTR), a chloride and bicarbonate transporter. Early diagnosis and access to therapies provides benefits in nutrition, pulmonary health, and cognitive ability. Several screening and diagnostic tests are available to support a diagnosis. We discuss the characteristics of screening and diagnostic tests for CF and guideline-based algorithms using these tools to establish a diagnosis. We discuss classification and management of common "diagnostic dilemmas," including the CFTR-related metabolic syndrome and other CFTR-associated diseases.

The diagnosis of cystic fibrosis (CF) is being made with increasing frequency in adults. Patients with CF diagnosed in adulthood typically present with respiratory complaints, and often have recurrent or chronic airway infection. At the time of initial presentation individuals may appear to have clinical manifestation limited to a single organ, but with subclinical involvement of the respiratory tract. Adult-diagnosed patients have a good response to CF center care, and newly available cystic fibrosis transmembrane receptor–modulating therapies are promising for the treatment of residual function mutation, thus increasing the importance of the diagnosis in adults with unexplained bronchiectasis.

Observations from studies during the last decade have changed the conventional view of cystic fibrosis (CF) microbiology, which has traditionally focused on a limited suite of opportunistic bacterial pathogens. It is now appreciated that CF airways typically harbor complex microbial communities, and that changes in the structure and activity of these communities have a bearing on patient clinical condition and lung disease progression. Recent studies of gut microbiota also suggest that disordered bacterial ecology of the CF gastrointestinal tract is associated with pulmonary outcomes. These new insights may alter future clinical management of CF.

There is a high prevalence of *Pseudomonas aeruginosa* in patients with cystic fibrosis and clear epidemiologic links between chronic infection and morbidity and mortality exist. Prevention and early identification of infection are critical, and stand to improve with the advent of new vaccines and laboratory methods. Once the organism is identified, a variety of treatment options are available. Aggressive use of antipseudomonal antibiotics is the standard of care for acute pulmonary exacerbations in cystic fibrosis, and providers must take into account specific patient characteristics when making treatment decisions related to antibiotic selection, route and duration of administration, and site of care.

Nontuberculous mycobacteria (NTM) are important emerging cystic fibrosis (CF) pathogens, with estimates of prevalence ranging from 6% to 13%. Diagnosis of NTM disease in patients with CF is challenging, as the infection may remain indolent in some, without evidence of clinical consequence, whereas other patients suffer significant morbidity and mortality. Treatment requires prolonged periods of multiple drugs and varies depending on NTM species, resistance pattern, and extent of disease. The development of a disease-specific approach to the diagnosis and treatment of NTM infection in CF patients is a research priority, as a lifelong strategy is needed for this high-risk population.

The importance of maintaining adequate nutrition in patients with cystic fibrosis has been well known for the past 3 decades. Achieving normal growth and maintaining optimal nutrition is associated with improved lung function. Comprehensive and consistent nutritional assessments at regular intervals can identify those at risk of nutritional failure and uncover micronutrient deficiencies contributing to malnutrition. Management of malnutrition in cystic fibrosis should follow a stepwise approach to determine the causes and comorbidities and to develop a nutritional plan. Nutritional management is crucial at every stage in a person's life with cystic fibrosis and remains a cornerstone of management.

Gastrointestinal (GI) manifestations commonly complicate the care of patients with cystic fibrosis (CF). Despite recent approval of CF transmembrane conductance regulator modulating agents that can improve pulmonary function, GI disorders continue to be relevant and require innovative therapies. This article discusses the most common GI complications of CF, including reflux, pancreatic insufficiency, small bowel intestinal overgrowth, distal intestinal obstruction syndrome, and GI malignancy, with emphasis on clinical presentation and management.

Advances in cystic fibrosis (CF) care transformed the condition from one considered lethal by age 7 into a chronic illness (median lifespan, >40 years). With the growing numbers of adults with CF voicing their preference for care in age appropriate settings, the CF community met the challenge by developing an adult-focused care system modeled on the highly successful pediatric CF centers. Adult CF programs ensure lifelong CF specialty care. Preparation for transfer occurs in a process of "transition." This article reviews progress in transition-related care and provides recommendations for research and clinical practice to improve the transition process.

Lung transplantation is a viable option for many patients with cystic fibrosis (CF) and end-stage lung disease. Criteria for transplant in patients with CF vary widely among transplant centers in terms of acceptable comorbidities; referral to multiple centers may be necessary to maximize patient opportunity for this potentially life-prolonging intervention. Early referral is critical to patient education and modification of risk factors associated with worse outcomes. If transplant evaluation has been completed, patients with CF and respiratory failure requiring mechanical ventilation and extracorporeal membrane oxygenation may remain viable candidates for transplant with outcomes comparable to other individuals with CF.

Non-cystic fibrosis bronchiectasis (NCFB) is an increasingly prevalent disease that places a significant burden on patients and health systems globally. Although many of the therapies used to treat NCFB were originally developed as cystic fibrosis (CF) therapies, not all of them have been demonstrated to be efficacious in NCFB and some may even be harmful. This article explores the evidence for which therapeutic strategies used to treat CF have been translated into the care of NCFB. The conclusion is that therapies for adult NCFB cannot be simply extrapolated from CF clinical trials, and in some instances, doing so may actually result in harm.

Chronic obstructive pulmonary disease (COPD) is a major public health problem. No therapies alter the natural history of the disease. Chronic bronchitis is perhaps the most clinically troublesome phenotype. Emerging data strongly suggest that cigarette smoke and its components can lead to acquired cystic fibrosis transmembrane conductance regulator (CFTR) dysfunction. Findings in vitro, in animal models, and in smokers with and without COPD also show acquired CFTR dysfunction, which is associated with chronic bronchitis. This abnormality is also present in extrapulmonary organs, suggesting that CFTR dysfunction may contribute to smoking-related systemic diseases.

PROGRAM OBJECTIVE

The goal of the *Clinics in Chest Medicine* is to provide practitioners with state-of-the-art information that is clinically useful, concise, well referenced, and comprehensive.

TARGET AUDIENCE

All practicing physicians and healthcare professionals who provide patient care utilizing findings from *Chest Medicine Clinics of North America*.

LEARNING OBJECTIVES

Upon completion of this activity, participants will be able to:
1. Review the genetics and epidemiology of cystic fibrosis.
2. Discuss the management of gastrointestinal, nutritional, and other side effects of cystic fibrosis.
3. Review issues in and strategies for lifelong management of cystic fibrosis.

ACCREDITATION

The Elsevier Office of Continuing Medical Education (EOCME) is accredited by the Accreditation Council for Continuing Medical Education (ACCME) to provide continuing medical education for physicians.

The EOCME designates this enduring material for a maximum of 15 *AMA PRA Category 1 Credit*(s)™. Physicians should claim only the credit commensurate with the extent of their participation in the activity.

All other health care professionals requesting continuing education credit for this enduring material will be issued a certificate of participation.

DISCLOSURE OF CONFLICTS OF INTEREST

The EOCME assesses conflict of interest with its instructors, faculty, planners, and other individuals who are in a position to control the content of CME activities. All relevant conflicts of interest that are identified are thoroughly vetted by EOCME for fair balance, scientific objectivity, and patient care recommendations. EOCME is committed to providing its learners with CME activities that promote improvements or quality in healthcare and not a specific proprietary business or a commercial interest.

The planning committee, staff, authors and editors listed below have identified no financial relationships or relationships to products or devices they or their spouse/life partner have with commercial interest related to the content of this CME activity:

David N. Assis, MD; Tracey L. Bonfield, PhD, D(ABMLI); Molly Bozic, MD; John Brewington, MD; Emanuela M. Bruscia, PhD; Douglas J. Conrad, MD; Pamela B. Davis, MD, PhD; Marie E. Egan, MD; Wael ElMaraachli, MD; Anjali Fortna; Steven D. Freedman, MD, PhD; Yvonne J. Huang, MD; Mary Ellen Kleinhenz, MD; Jonathon L. Koff, MD; John J. LiPuma, MD; Patrick Manley; Stacey L. Martiniano, MD; Matthew R. Morrell, MD; Thomas S. Murray, MD, PhD; Palani Murugesan; Jerry A. Nick, MD; Megumi J. Okumura, MD, MAS; Steven M. Rowe, MD, MSPH; Erin Scheckenbach; George M. Solomon, MD; Missale Solomon, MD; Kimberly A. Spoonhower, MD; Jaideep S. Talwalkar, MD; S. Vamsee Raju, B.Pharm, Phd; Angela C.C. Wang, MD.

The planning committee, staff, authors and editors listed below have identified financial relationships or relationships to products or devices they or their spouse/life partner have with commercial interest related to the content of this CME activity:

J.P. Clancy, MD is on the speakers' bureau for Genentech, Inc., has research support from Vertex Pharmaceuticals Incorporated; Nivalis Therapeutics; Gilead; and ProQR Therapeutics.
Charles L. Daley, MD has an employment affiliation with Insmed Incorporated.
Mark T. Dransfield, MD is a consultant/advisor for GSK group of companies, and has research support from GSK group of companies; Astra Zeneca; Novartis AG, Boehringer Ingelheim GmbH; the National Institutes of Health; U.S. Department of Defense; Yungjin Pharm; Pulmonx; and PneumoRx, a BTG International group company.
Maria R. Mascarenhas, MBBS is a consultant/advisor for Cystic Fibrosis Foundation.
David P. Nichols, MD has research support from Gilead and Vertex Pharmaceuticals Incorporated.
Joseph M. Pilewski, MD is a consultant/advisor for Vertex Pharmaceuticals Incorporated.

UNAPPROVED/OFF-LABEL USE DISCLOSURE

The EOCME requires CME faculty to disclose to the participants:
1. When products or procedures being discussed are off-label, unlabelled, experimental, and/or investigational (not US Food and Drug Administration [FDA] approved); and
2. Any limitations on the information presented, such as data that are preliminary or that represent ongoing research, interim analyses, and/or unsupported opinions. Faculty may discuss information about pharmaceutical agents that is outside of FDA-approved labelling. This information is intended solely for CME and is not intended to promote off-label use of these medications. If you have any questions, contact the medical affairs department of the manufacturer for the most recent prescribing information.

TO ENROLL

To enroll in the *Chest Medicine Clinics* Continuing Medical Education program, call customer service at 1-800-654-2452 or sign up online at http://www.theclinics.com/home/cme. The CME program is available to subscribers for an additional annual fee of USD $225.

METHOD OF PARTICIPATION

In order to claim credit, participants must complete the following:

1. Complete enrolment as indicated above.
2. Read the activity.
3. Complete the CME Test and Evaluation. Participants must achieve a score of 70% on the test. All CME Tests and Evaluations must be completed online.

CME INQUIRIES/SPECIAL NEEDS

For all CME inquiries or special needs, please contact elsevierCME@elsevier.com.

CLINICS IN CHEST MEDICINE

THE CLINICS ARE AVAILABLE ONLINE!
Access your subscription at:
www.theclinics.com

Preface
Cystic Fibrosis

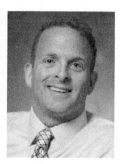

Jonathan L. Koff, MD

Editor

Tremendous progress has been made for individuals with cystic fibrosis since the last issue of *Clinics in Chest Medicine* on cystic fibrosis, which was published nearly a decade ago. Cystic fibrosis is a common genetic disease that is caused by mutations in the cystic fibrosis transmembrane regulator gene. Since this discovery in 1989, we now recognize that there are approximately 2000 genetic variations, which provide an increased appreciation for differences in disease genotype-phenotype relationships. Most importantly is the continued progress in patient outcomes. Improvements in survival have translated into more individuals with cystic fibrosis older than 18 years of age than children, which will prompt a transition in the focus of this disease from a life-shortening pediatric disease to an adult chronic disease.

In the United States, median survival is more than 40 years for individuals with cystic fibrosis. In fact, estimates suggest that children born with cystic fibrosis in 2010 will live into their 50s, and this conservative calculation does not account for some recent and future therapies. There are several reasons for this success. Universal newborn screening provides earlier diagnosis, which allows for initiation of therapies to attenuate disease progression. Once diagnosed, treatment for cystic fibrosis is organized at specialized centers, accredited by the Cystic Fibrosis Foundation, which provide multidisciplinary team-based care that is a model for clinical care delivery for chronic diseases. In addition, an emphasis on the quality improvement process has also driven center-based improvements independent of randomized

clinical trials, which are often challenging given the size of this patient population. Working closely with each cystic fibrosis center, the Cystic Fibrosis Foundation maintains a patient registry database that provides metrics for each center's adherence to established clinical care guidelines. This provides a best-practice model to benchmark each program's outcomes, and an opportunity for quality improvement initiatives to target areas of need. Perhaps most importantly, successful changes can be implemented at other centers. Finally, research has translated into effective therapies for individuals with cystic fibrosis. These include pancreatic enzyme replacement therapy, inhaled mucolytics, and antibiotics. Recently, cystic fibrosis therapies have provided cutting-edge examples of personalized medicine. The first drug received approval by the US Food and Drug Administration (FDA) in 2012, and more recently, the FDA approved a combination therapy in 2015. These oral medications directly target specific gene mutations to improve their function for more than 30% of individuals with cystic fibrosis in the United States. Currently, intense efforts are underway to identify similar therapies for the remainder of the cystic fibrosis population.

The introduction of personalized medicine to available cystic fibrosis therapies, in addition to a robust therapeutic pipeline, provides significant optimism that outcomes will continue to improve. This issue of the *Clinics in Chest Medicine* synthesizes the recent progress in our understanding of the epidemiology, genetics, pathobiology, and lung "microbiome" of cystic fibrosis by experts in

Clin Chest Med 37 (2016) xv–xvi
http://dx.doi.org/10.1016/j.ccm.2015.12.001
0272 5231/16/$ – see front matter © 2016 Published by Elsevier Inc.

the field. Next, our experts focus on the approach to treatment for *Pseudomonas* and nontuberculous mycobacteria, which are challenging pathogens in this population. As more individuals with cystic fibrosis reach adulthood with better lung function, we recognize the effect of comorbidities on patient outcomes. The next group of experts highlights the importance of nutrition to maintain good clinical outcomes and identifies the many manifestations of gastrointestinal disease in cystic fibrosis with an eye toward novel therapeutic approaches. The final group of experts provides an opportunity for cystic fibrosis to inform us about improving care, and identifying novel therapies, in other diseases. I would like to thank the authors for contributing outstanding articles to this issue as well as the publisher for their assistance with this issue.

Jonathan L. Koff, MD
Department of Medicine
Yale University
300 Cedar Street
New Haven, CT 06520, USA

Adult Cystic Fibrosis Program
Yale University
789 Howard Avenue, 2nd Floor
New Haven, CT 06519, USA

E-mail address:
jon.koff@yale.edu

Epidemiology of Cystic Fibrosis

Kimberly A. Spoonhower, MD[a], Pamela B. Davis, MD, PhD[b],*

KEYWORDS

- Cystic fibrosis • Cystic fibrosis epidemiology • Cystic fibrosis diagnosis • Review

KEY POINTS

- The prognosis of cystic fibrosis has improved substantially so that now more than half of the patient population is in the adult age range.
- Further improvements are expected because allele-specific therapies targeting the basic defect are being developed and reaching approval for use in the United States and other countries.
- Although identification by newborn screening is now available in all 50 states by pancreatic function markers and mutation detection, the diagnosis remains a clinical diagnosis.

Cystic fibrosis (CF) arises from genetic defects in a single gene, which encodes the cystic fibrosis transmembrane conductance regulator (CFTR),[1] a chloride channel that is widely distributed in epithelial surfaces. Epithelia in the airway, paranasal sinuses, pancreas, gut, biliary tree, vas deferens, and sweat ducts express CFTR and depend on it for normal function.[2] Defects in CFTR function in these organs give rise to lung infection and bronchiectasis, leading eventually to respiratory failure; pancreatic insufficiency with malabsorption; episodic intestinal obstruction; liver disease in some patients; and male infertility. Failure of CFTR-mediated chloride transport in the sweat ducts gives rise to a markedly elevated concentration of chloride in sweat, which is the basis for the definitive diagnostic test for CF.[3]

The early pathophysiology of CF has been difficult to study in human infants. Genetically engineered mouse models do not replicate the structure of the human lung or the pathobiology of CF in other organs with great fidelity, but the recent development of the pig model of CF, which closely replicates the human pathobiology of CF in most organs,[4] has given insight into early changes in CF. In the neonatal CF pig pancreas, secreted fluid contains reduced bicarbonate content and higher protein concentration, and fluid secretion fails to respond normally to secretin stimulation.[5] Patchy inflammatory changes and fibrotic remodeling are also observed.[6] Progression to pancreatic destruction can be envisioned from this origin. In the airway, failure of CFTR to secrete bicarbonate (as well as chloride) leads to low pH of airway surface liquid, which impairs bacterial killing.[7] This effect incites inflammatory responses and initiates the vicious cycle of airway damage, vulnerability to infection, and recruitment of destructive inflammatory cells.[7] Airway plugging appears to occur in the infant CF pig because of glandular secretion of mucus with abnormal properties that remains tethered to the submucosal glands is not released, and therefore, is difficult to clear.[8] This mucus also traps bacteria and contributes to the cycle of infection, inflammation, and damage. In the pig CF model, periciliary fluid depth is not reduced.[8] Rather, the reduced pH of airway surface liquid and the abnormalities of glandular mucus dominate the very early pathophysiology. Progression to chronic infection and bronchiectasis occurs in the pig model as it does in the human.

Disclosure Statement: The authors have no industry connections or conflicts to declare.
[a] Department of Pediatrics (retired), Case Western Reserve University School of Medicine, 2109 Adelbert Road, Cleveland, OH 44106, USA; [b] Case Western Reserve University School of Medicine, Dean's Office, 2109 Adelbert Road, Cleveland, OH 44106, USA
* Corresponding author.
E-mail address: pbd@case.edu

chestmed.theclinics.com

Despite the extensive multiorgan pathobiology of CF, in the twenty-first century, improved quality of care and rapidly emerging therapeutic strategies to restore chloride transport profoundly impact the epidemiology and pathobiology of CF. Outcomes are steadily improving, and CF now serves as a model for chronic illness management, continuous quality improvement via registry data, and a seamless link between basic science research, translational studies, clinical trials, and subsequent outcomes research to enable rapid expansion of treatment options.

CHANGES IN INCIDENCE AND PREVALENCE

CF was first formally described in 1938 by Dr Dorothy Andersen[9] and evolved from a disease of malnutrition and death in early childhood to one in which there is considerable demand for adult care providers for middle-aged patients with CF. The 2013 median predicted survival of 40.7 years reflects decades of improved care delivery, and even now, the impact of newly approved CFTR modulating therapies is yet to be felt.[10] Widely implemented newborn screening programs, therapies aimed at restoring chloride transport, a robust model of quality care delivery, and rapidly evolving new therapies are changing the epidemiology of CF.

One might have expected that the availability of DNA-based diagnosis of CF might change the incidence, and eventually, the prevalence of CF. Strategies to test prospective parents for heterozygosity for CF alleles, followed by prenatal diagnosis of the fetus,[11] might have been expected to reduce the number of births of children with CF if parents elected to terminate affected pregnancies. Nevertheless, estimates of the prevalence of CF in Caucasians in California in 2004, about 1 in 2577 live births,[12] are not dissimilar from the 1 in 3419 determined in early neonatal screening in Wisconsin more than 20 years ago.[13] Whether prenatal diagnosis is not yet sufficiently prevalent to make a difference, or whether the remarkable improvement in prognosis for patients with CF has encouraged parents to continue pregnancies known to have CF infants, or whether we are at the cusp of a decline in incidence, as is now being observed in Massachusetts for babies homozygous for the most frequent mutation in American patients with CF, Phe508del,[14] is not clear.

Broad implementation of newborn screening programs has resulted in earlier diagnosis of CF. Studies suggest that patients diagnosed before the onset of symptomatic lung disease have improved nutrition and pulmonary outcomes later in life.[15] Newborn screening programs have been implemented in all 50 states in the United States since 2010 and exist in the United Kingdom, Australia, and many countries in Europe. The specific protocol for testing varies among countries, and even among states in the United States.

In the US Cystic Fibrosis Foundation Patient Registry, the number of newly diagnosed patients detected by newborn screen increased from 5.7% in 1998 to 62% by 2013.[2] The 2013 median age at diagnosis was 4 months.[10] Newborn screening programs in London and South East England noted a reduced age at diagnosis following implementation of newborn screening programs from 2.4 years to 3 weeks.[16]

Data from the California state newborn screening program offered insight into the birth prevalence of CF disease among varied racial and ethnic minorities, as approximately 50% of the overall population in that state identify as a racial or ethnic minority. From the California program, the overall birth prevalence for infants with CF was 19.9 per 100,000.[12] The birth prevalence for Native American, white, and black was reported as 37.2, 38.8, and 17.1 per 100,000, respectively, and those identified as being of Asian origin had very low prevalence.[12] Thus, the incidence and prevalence of CF vary by race, with those of Asian origin having the least prevalence, and African Americans having lower prevalence than Native Americans or Caucasian patients.

CYSTIC FIBROSIS–RELATED CONDITIONS

The diagnostic category of Cystic Fibrosis Related Metabolic Syndrome (CRMS) was added to the US Patient Registry in 2010 for those infants identified at risk for CF through newborn screening with an indeterminate sweat chloride ($\geq$30–59 mmol/L), and less than 2 known disease-causing mutations in CFTR (the gene that causes CF). In 2013, data for 502 patients with CRMS were recorded, accounting for 8.4% of all patients recorded in the US Patient Registry.[2] An additional diagnostic category of CFTR-related disorder has also been available in the Registry since 2010. These patients do not meet diagnostic criteria for CF, but have an isolated CF-related condition, such as congenital bilateral absence of the vas deferens (CBAVD), and may have mutations in the CFTR gene.[17]

Ongoing data collection and analysis for these separate groups of individuals with CFTR-related disorders are important for better understanding genotype-phenotype relationships as new mutations in the CFTR gene are described. Most individuals with CRMS carry one copy of Phe508del

(62.5%) or Arg117His (32.4%), which may have important implications for treatment if signs or symptoms of disease develop later in life.[10]

DIAGNOSIS

Although newborn screening identifies a significant proportion of new diagnoses, CF remains primarily a clinical diagnosis. The CF Foundation–published guidelines for the diagnosis of CF state that the diagnosis should be based on the following: one or more clinical features, history of CF in a sibling, or a positive newborn screen plus laboratory evidence of an abnormality in the CFTR gene or protein.[10] The gold standard for demonstrating an abnormality in the CFTR protein remains the sweat chloride test performed according to CF Foundation guidelines.[3,18] Sweat chloride values of 60 mmol/L or greater are diagnostic of CF, whereas values 40 to 59 mmol/L for individuals 6 months of age or older, and values 30 to 59 mmol/L for infants under the age of 6 months warrant further evaluation with CFTR mutation analysis.[18]

CFTR mutation analysis and genotyping are increasingly important not just for diagnosis but also for prognosis, and to guide treatment in the era of new genotype-specific therapies. The most common CFTR mutation is Phe508del, with 86.4% of patients in the 2013 US Registry having at least one copy of this mutation.[10] Of these, 46.5% of patients are homozygous for the Phe508del mutation, and 39.9% are heterozygous.[10] The proportion of patients without at least one copy of Phe508del is increasing over time,[14] and some have suggested that this is a result of gradual application of guidelines for prenatal screening put forth by the American College of Obstetrician and Gynecologists and other organizations.[11]

Despite the early diagnosis afforded by neonatal or prenatal screening, about 10% of patients are still identified when they are more than 18 years of age,[10] because the current cohort of teenagers and adults was born before neonatal screening was prevalent. Often, these individuals have mild disease as a consequence of having at least one mutant allele that entrains milder lung disease and retained pancreatic function, so they do not attract medical attention early in life. These individuals may present with other CF complications, such as male infertility, intestinal obstruction, pancreatitis, chronic sinusitis, or heat prostration. Therefore, internists as well as pediatricians continue to need to be alert to CF manifestations, even if they present in otherwise healthy-appearing adults. Over time, the number of previously unidentified CF patients who reach adulthood will decrease with the universal application of neonatal screening.

CLASSIFICATION OF MUTANT FORMS OF CYSTIC FIBROSIS TRANSMEMBRANE CONDUCTANCE REGULATOR AND THEIR IMPLICATIONS

Classification of the mutant form of CFTR in each patient is important, because allele-specific therapeutic options are becoming available for patients with CF. There are 6 classes of mutations.[19–21] Class I mutations encode a premature stop codon and result in truncated and nonfunctional CFTR. Class II mutants produce protein that does not fold properly and is recognized and destroyed by the cell's quality control machinery. Therefore, most CFTR from class II mutants do not reach the cell surface. Phe508del, a class II mutation, is the most common CF mutation. The few Phe508del molecules that do reach the surface do not open to the same extent as normal CFTR and are also retrieved from the surface much more rapidly than normal CFTR.[22] Thus, the errors for any given mutation may not be confined to a single class. Class III mutations reach the cell surface but fail to activate channel opening. Class IV mutants have abnormal channel function. Class V mutants are splice variations in which an abnormal protein is produced because the splicing of the mRNA is defective. Class VI mutants are recovered from the cell surface much more rapidly than normal.

Although wide phenotypic variation exists among individuals with the same genotype, patients who have 2 alleles from classes I–III most often have early manifestation of pancreatic insufficiency and more severe pulmonary disease than patients with mutation classes V and VI (and some members of class IV) in which there may be some small residual amount of CFTR function.[23]

TREATMENTS DIRECTED AT THE BASIC DEFECT

Exciting results have been obtained for a small molecule, ivacaftor, in class III and IV mutations that reach the surface but fail to open properly. Tested first in patients with the Gly551Asp mutation, ivacaftor treatment resulted in substantial increases in pulmonary function, reduced pulmonary exacerbations, significant weight gain, and normalization of the sweat chloride.[24,25] The approval of ivacaftor by the US Food and Drug Administration (FDA) in 2012 has led to sustained improvements in lung function, growth and nutrition parameters, and quality of life.[26] Ivacaftor, a

CFTR potentiator, increases the likelihood that the CFTR protein channel at the cell surface will open to facilitate chloride transport[26] and is available as capsules or granules to be taken orally twice daily. Recently, FDA approval was extended to patients heterozygous for additional mutations including Arg117His, and other gating mutations in patients with CF aged 2 years and older. If allele-specific therapies can be as successful as ivacaftor appears to be and can be instituted before structural damage occurs in the critical organ systems, they have the potential to change the face of the disease for life.

However, patients heterozygous for gating mutations only account for approximately 4% of patients in the United States.[10] To target most patients who carry at least one copy of Phe508del, the combination of ivacaftor with a corrector, lumacaftor, has been studied. The Phe508del mutation, a class II protein misfolding mutation, limits the amount of functional CFTR that reaches the cell surface and is thus available to transport chloride.[27] Corrector compounds such as lumacaftor, and others in development, improve the trafficking of CFTR to the cell surface. The addition of a potentiator, such as ivacaftor, increases CFTR channel opening at the cell surface.[19,28,29] Phase II studies of the lumacaftor/ivacaftor combination demonstrated improved lung function as measured by forced expiratory volume in the first second of expiration (FEV$_1$)% predicted, and decreased sweat chloride concentration in subjects homozygous for the Phe508del mutation (but not those heterozygous for this mutation), although the improvement is modest.[28] A subsequent phase III study demonstrated sustained, although modest, improvement in lung function and quality of life in CF patients homozygous for the Phe508del mutation,[29] and the combination drug, trade-named Orikambi, was approved by the FDA for these patients. However, lumacaftor plus ivacaftor in a single fixed dose combination almost surely can be improved for treatment of Phe508del.[30] A fixed combination may not be appropriate for all patients because one drug is an inhibitor of CYP3A and the other is metabolized by it.[31] Moreover, recent data indicate that ivacaftor, over time, interferes with the therapeutic effect of lumacaftor.[32,33] Investigations of additional compounds that can potentiate and correct Phe508del CFTR continue and eventually will target other class II CFTR mutants, and patients heterozygous for Phe508del.

Class I or nonsense mutations, characterized by a premature stop codon that results in a truncated, nonfunctional CFTR protein,[34] are the target of phase 3 clinical trials of Ataluren, a compound structurally similar to aminoglycoside antibiotics.[35] There was no difference in relative change in lung function or number of pulmonary exacerbations between treatment and placebo groups.[35] However, post-hoc analysis of a subgroup of subjects not using inhaled tobramycin did show improvements in lung function and decreased number of pulmonary exacerbations, which has prompted further studies.[35]

CLINICAL MANIFESTATIONS OF CYSTIC FIBROSIS

Despite advances in CFTR mutation analysis, 1.1% of patients in the US Registry have one or more unknown alleles.[10] Thus, the cornerstone of diagnosis remains the clinical signs and symptoms. These signs and symptoms include pulmonary manifestations, gastrointestinal manifestations, and other organ systems affected by CFTR dysfunction.

Pulmonary manifestations include persistent infection with typical CF pathogens, such as *Staphylococcus aureus*, nontypeable *Hemophilus influenzae*, *Pseudomonas aeruginosa*, *Stenotrophomonas maltophilia*, and *Burkholderia cepacia*.[2,27] In the United States, the prevalence of *P aeruginosa* decreased since 2003, but the prevalence of methicillin-sensitive and methicillin-resistant *S aureus* species, and *Stenotrophomonas maltophilia*, increased in the same time period.[10] The CF Foundation published revised infection control and prevention guidelines to decrease the exposure to CF pathogens in the health care setting.[36]

Additional pulmonary manifestations include chronic cough and sputum production, chronic wheeze, digital clubbing, and persistent abnormalities such as bronchiectasis, atelectasis, and infiltrates on chest radiographs.[2,18] Furthermore, sinopulmonary complications of CF such as nasal polyps and paranasal sinus abnormalities on radiographic imaging of the sinuses should also prompt evaluation for CF.[2,18]

Gastrointestinal manifestations of CF include meconium ileus in the newborn period, distal intestinal obstructive syndrome (DIOS), and rectal prolapse.[27] Pancreatic manifestations include steatorrhea, malabsorption resulting in failure to thrive, and chronic pancreatitis. The prevalence of pancreatitis as a complication of CF has been increasing over time and is likely a result of the increased number of CF patients diagnosed with class IV and V mutations.[10] The prevalence of pancreatitis in patients with class I–III mutations is 0.4%, but 8.3% for patients with class IV and V mutations.[10]

Additional gastrointestinal manifestations of CF include hepatic disease such as prolonged neonatal jaundice, and clinical or histologic evidence of focal biliary cirrhosis or multilobar cirrhosis.[18] Other clinical manifestations of CF that should prompt diagnostic evaluation include salt loss syndromes and male genital abnormalities, such as CBAVD.[18]

Complications of CF include CF-related diabetes (CFRD), osteopenia, osteoporosis, arthritis, and depression. The prevalence of these complications is increasing both as the CF population ages and as screening for these complications improves across centers. The prevalence of DIOS, allergic bronchopulmonary aspergillosis, and osteoporosis has remained relatively stable with approximately 5% of patients experiencing each.[10] The prevalence of depression, however, increased from approximately 5% in 2003 to 12.3% in 2013.[10] Aggressive screening efforts, and increasing awareness of the impact of chronic illness on mental health, may account for this increase. Similarly, the prevalence of CFRD in patients aged 18 years and older is 34.3%, but only 6.5% in children, so overall prevalence increases with the aging of the CF population.[2] For CFRD and depression, prevalence varies by center. Quality improvement initiatives may enable the rapid, systematic application of best practices in screening[37] and reduce variation.

OUTCOMES IN CYSTIC FIBROSIS: IMPROVEMENTS AND CHALLENGES

Pulmonary and nutrition outcomes, as measured by FEV_1% predicted and body mass index (BMI), respectively, have improved over the last decade across US Care Centers. These improvements are the result of an increasing armamentarium of treatments, robust registry data collection and analysis, and the regular application of evidence-based care guidelines through quality improvement initiatives.[37] Lung function as measured by FEV_1% predicted remains an important indicator of health and disease progression. The proportion of patients 18 years old with an FEV_1% predicted of 70% or greater (normal/mild) increased from 34.8% in 1987 to 71.9% in 2013, and the proportion of those 18 years old with an FEV_1% predicted less than 40% (severe) decreased from 31.6% to 7.2% over the same time period.[10] Although there is significant variation in pulmonary outcomes by center and birth cohort in both children and adults, there is also variation based on mutation class, with class IV and V mutations demonstrating better lung function than those with class I–III mutations.[10,23]

Nutrition outcomes are increasingly recognized as important indicators of health and disease progression. Nutritional status and growth in early life

are predictive of lung function later in life[38] as well as survival.[39] Although outcomes vary by center, CFRD status, birth cohort, and mutation class, overall indicators of nutrition, such as BMI and BMI percentile, have improved over the last decade. The median BMI percentile for patients aged 2 to 19 years by center is 53.4, and the median BMI for adult men and women is 22.8 and 21.6, respectively.[10] Despite these improvements and aggressive nutritional therapies, the median percentage of patients who did not reach nutrition goals set forth by published guidelines[40] remains 45.3% for children aged 2 to 19, and 52.6% for adults.[2]

Accredited Centers for the care of patients with CF pride themselves (and are accredited on the basis of) on the universally applied evidence-based practice. Moreover, the CF Foundation has taken leadership in making many new drugs available to patients with CF, regardless of the patient's ability to pay. Despite these measures, socioeconomic, racial, and ethnic disparities exist in outcomes for CF, as they do for nearly all chronic diseases. In a study of pediatric patients with CF using Medicaid status as a proxy for socioeconomic status (SES), patients with Medicaid had worse pulmonary outcomes, worse nutritional outcomes, and an adjusted risk of death 3.65 times higher (95% confidence interval: 3.03–4.40) than non-Medicaid patients.[41] Both the Medicaid and the non-Medicaid populations had a similar number of visits to CF care centers,[41] suggesting that access to subspecialty care per se may not explain these results. Another study reported worse nutritional outcomes in African American patients with CF than non-Hispanic white patients.[42] A study of adolescents and adults with CF examined the impact of SES and minority status on health-related quality of life and found that low SES was associated with significantly lower quality-of-life scores across several domains for children, parents, and adults.[43] African American and Hispanic children and adolescents had worse lung function, lower weight and height scores, and a greater likelihood of P aeruginosa colonization compared with their Caucasian counterparts.[43] In addition, poorer patient-reported outcomes of quality of life across many domains, such as body image, physical functioning, social functioning, and respiratory symptoms, were also associated with low SES and minority status.[43] The proportions of patients in the 2013 US Patient Registry who received Medicaid or other state insurance program were 53.8% of patients less than 18 years of age, 41% of patients aged 18 to 26 years, and 27.1% of patients aged greater than 26 years of age.[10,43]

INCREASING ADULT POPULATION OF CYSTIC FIBROSIS PATIENTS

As pulmonary and nutrition outcomes improve overall, one of the most significant changes in the epidemiology of CF is the increasing adult population. The median age of people with CF in the US Registry is 17.9 years, and patients range up to age 85 years.[10] The proportion of adult patients, defined as aged 18 years and older, increased from 29.2% in 1986 to 49.7% in 2013.[10] This demographic shift creates significant challenges to CF care centers to provide care teams with age-appropriate training and board certification. Adults with CF require care for the multisystem manifestations of CF in accordance with CF guidelines, but they also require care providers who are able to manage adult medical issues such as reproduction, routine health maintenance screenings, and issues related to palliative care and end of life.[44] For example, the number of pregnancies in women with CF has increased since the 1990s and is now approximately 4 pregnancies per 100 women with CF per year.[10] The incidence of gastrointestinal cancer is markedly increased in patients with CF and, as the population ages, is expected to increase.[45] The incidence of cancer increases, too, with immunosuppressive treatment for transplantation, which is also on the increase.[46] This increase will affect the epidemiology of CF in the years to come.

CYSTIC FIBROSIS CENTERS: IMPACT ON OUTCOMES

The CF care center remains the model of care delivery for both children and adults with CF, which focuses on delivering optimal care, providing access to clinical trials and to basic science research, and training future CF care providers.[37] The role of the CF Center is to provide comprehensive care throughout all stages of life, focusing on the patient and family as a whole, and requires ongoing, reliable communication among the CF Care Team, other subspecialists, and primary care physicians. The national US CF Patient Registry assists centers in delivering high-quality care by providing annual Center outcome metrics, which inform continuous quality improvement at the Center level as well as care at the individual patient level. A model for chronic disease management, the use of a patient registry, evidence-based guidelines for care, and the rapid, systematic application of innovative therapies provide a foundation for a collaborative network of care improvement. This model for care delivery and improvement has been applied in many other chronic illnesses, such as asthma, inflammatory bowel disease, and perinatal care, with similar improvements in outcomes.[47,48]

The innovations in diagnosis and treatment of CF, from widespread institution of neonatal screening, to discovery and testing of new drugs and formulations, to implementation of coordinated care across an individual's lifespan, have positioned patients with CF to live longer and more satisfying lives. Now, innovative therapies aimed at restoring CFTR protein function based on functional mutation class may fundamentally alter the demographics of CF by changing the underlying cause and course of the disease.

Although the long-term impact of CFTR modulating therapies remains under investigation, hope remains that a robust clinical care and research network will continue to improve outcomes and survival in CF. Through these efforts, CF transitions from a disease fatal in childhood to a chronic illness managed effectively throughout the lifespan of a thriving adult population.

REFERENCES

1. Riordan JR, Rommens JM, Kerem B, et al. Identification of the cystic fibrosis gene: cloning and characterization of complementary DNA. Science 1989; 245(4922):1066–73 [Erratum appears in Science 1989;245(4925):1437].
2. Davis PB. Cystic fibrosis since 1938. Am J Respir Crit Care Med 2006;173(5):475–82.
3. LeGrys V, Yankaskas J, Quittell L, et al. Diagnostic sweat testing: the Cystic Fibrosis Foundation guidelines. J Pediatr 2007;151:85–9.
4. Ostedgaard LS, Meyerholz DK, Chen JH, et al. The ΔF508 mutation causes CFTR misprocessing and cystic fibrosis-like disease in pigs. Sci Transl Med 2011;3(74):74ra24.
5. Uc A, Giriyappa R, Meyerholz DK, et al. Pancreatic and biliary secretion are both altered in cystic fibrosis pigs. Am J Physiol Gastrointest Liver Physiol 2012;303(8):G961–8.
6. Abu-El-Haija M, Ramachandran S, Meyerholz DK, et al. Pancreatic damage in fetal and newborn cystic fibrosis pigs involves the activation of inflammatory and remodeling pathways. Am J Pathol 2012;181(2):499–507.
7. Pezzulo AA, Tang XX, Hoegger MJ, et al. Reduced airway surface pH impairs bacterial killing in the porcine cystic fibrosis lung. Nature 2012; 487(7405):109–13.
8. Hoegger MJ, Fischer AJ, McMenimen JD, et al. Impaired mucus detachment disrupts mucociliary transport in a piglet model of cystic fibrosis. Science 2014;345(6198):818–22.
9. Andersen D. Cystic fibrosis disease of the pancreas and its relation to celiac disease. Am J Dis Child 1938;56:344–99.

10. Cystic Fibrosis Foundation. Cystic Fibrosis Foundation Patient Registry 2013 Annual Data Report. Bethesda (MD): 2014.
11. Committee on Genetics, American College of Obstetricians and Gynecologists. Update on carrier screening for cystic fibrosis ACOG Committee Opinion Number 325, American College Obstetrics and Gynecologists. Obstet Gynecol 2005;106: 1465–8.
12. Feuchtbaum L, Carter J, Dowray S, et al. Birth prevalence of disorders detectable through newborn screening by race/ethnicity. Genet Med 2012;14: 937–45.
13. Korosok M, Wei W, Farrell P. The incidence of cystic fibrosis. Stat Med 1996;15(5):15449–62.
14. Hale J, Parad R, Comeau A. Newborn screening showing decreasing incidence of cystic fibrosis. N Engl J Med 2008;358:973–4.
15. Borowitz D, Robinson K, Rosenfeld M, et al. Cystic Fibrosis Foundation evidence-based guidelines for management of infants with cystic fibrosis. J Pediatr 2009;155:S73–93.
16. Lim M, Wallis C, Price J, et al. Diagnosis of cystic fibrosis in London and South East England before and after the introduction of newborn screening. Arch Dis Child 2014;99:197–202.
17. Cystic Fibrosis Foundation, Borowitz D, Parad R, et al. Cystic Fibrosis Foundation practice guidelines for the management of infants with cystic fibrosis transmembrane conductance regulator-related metabolic syndrome during the first two years of life and beyond. J Pediatr 2009;155:S106–16.
18. Farrell P, Rosenstein B, White T, et al. Guidelines for diagnosis of cystic fibrosis in newborns through older adults. J Pediatr 2008;153:S4–14.
19. Rogan M, Stoltz D, Hornick D. Cystic fibrosis transmembrane conductance regulator intracellular processing, trafficking, and opportunities for mutation-specific treatment. Chest 2011;139:1480–90.
20. Welsh M, Smith A. Molecular mechanisms of CFTR chloride channel dysfunction in cystic fibrosis. Cell 1993;73(7):1251–4.
21. Castellani C, Cuppens H, Macek M, et al. Consensus on the use and interpretation of cystic fibrosis mutation analysis in clinical practice. J Cyst Fibros 2008;7(3):179–96.
22. Goor FV, Straley K, Cao D, et al. Rescue of DeltaF508-CFTR trafficking and gating in human cystic fibrosis airway primary cultures by small molecules. Am J Physiol Lung Cell Mol Physiol 2006; 290:L1117–30.
23. McCone E, Goss C, Aitken M. CFTR genotype as a predictor of prognosis in cystic fibrosis. Chest 2006; 130:1441–7.
24. Accurso F, Rowe S, Clancey J, et al. Effect of VX-770 in persons with cystic fibrosis and the G551D-CFTR mutation. N Engl J Med 2011;363:1991–2003.
25. Ramsey B, Davies J, McElvaney J, et al. A CFTR potentiator in patients with cystic fibrosis and the G551D mutation. N Engl J Med 2011;365:1663–72.
26. Kotha K, Clancy J. Ivacaftor treatment of cystic fibrosis patients with the G551D mutation. Ther Adv Respir Dis 2013;7:288–96.
27. O'Sullivan B, Freedman S. Cystic fibrosis. Lancet 2009;373:1991–2004.
28. Boyle M, Bell S, Konstan M, et al. A CFTR corrector (lumacaftor) and a CFTR potentiator (ivacaftor) for treatment of patients with cystic fibrosis who have a Phe508del CFTR mutation. Lancet Respir Med 2014;2:527–38.
29. Wainwright CE, Elborn JS, Ramsey BW, et al, TRAFFIC Study Group, TRANSPORT Study Group. Lumacaftor with ivacaftor in CF patients homozygous for Phe508-del-CFTR. N Engl J Med 2015; 373(3):220–31.
30. Davis PB. Another beginning for cystic fibrosis therapy. N Engl J Med 2015;373(3):274–6.
31. Roberston SM, Luo X, Dubey N, et al. Clinical drug-drug interaction assessment of ivacaftor as a potential inhibitor of cytochrome P450 and P-glycoprotein. J Clin Pharmacol 2015;55(1):56–62.
32. Cholon D, Quinney N, Fulcher M, et al. Potentiator ivacafor abrogates pharmacological correction of deltaF508 CFTR in cystic fibrosis. Sci Transl Med 2014;6:246ra96.
33. Veit G, Avramescu RG, Perdomo D, et al. Some gating potentiators, including VX-770, diminish ΔF508-CFTR functional expression. Sci Transl Med 2014;6(246):246ra97.
34. Welch E, Barton E, Zhuo J, et al. PTC124 targets genetic disorders caused by nonsense mutations. Nature 2007;447:87–91.
35. Kerem E, Konstan M, DeBoeck K, et al. Ataluren for the treatment of nonsense-mutation cystic fibrosis: a randomised, double-blind, placebo-controlled phase 3 trial. Lancet Respir Med 2014;2:539–47.
36. Saiman L, Siegel J, LiPuma J, et al. Infection prevention and control guidelines for cystic fibrosis. Infect Control Hosp Epidemiol 2014;35:S1–67.
37. Mogayzel P, Dunitz J, Marrow L, et al. Improving care delivery and outcomes: the impact of the cystic fibrosis care network. BMJ Qual Saf 2014;23:i3–8.
38. Konstan M, Butler S, Wohl M, et al. Growth and nutritional indexes in early life predict pulmonary function in cystic fibrosis. J Pediatr 2003;142:624–30.
39. Yen E, Quinton H, Borowitz D. Better nutritional status in early childhood is associated with improved clinical outcomes and survival in patients with cystic fibrosis. J Pediatr 2013;162:530–5.
40. Stalings V, Stark L, Robinson K, et al, Clinical Practice Guidelines on Growth and Nutrition Subcommittee, Ad Hoc Working Group. Evidence-based practice recommendations for nutrition-related management of children and adults with cystic fibrosis

and pancreatic insufficiency: results of a systematic review. J Am Diet Assoc 2008;108:832–9.

41. Schecter M, Shelton B, Margolis P, et al. The association of socioeconomic status with outcomes in cystic fibrosis patients in the United States. Am J Respir Crit Care Med 2001;163:1331–7.

42. Hamosh A, FitzSimmons S, Macek M, et al. Comparison of the clinical manifestations of cystic fibrosis in black and white patients. J Pediatr 1998;132:255–9.

43. Quittner A, Schecter M, Rasouliyan L, et al. Impact of socioeconomic status, race, and ethnicity on quality of life in patients with cystic fibrosis in the United States. Chest 2010;137:642–50.

44. Yankaskas J, Marshall B, Sufian B, et al. Cystic fibrosis adult care. Chest 2004;125:1S–39S.

45. Neglia J, FitzSimmons S, Maisonneuve P, et al. The risk of cancer among patients with CF. N Engl J Med 1995;332:494–9.

46. Meyer K, Francois M, Thomas H, et al. Colon cancer in lung transplant recipients with CF: increased risk and results of screening. J Cyst Fibros 2011;10: 366–9.

47. Billett A, Colletti R, Mandel K, et al. Exemplar pediatric collaborative improvement networks: achieving results. Pediatrics 2013;2013:196–203.

48. Crandall W, Margolis P, Kappelman M, et al. Improved outcomes in a quality improvement collaborative for pediatric inflammatory bowel disease. Pediatrics 2012;129:e1030–41.

Genetics of Cystic Fibrosis
Clinical Implications

Marie E. Egan, MD

KEYWORDS

- Cystic fibrosis transmembrane conductance regulator protein mutation • Potentiator • Corrector
- Read through agent • Genetic modifier

KEY POINTS

- Understanding the consequence of cystic fibrosis transmembrane conductance regulator protein (CFTR) mutations is essential for prescribing appropriate drugs and providing optimal patient care.
- It is important to know the class of CFTR mutation an individual patient carries; newly approved drugs target specific gene alterations, and additional therapies are being developed.
- Pulmonary phenotype is greatly influenced by modifier genes that are distinct from CFTR.
- Some individuals with mutations of both CFTR genes may not be identified until adulthood. Cystic fibrosis should be considered when patients present with pancreatitis, sinusitis, diffuse bronchiectasis, or male infertility.

INTRODUCTION

Cystic fibrosis (CF) is a common life-shortening autosomal recessive genetic disorder that is characterized by eccrine (sweat) gland dysfunction, chronic obstructive lung disease, and exocrine pancreatic dysfunction. Mutations in the gene that encodes for the CF transmembrane conductance regulator protein (CFTR), which is located on chromosome 7, underlie this multisystem disorder.[1] CFTR is a large glycoprotein and a member of the adenosine triphosphate (ATP)-binding cassette superfamily of proteins. CFTR is expressed in many cell types, with phenotypic alterations primarily identified in epithelial cells of airways, sinuses, the gastrointestinal tract (including the pancreas and biliary system), the sweat glands, and the genitourinary system. Dysfunction of CFTR leads to a wide and variable array of presenting manifestations and complications.[1]

CYSTIC FIBROSIS TRANSMEMBRANE CONDUCTANCE REGULATOR PROTEIN MUTATIONS AND THE DISEASE SPECTRUM

CF occurs most frequently in persons of European descent. The prevalence in the Caucasian populations of Europe, North America, Australia, and New Zealand varies, but approximates 1 out of every 2800 to 1 out of every 3500 live births.[1] Although less common, the disorder exists in many other populations including African, Hispanic, Middle Eastern, South Asian, and eastern Asian populations.[1,2]

Many CFTR variants have been identified, and they have been grouped into 5 or 6 mutation classes. The clinical consequence of all variants has not been determined. In fact, only a few of these mutations account for 85% of the disease burden.[1,2] These mutations are often used in diagnostic screening panels.[1,2] In addition to disease-causing mutations, there is increased complexity, because some alterations in the gene are thought to be of little or no clinical consequence.[1,2]

Although more likely to be diagnosed during infancy, some individuals with mutations of both CFTR genes may not be identified until adulthood. Often their clinical course appears to be relatively mild (compared with individuals diagnosed in infancy), and their clinical symptoms are often attributed to other disease states. Ultimately the diagnosis of CF is considered when individuals present with pancreatitis, sinusitis, diffuse

Disclosure: None.
Department of Pediatrics, Yale School of Medicine, 333 Cedar Street, Fitkin 526, New Haven, CT 06520, USA
E-mail address: marie.egan@yale.edu

Clin Chest Med 37 (2016) 9–16
http://dx.doi.org/10.1016/j.ccm.2015.11.002

bronchiectasis, or male infertility. Clearly, the relationship between CFTR genotype and clinical phenotype is highly complex, and is not predictable for individual patients.[1,2] However, as a general rule, mutations categorized as severe are associated almost uniformly with high sweat chloride values, pancreatic insufficiency, and generally with more rapid progression of lung disease. There are exceptions to that rule, such as patients who carry 3849 + 10kbC→T, as they often have borderline sweat chloride concentrations and pancreatic sufficiency. However, these individuals do develop chronic lung disease and are colonized with *Pseudomonas aeruginosa* as frequently as patients who carry F508del.[1,2]

The most common CFTR mutation is the deletion of a single phenylalanine residue at amino acid 508 (F508del, Phe508del). This mutation is responsible for the high incidence of CF in European populations. Approximately 80% of individuals with CF of northern European descent carry at least 1 copy of the F508del mutation, and nearly half of patients are homozygous for this mutation.[1,2] Although F508del is present in other populations, its prevalence is much lower. It should be noted that in certain populations the prevalence of mutations other than F508del could be quite high.[1]

CYSTIC FIBROSIS TRANSMEMBRANE CONDUCTANCE REGULATOR PROTEIN MUTATIONS DIVIDED INTO FUNCTIONAL CLASSES

To date, almost 2000 CFTR mutations have been identified. These mutations affect the CFTR protein either by reducing the amount of protein that reaches the cell membrane surface, or by reducing the function of CFTR as a chloride channel.[2] CFTR mutations are grouped into 5 to 6 classes based on their functional effects (**Fig. 1**).[3–7] Class I, II, III, and VI mutations result in essentially no functional CFTR at the cell surface. Class IV and V mutations allow some CFTR to reach the surface, and are often associated with residual function.[7]

Each mutation class will be discussed separately.

Class I mutations are nonsense mutations, which introduce premature stop codons that prevent the translation machinery from producing full-length CFTR. These mutations appear in 10% of CF patients.[3,6,7]

Class II mutations lead to misfolded, or improperly processed CFTR protein. Most of this protein is degraded by cellular quality control mechanisms.[5,6,8] F508del or Phe508del (a deletion of phenylalanine at position 508), the most common CFTR mutation, is a class II mutation.[5,6,9] F508del leads to misfolded CFTR protein, the majority of which is degraded by cellular quality control mechanisms.[5,6,8] Of note, the F508del mutation has additional consequences that affect other aspects of channel function, demonstrating that some mutations may actually fit into more than one mutational class.

Class III gating mutations result in a full-length CFTR protein that has difficulties with activating/gating. These mutations are present in a minority of individuals with CF (4%). The G551D mutation is part of this class.[3,8]

Class IV mutations affect chloride conductance, which is the movement of chloride through the pore of the channel.[3] These mutations are also quite rare. One of the most common class IV

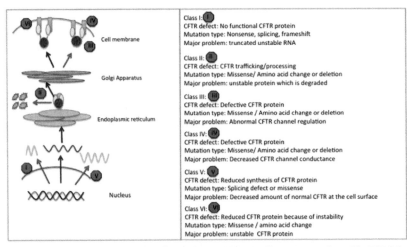

Fig. 1. Mutational classes I. Class I mutations Gly542X, Trp1282X II. Class II mutations Phe508del, Asn1303Lys III. Class III Gly551Asp, Gly551Ser IV. Class IV mutations ArgR117His, Arg347Pro, V. Class V mutations 3849 + 10kbC→T, 5T VI. Class VI mutations Gln1412X, 4279insA.

mutations, arginine 117 changed to histidine (R117H), appears in only 2% of CF cases worldwide.[4]

Class V mutations result in decreased amounts of CFTR protein produced, which is often due to a splicing defect, or a missense mutation. There is often residual detectable CFTR function. 3849 + 10kbC→T is a mutation that belongs to this class. The CFTRs that are produced by these mutations function normally.

Class VI mutations produce unstable CFTR, which results in reduced amounts of protein at the cell surface membrane.

Of note, in the past, understanding a patient's CFTR mutation had little to no effect on clinical care, as therapies were not available to alter dysfunctional CFTR protein. However, at this time, it is important to know the class of mutation one's patients carry, as newly approved drugs, and additional drugs in development, target specific gene alterations. Therefore, knowing which mutation patients carry, and understanding the consequence of those mutations, are essential for prescribing appropriate drugs and providing optimal patient care.

MODIFIERS

Cutting and colleagues showed that genotype alone accounts for a modest portion of the respiratory phenotype, which led to further studies focusing on the environment and modifier genes.[2] Non-CFTR modifier gene polymorphisms appear to be responsible for much of the variation in the progression of lung disease.[2] Genome wide association studies (GWAS) identified a few regions of interest with regard to severity of lung disease. One region is located on chromosome 11 in a region between EHF (an epithelial transcription factor) and APIP (an inhibitor of apoptosis). In addition, there is a region on chromosome 20 that encompasses several genes (MC3R, CASS4, AURKA), which are thought to contribute to lung host defense.[2] GWAS analyses also identified genetic regions that predispose to risk for liver disease, CF-related diabetes, and meconium ileus (Table 1).[2]

GENETICS AND DIAGNOSIS

The diagnosis of CF is usually made, and confirmed, with sweat testing collected by quantitative pilocarpine iontophoresis. However, genetic testing plays an ever-growing role in the CF diagnosis at all ages (newborns through adults).[1] Since 2009, neonatal screening for CF has been universal in the United States. Testing protocols vary

Table 1
Genetic modifiers

Clinical Feature	Gene/Locus
Obstructive Lung disease	TGFβ1, MBL2, EHF, APIP, Chromosome 20q13.2, SLC9A3, SLC6A14
Intestinal Obstruction	MSRA, SLC6A14, SLC9A3
Diabetes (CFRD)	TCF7L2, CDKAL1, CDKN2A/B, IGF2BP2, SLC26A9
Infection with Pseudomonas aeruginosa	MBL2, DCTN4, SLC6A14
BMI (low)	Chr1p36.1 and Chr5q14

from state to state, but most screening programs rely on genetic evaluation as part of the screening process. Most protocols include genetic evaluation of all newborn screening samples that are identified by immunoreactive trypsinogen (IRT) as high risk. This evaluation often tests for the most common CFTR mutations. However, the exact screening panel varies from state to state. In California, newborn screening relies solely on genetic screening.[1,2]

By probing for 40 of the most common mutations, the genotype of 80% to 90% of Americans with CF can be determined. This approach is quick, and less costly than more comprehensive sequencing.[1,2] In certain cases, sequencing the entire CFTR gene is necessary to establish the genotype and diagnosis. This procedure is also available commercially, and although it is relatively expensive, sequencing can identify polymorphisms and unique mutations of unknown clinical importance.

GENETICS AND THERAPIES
Gene Therapy: Replacement or Edit

Gene therapy has remained an elusive target in CF, because of challenges of in vivo delivery. In recent years, there have been many advances in gene therapy for treatment of diseases involving the hematolymphoid system, where harvest and ex vivo manipulation of cells for autologous transplantation is possible. This is not an option in CF because of involvement of the lung and other internal organs. Many clinical trials have used viral vectors for delivery of the CFTR gene, or CFTR expression plasmids that are compacted by polyethylene glycol-substituted lysine 30-mer peptides, with limited success.[10] Moreover, delivery of plasmid DNA for gene addition, without targeted insertion, does not result in correction of the endogenous gene, and is not subject to normal CFTR gene regulation. A concern of previous viral delivery systems is that virus-mediated integration of the CFTR cDNA could introduce the risk of nonspecific integration into important genomic sites. More recently, the UK Cystic Fibrosis Gene Therapy Consortium has tested liposomes to deliver plasmids containing cDNA-encoding CFTR to the lung.[11] This study showed some benefit, as there was a lessening of the pulmonary decline that resulted in a very modest improvement in FEV1.[11] Overall, although these recent results are encouraging, they suggest that new gene delivery vectors will need to be designed if this therapy is to be used clinically.

An attractive approach for CF gene therapy would be site-specific gene editing. Unlike the delivery of plasmids containing CFTR, which would be transiently expressed, or the use of nonspecific viral integration, site-specific gene editing would correct CFTR at its endogenous site. This would result in permanent gene modification under normal regulatory control. Current approaches for site-specific gene editing include:

Short fragment homologous recombination using DNA fragments containing the correct CFTR sequence that can recombine with F508del *CFTR* genomic DNA, and result in gene correction,[12–14]

Zinc finger nucleases (ZFNs),[15] which have been used to insert a CFTR transgene at the *CCR5* locus[16]

CRISPR/Cas-9 technology has been used to correct F508del in intestinal organoids from CF patients in culture,[17] but this has been complicated by a high number of off-target effects. Lastly, the efficiency of gene modification is low, and in vivo delivery remains an important challenge.

SMALL MOLECULES DIRECTED AT FIXING MUTANT CFTR

As new CF therapies emerge that directly target mutant CFTR, it is increasingly important to know an individual's genotype. In addition, the distribution of various CFTR mutations can aid in identifying individuals most likely to benefit from certain emerging therapies.[4] High-throughput screening has led to the identification of many classes of CFTR correctors and potentiators (**Fig. 2**) that address defects in the cellular processing, or chloride channel function of mutant CFTR.[5] **Correctors** aim to correct the folding and trafficking defects of F508del-CFTR and other class II mutants to increase the amount of CFTR on the cell surface membrane.[3,5] **Potentiators** activate, or enhance chloride channel activity of mutant CFTR, which is present at the cell surface (eg, Class III possibly Class IV mutations[3,5,7,8]).

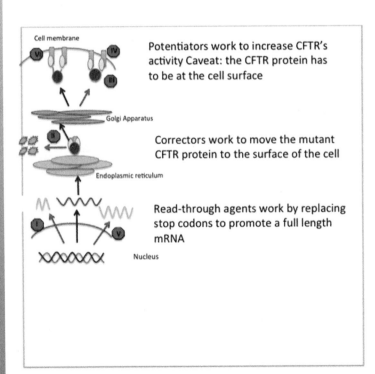

Potentiators work to increase CFTR's activity Caveat: the CFTR protein has to be at the cell surface

Correctors work to move the mutant CFTR protein to the surface of the cell

Read-through agents work by replacing stop codons to promote a full length mRNA

Cell membrane

Golgi Apparatus

Endoplasmic reticulum

Nucleus

Fig. 2. Correctors, potentiators, read-through agents. Schema demonstrating which defects are treated by the different categories of small molecules.

Another class of compounds, **read-through agents**, forces the translation machinery to ignore the premature stop codons introduced by class I mutations, resulting in production of full-length CFTR.[8] In this section, US Food and Drug Administration (FDA)-approved agents will be discussed to illustrate the potential of personalized medicine. Highlighting these new small molecules is not an endorsement of any particular therapy.

APPROVED AGENTS: (IVACAFTOR AND IVACAFTOR/LUMACAFTOR)
Ivacaftor

Ivacaftor (VX-770), the first approved drug targeting the underlying cause of CF, is a potentiator with high potency and efficacy.[3,5]

Individuals with the G551D CFTR mutation

A phase III study assessed ivacaftor in patients aged 12 years and older with at least 1 copy of the glycine 551→aspartate (G551D) mutation, a class III gating mutation.[3,18,19] In this study, treatment with ivacaftor for 24 weeks improved lung function, as assessed by change in percent predicted force expiratory volume in 1 second (FEV$_1$), an effect that was sustained through 48 weeks.[19] Treatment with ivacaftor also improved CFTR chloride channel function, as assessed by sweat chloride concentrations, and was associated with a lower proportion of patients experiencing pulmonary exacerbations.[19]

Similar results were observed in a study, which assessed ivacaftor treatment for 48 weeks in patients aged 6 to 11 years.[20] In addition, weight gain was significantly greater among patients taking ivacaftor, compared with the placebo group. However, there were no differences between groups in the rate of pulmonary exacerbations.[20] Extension studies that assessed long-term use of ivacaftor found sustained improvements in FEV$_1$, weight, and patient-reported symptoms during an additional 96 weeks of ivacaftor treatment.[18] This included a consistent safety profile.[18]

The FDA approved ivacaftor in 2012 as therapy for patients aged 6 years and older with at least 1 copy of the G551D gating mutation.[3,5,8] Subsequently ivacaftor has been approved for use in children as young as 2 years of age.

Individuals with non-G551D gating mutations and class IV mutations

Ivacaftor treatment was subsequently studied in individuals with non-G551D gating mutations. In this study this drug was shown to improve FEV$_1$, sweat chloride concentration, body mass index, and patient-reported symptoms for up to 24 weeks among patients aged 6 years and older with a number of any of non-G551D class III gating mutations. On the basis of these findings, the FDA expanded the indication label for ivacaftor to include those additional mutations.[3]

Ivacaftor was studied in subjects who carry class IV and V mutations, as both groups result in protein at the cell surface.[8] Trials assessed the efficacy and safety of ivacaftor in 69 patients, aged 6 years or older, with the class IV R117H mutation that affects chloride conductance.[4,5,21] These studies led the FDA to approve ivacaftor for patients with the R117H mutation who are 2 years of age or older. In the overall analysis, after 24 weeks, treatment with ivacaftor significantly improved sweat chloride concentrations and patient-reported symptoms in the overall cohort, but there were no significant difference between ivacaftor and placebo in absolute change in percent predicted FEV$_1$.[21] However, when these data are examined more closely, and stratified into 2 groups (children under 18 years of age and adults 18 years and older), the results are significantly different. Ivacaftor treatment significantly improved FEV$_1$ among patients aged 18 years or older.[21] It is hypothesized that the younger age group has preserved lung function with this milder mutation, making it difficult to observe a significant improvement in FEV1 prior to adulthood.

Ivacaftor and F508del Mutation

Although ivacaftor was developed primarily for class III mutations, it has shown some activity against the class II mutation F508del in vitro.[4] However, the trafficking defect associated with F508del is more severe than the gating defect,[8] and because so little F508del reaches the surface, potentiators targeting the gating defect associated with F508del are unlikely to have clinical benefit.[4,5] This expectation was borne out in a phase II study, which evaluated the safety and efficacy of ivacaftor in CF patients, aged 12 years or older, with 2 copies (homozygous) of F508del.[22] This was a trial in 140 patients, comprising a 16-week treatment period followed by a 96-week, open-label extension study.[22] Although ivacaftor treatment was associated with a statistically significant improvement in sweat chloride concentration during the 16-week period, there were no significant differences between ivacaftor and placebo in changes in FEV$_1$, patient-reported health, pulmonary exacerbations, or antibiotic treatment.[22] Thus, treatment with ivacaftor alone offers no clinical benefit in patients homozygous for F508del.[22]

Safety of Ivacaftor

Ivacaftor is generally well tolerated, even in children aged 2 to 5 years.[3,20,23] However, some patients have experienced elevated transaminase levels while on therapy.[3] Therefore, transaminase levels should be monitored every 3 months for the first year, then annually thereafter, and ivacaftor should be discontinued in patients with transaminase levels higher than 3 times the upper limit of normal.[3] Results from animal studies also suggest an ocular risk in juvenile patients.[3] However, no ophthalmologic effects, such as cataracts, were observed in a study, which is the clinical trial that assessed the ocular safety of ivacaftor in patients aged 11 years or younger.

Although most studies assessing the efficacy and safety of ivacaftor have enrolled patients with FEV_1 at 40% predicted or higher, ivacaftor use in patients with more severe disease has been studied.[24] Ivacaftor treatment improved FEV_1, forced vital capacity (FVC), and body weight.[24] In addition, intravenous antibiotic use significantly decreased, suggesting that ivacaftor is effective in individuals with the G551D mutation, and severe pulmonary disease.[24]

Lumacaftor Plus Ivacaftor: Challenges with Correcting F508del

Lumacaftor (VX-809) was the first CFTR corrector to be tested in individuals with CF.[3,5] In vitro, lumacaftor improves F508del maturation and F508del-mediated chloride ion transport by fivefold.[25] It also increases cell surface stability of F508del to a level seen with normal CFTR.[25] When lumacaftor was taken to clinical trial, its effects on F508del were marginal.[4,26] Patients homozygous for F508del and over 18 years of age were given lumacaftor monotherapy for 28 days, and this resulted in a modest reduction in sweat chloride concentrations.[4,26,27] However, there were no significant differences between lumacaftor and placebo in cough, pulmonary exacerbations, changes in FEV_1, or patient-reported symptoms.[26] Taken together, it was clear that as a single agent lumacaftor was not going to be clinically efficacious for patients with F508del.

The efficacy of lumacaftor monotherapy is limited, in part, because of the functional complexity of F508del.[5,8] Full correction of F508del will likely require combination strategies.[28] One combination approach combines a corrector, which would help F508del reach the cell surface, and a potentiator, which would aid in keeping the ion channel open.[3–5] This approach was tested in clinical trials that combined lumacaftor with ivacaftor, and provided the basis for the FDA approval of this combination agent for patients 12 years and older who are homozygous for the F508del mutation in 2015.

Both phase II and III studies have been conducted using the combination therapy. The phase III studies assessed the efficacy and safety of 24 weeks treatment with 400 mg lumacaftor daily or 600 mg lumacaftor every 12 hours, combined with 250 mg ivacaftor every 12 hours in 1122 individuals aged 12 years and older who are homozygous for F508del.[29] In one study (N = 559), the mean absolute change from baseline in percent predicted FEV_1 was 2.6% to 4.0% points (P<.001).[29] The mean relative difference from baseline was 4.3% to 6.7% (P<.001).[29] In the parallel study (N = 563), the changes in lung function were similar to the above mentioned study results.[29] Treatment with the lumacaftor–ivacaftor combination significantly reduced the rate of pulmonary exacerbations by 30% to 39%.[29] On the basis of these results, the FDA approved a coformulated combination of lumacaftor (400 mg every 12 hours) and ivacaftor (250 mg every 12 hours) in July of 2015.

ADVERSE EVENTS

The most commonly reported adverse events with lumacaftor monotherapy were cough, pulmonary exacerbation, headache, productive cough, upper respiratory tract infection, and chest tightness.[27] Lumacaftor monotherapy actually increased the occurrence of chest tightness and dyspnea, suggesting a need to monitor for these events in other trials of lumacaftor/ivacaftor combination therapy.[27] The combination of lumacaftor and ivacaftor was well tolerated in the reported study. The number of individuals reporting adverse events was similar between the placebo and lumacaftor–ivacaftor treatment groups.[4,27,29] Once again, the most commonly reported adverse events were cough, pulmonary exacerbation, and headache.[27,29] The most commonly reported adverse events in the lumacaftor–ivacaftor groups were mild-to-moderate respiratory events, including dyspnea and chest tightness.[29]

Although the combination of lumacaftor and ivacaftor yielded significant clinical improvements among individuals homozygous for F508del, the improvement was not as robust as that seen with ivacaftor monotherapy in individuals with G551D mutations.[23] In addition, because of drug–drug interactions, combination therapy requires a higher dose of ivacaftor, which can lead to problems when individuals are given other drugs commonly used to treat CF.[23] Two in vitro studies have shown that prolonged exposure to ivacaftor limits the efficacy of lumacaftor and another corrector, VX-661, by destabilizing the corrected F508del.[30–32] Although it is not clear whether ivacaftor exerts similar effects in vivo,[23] a change in dose might be needed to improve the efficacy of regimens combining ivacaftor with correctors.[30] More effective combination therapy may require personalized dosage combinations.[23]

EMERGING THERAPIES

There are a number of additional potentiators and correctors under development. These small molecules include QBW251, which is a potentiator targeting the gating defect of F508del and class III mutations. There is an investigational corrector, VX-661.[3,7,8] In vitro studies, VX-661, like lumacaftor, improves processing and trafficking of F508del when combined with ivacaftor. In addition, VX-661 increases chloride transport, both in homozygous F508del, and in heterozygous G551D/F508del cells. In a phase II study of 128 F508del homozygous patients aged 18 years or older, treatment with VX-661 for 28 days induced modest reductions in sweat chloride concentrations, and significantly improved FEV_1 with minimal adverse events. There are ongoing clinical trials of VX-661 and ivacaftor.

EMERGING READ-THROUGH AGENTS: ATALUREN

Ataluren (PTC-124) is a read-through agent that selectively overrides premature stop codons introduced by class I CFTR mutations.[3,7,33] In a phase II proof-of-concept study in patients 18 years and older with at least one nonsense CFTR mutation, Ataluren was well-tolerated and improved electrophysiologic abnormalities caused by CFTR dysfunction.[7] Two additional phase II studies found that treatment with Ataluren improved total chloride ion transport, as assessed by nasal potential difference (NPD), in both children and adults with nonsense mutations.[6,7,34] On the basis of these studies, a phase III trial assessed Ataluren treatment for 48 weeks in 232 patients aged 6 years or older with nonsense CFTR mutations.[33] The study found no significant differences between Ataluren and placebo in changes in FEV_1 or sweat chloride concentration.[33] However, a post hoc analysis found a statistically significant treatment effect on pulmonary function and pulmonary exacerbations in patients who were not using inhaled tobramycin.[3,33] Importantly, Ataluren was associated with increased creatinine concentrations, particularly in dehydrated patients and those receiving nephrotoxic, systemic antibiotics for pulmonary exacerbations.[33] A phase III clinical trial is underway assessing 48-week Ataluren treatment in patients aged 6 years and older who are not receiving chronic inhaled aminoglycosides.

SUMMARY

There was significant optimism that the promise of the identification, in 1989, of the genetic defect that causes cystic fibrosis would quickly translate into novel therapies. However, that revolution has taken time. Until recently, the treatment for all patients with CF was driven by symptoms. With proactive care plans that were designed to address patient symptoms, the quality of life and life expectancy have improved significantly. At this time, the first treatment based on a specific genetic mutation, which is an incredible example of personalized medicine, has only been FDA approved for 3 years. Many future treatments for CF are likely to be tailored to an individual patient's specific genotype, thus making understanding genotype essential for patient care. However, these therapies form only 1 component in comprehensive care of individuals with /CF. Patients will still require therapies for their symptoms, and they will still need to work with their care teams to design the best care strategies.

REFERENCES

1. O'Sullivan BP, Freedman SD. Cystic fibrosis. Lancet 2009;373(9678):1891–904.
2. Cutting GR. Cystic fibrosis genetics: from molecular understanding to clinical application. Nat Rev Genet 2015;16(1):45–56.
3. Pettit RS, Fellner C. CFTR modulators for the treatment of cystic fibrosis. P T 2014;39(7):500–11.
4. Boyle MP, De Boeck K. A new era in the treatment of cystic fibrosis: correction of the underlying CFTR defect. Lancet Respir Med 2013;1(2):158–63.
5. Rowe SM, Verkman AS. Cystic fibrosis transmembrane regulator correctors and potentiators. Cold Spring Harb Perspect Med 2013;3(7):1–15.
6. Wilschanski M, Miller LL, Shoseyov D, et al. Chronic ataluren (PTC124) treatment of nonsense mutation cystic fibrosis. Eur Respir J 2011;38(1):59–69.
7. Wilschanski M. Novel therapeutic approaches for cystic fibrosis. Discov Med 2013;15(81):127–33.
8. Galietta LJ. Managing the underlying cause of cystic fibrosis: a future role for potentiators and correctors. Paediatr Drugs 2013;15(5):393–402.
9. Davis PB. Another beginning for cystic fibrosis therapy. N Engl J Med 2015;373(3):274–6.
10. Griesenbach U, Pytel KM, Alton EW. Cystic fibrosis gene therapy in the UK and elsewhere. Hum Gene Ther 2015;26(5):266–75.

11. Alton EW, Armstrong DK, Ashby D, et al. Repeated nebulisation of non-viral CFTR gene therapy in patients with cystic fibrosis: a randomised, double-blind, placebo-controlled, phase 2b trial. Lancet Respir Med 2015;3(9):684–91.

12. Goncz KK, Kunzelmann K, Xu Z, et al. Targeted replacement of normal and mutant CFTR sequences in human airway epithelial cells using DNA fragments. Hum Mol Genet 1998;7(12):1913–9.

13. Goncz KK, Colosimo A, Dallapiccola B, et al. Expression of DeltaF508 CFTR in normal mouse lung after site-specific modification of CFTR sequences by SFHR. Gene Ther 2001;8(12):961–5.

14. Bruscia E, Sangiuolo F, Sinibaldi P, et al. Isolation of CF cell lines corrected at DeltaF508-CFTR locus by SFHR-mediated targeting. Gene Ther 2002;9(11):683–5.

15. Beumer K, Bhattacharyya G, Bibikova M, et al. Efficient gene targeting in Drosophila with zinc-finger nucleases. Genetics 2006;172(4):2391–403.

16. Ramalingam S, Daughtridge GW, Johnston MJ, et al. Distinct levels of Sox9 expression mark colon epithelial stem cells that form colonoids in culture. Am J Physiol Gastrointest Liver Physiol 2012;302(1):G10–20.

17. Schwank G, Koo BK, Sasselli V, et al. Functional repair of CFTR by CRISPR/Cas9 in intestinal stem cell organoids of cystic fibrosis patients. Cell Stem Cell 2013;13(6):653–8.

18. McKone EF, Borowitz D, Drevinek P, et al. Long-term safety and efficacy of ivacaftor in patients with cystic fibrosis who have the Gly551Asp-CFTR mutation: a phase 3, open-label extension study (PERSIST). Lancet Respir Med 2014;2(11):902–10.

19. Ramsey BW, Davies J, McElvaney NG, et al. A CFTR potentiator in patients with cystic fibrosis and the G551D mutation. N Engl J Med 2011;365(18):1663–72.

20. Davies JC, Wainwright CE, Canny GJ, et al. Efficacy and safety of ivacaftor in patients aged 6 to 11 years with cystic fibrosis with a G551D mutation. Am J Respir Crit Care Med 2013;187(11):1219–25.

21. Moss RB, Flume PA, Elborn JS, et al. Efficacy and safety of ivacaftor in patients with cystic fibrosis who have an Arg117His-CFTR mutation: a double-blind, randomised controlled trial. Lancet Respir Med 2015;3(7):524–33.

22. Flume PA, Liou TG, Borowitz DS, et al. Ivacaftor in subjects with cystic fibrosis who are homozygous for the F508del-CFTR mutation. Chest 2012;142(3):718–24.

23. Davies JC. The future of CFTR modulating therapies for cystic fibrosis. Curr Opin Pulm Med 2015;21(6):579–84.

24. Barry PJ, Plant BJ, Nair A, et al. Effects of ivacaftor in patients with cystic fibrosis who carry the G551D mutation and have severe lung disease. Chest 2014;146(1):152–8.

25. Van Goor F, Hadida S, Grootenhuis PD, et al. Correction of the F508del-CFTR protein processing defect in vitro by the investigational drug VX-809. Proc Natl Acad Sci U S A 2011;108(46):18843–8.

26. Clancy JP, Rowe SM, Accurso FJ, et al. Results of a phase IIa study of VX-809, an investigational CFTR corrector compound, in subjects with cystic fibrosis homozygous for the F508del-CFTR mutation. Thorax 2012;67(1):12–8.

27. Boyle MP, Bell SC, Konstan MW, et al. A CFTR corrector (lumacaftor) and a CFTR potentiator (ivacaftor) for treatment of patients with cystic fibrosis who have a phe508del CFTR mutation: a phase 2 randomised controlled trial. Lancet Respir Med 2014;2(7):527–38.

28. Farinha CM, King-Underwood J, Sousa M, et al. Revertants, low temperature, and correctors reveal the mechanism of F508del-CFTR rescue by VX-809 and suggest multiple agents for full correction. Chem Biol 2013;20(7):943–55.

29. Wainwright CE, Elborn JS, Ramsey BW, et al. Lumacaftor-Ivacaftor in patients with cystic fibrosis homozygous for Phe508del CFTR. N Engl J Med 2015;373(3):220–31.

30. Mall MA, Sheppard DN. Chronic ivacaftor treatment: getting F508del-CFTR into more trouble? J Cyst Fibros 2014;13(6):605–7.

31. Veit G, Avramescu RG, Perdomo D, et al. Some gating potentiators, including VX-770, diminish DeltaF508-CFTR functional expression. Sci Transl Med 2014;6(246):246ra297.

32. Cholon DM, Quinney NL, Fulcher ML, et al. Potentiator ivacaftor abrogates pharmacological correction of DeltaF508 CFTR in cystic fibrosis. Sci Transl Med 2014;6(246):246ra296.

33. Kerem E, Konstan MW, De Boeck K, et al. Ataluren for the treatment of nonsense-mutation cystic fibrosis: a randomised, double-blind, placebo-controlled phase 3 trial. Lancet Respir Med 2014;2(7):539–47.

34. Sermet-Gaudelus I. Ivacaftor treatment in patients with cystic fibrosis and the G551D-CFTR mutation. Eur Respir Rev 2013;22(127):66–71.

Innate and Adaptive Immunity in Cystic Fibrosis

Emanuela M. Bruscia, PhD[a],*,
Tracey L. Bonfield, PhD, D(ABMLI)[b],*

KEYWORDS

- Innate immunity • Adaptive immunity • Lung hyperinflammation • Bacterial infection

KEY POINTS

- Innate and adaptive immunity is dysregulated in individuals with cystic fibrosis (CF).
- Immune dysregulation in CF is driven by inherited and acquired factors.
- Both CF airway epithelium and CF immune cells contribute to immune dysregulation in CF.
- Therapies that reduce inflammation or boost the anti-inflammatory response may prevent the progression of CF lung disease.
- An effective, long-term therapy for CF should ameliorate the defective immune response.

INNATE IMMUNITY
Altered Barrier Function Impairs Host Defense in Cystic Fibrosis

The airway epithelium works as a physical barrier between the external environment and internal structures, which represent the lung's first defense against inhaled microorganisms. The barrier function of airway epithelium is accomplished by (1) mucociliary transport, which traps and removes inhaled foreign particles in the airways[1]; (2) secreted antimicrobial molecules that kill inhaled pathogens[2]; and (3) cell-cell connections that regulate epithelial paracellular permeability.[3] The integrity of the airway epithelium in individuals with cystic fibrosis (CF) is often disrupted at several levels, thus playing a central role in dysregulated innate immunity.

Reduced mucociliary clearance

The major macromolecular components of lung mucus are mucins, which are secreted by various cells of the conducting airway epithelium. Mucins are folded in an organized manner so as to reach a specific viscosity necessary for efficient release and transport. The cystic fibrosis transmembrane conductance regulator (CFTR) gene, which is defective in CF, produces a protein whose basic function regulates ion transport on the surface of the airways that contributes to mucus hydration and periciliary transport, which are altered on mucosal surfaces in CF.[4] Recent studies in the CF pig, which models the intrinsic human disease, revealed that CF mucosal properties (eg, elasticity and tenacity) are abnormal, leading to defective mucus detachment from the submucosal gland ducts of piglet tracheal tissues, thus impairing mucociliary transport. Alterations of mucosal proprieties are directly linked to reduced CFTR-dependent chloride and bicarbonate secretion,[5] which result in increased acidity of the airway surface liquid.[6] A similar scenario may compromise the gastrointestinal function.[7] As the disease

Disclosures: None.
[a] Section of Respiratory Medicine, Department of Pediatrics, Yale University School of Medicine, 330 Cedar Street, FMP, Room#524, New Haven, CT 06520, USA; [b] Division of Pulmonology, Allergy and Immunology, Department of Pediatrics, Case Western Reserve University School of Medicine, 0900 Euclid Avenue, Cleveland, OH 44106-4948, USA
* Corresponding authors.
E-mail addresses: emanuela.bruscia@yale.edu; Tracey.Bonfield@case.edu

Clin Chest Med 37 (2016) 17–29
http://dx.doi.org/10.1016/j.ccm.2015.11.010

progresses, increased absorption of sodium, via epithelial sodium channel (ENaC) will further contribute to airway surface liquid dehydration, decreased periciliary liquid transport, and impaired ciliary function, thus exacerbating defective mucociliary transport in CF airways.[8] The biophysical properties of CF mucus may also be altered because of epithelial production of adenosine,[9] and neutrophilic oxidative stress.[10]

A number of microorganisms (including *Staphylococcus aureus*, *Pseudomonas aeruginosa*, *Burkholderia cepacia*, *Haemophilus influenza* have been implicated in CF. These pathogens bind to mucins secreted by the respiratory tract, which normally is cleared by mucociliary clearance. However, it is clear that in a disease such as CF, in which mucociliary transport is altered, this essential and basic innate immune defense is compromised. Reduced mucociliary clearance and stagnating mucus will affect the innate immune response by several potential mechanisms including:

- Favoring the trapping of bacteria in the airways, which has been observed in lung tissue sections of patients with CF.[11]
- Altering the airway microenvironment (eg, oxygen tension, glucose, and iron concentrations), which may benefit bacterial adaptation. For example, *P aeruginosa* evolves from a nonmucoid to a mucoid strain, which is more resistant to antibiotics.
- Altering the behavior and function of lung immune cells. Impaired lung mucus may alter function of lung macrophages (MΦ),[12] compromising their production of anti-inflammatory and repair mediators (also discussed in the section on macrophages/monocytes, later in this article).

Intensive research is ongoing to identify novel drugs to improve mucus hydration and mucociliary clearance in CF. These therapies may also assist to reestablish basic barrier function in CF, which has additional therapeutic implications.

Altered airway surface liquid composition

There are several factors (summarized in the following sections) that have been linked to altered airway surface liquid (ASL) composition.

Airway surface liquid acidification The acidic pH of the CF ASL neutralizes the activity of several enzymes/peptides that normally provide protection against pathogens. The antimicrobial peptides β-defensin-3 and cathelicidin (LL-37) are downregulated in the lungs of pigs and patients with CF.[13] Lysozyme and lactoferrin are additional proteins that are abundantly secreted by lung epithelial cells and immune cells, and perform important host defense functions. Lactoferrin, which sequesters iron, may be low in CF.[14] As a consequence, iron may accumulate in the lavage and lungs of patients with CF, favoring microbial growth and viral infection.[15,16] Reduced concentrations of lactoferrin in CF lungs also may be a result of suboptimal degranulation of secondary and tertiary granules in CF neutrophils.[17]

In normal airways, the secreted protein Short Palate Lung and Nasal epithelial Clone 1 (SPLUNC1) plays an important role in innate immunity by binding bacterial products[18] and inhibiting sodium absorption in a pH-dependent manner.[19] Thus, in the CF airways, in which pH is lower, SPLUNC1 is inactive, further compromising innate immune functions.

Increased protease activity Increased lung neutrophil recruitment, which reflects persistent inflammation, is a hallmark of CF lung disease. In normal lung, neutrophils migrate to the airways in response to chemokines, and are activated, programmed for cell death, and removed from the airways by MΦ or by expectoration (see also the sections titled Neutrophils and Macrophages/monocytes). This coordinated process is altered in CF lungs, which results in lung neutrophilia causing the accumulation of neutrophil proteases. CF sputum has high concentrations of neutrophil elastase,[20] which correlates with more rapid decline in lung function in individuals with CF.[21] Elevated neutrophil elastase activity in the airways, degrades structural airway matrix proteins (eg, collagen and elastin)[22] and cleaves plasma membrane receptors/proteins involved in immune regulation. For example, the interleukin (IL)-8 receptor CXCR1,[23] MΦ phosphatidylserine that mediates apoptotic cell clearance[24] (see also the section Macrophages/monocytes), complement (C3, C5, and dC3bi), complement receptors (eg, CR1), and lymphocyte receptors (CD4 and CD8)[25] are all affected by elastase. Increased neutrophil elastase activity also has been associated with increased mucin expression, secretion,[26] and activation of Toll-like receptor (TLR)4 signaling.[27]

All of these changes exacerbate inflammation, interfere with efficient bacterial clearance, and compromise lung tissue integrity. Unfortunately, ivacaftor treatment, which improves mutation-specific CFTR function, is not associated with improvements in neutrophil elastase or sputum inflammation,[28] suggesting that anti-inflammatory therapies may still be necessary for patients with CF to reduce lung tissue damage over time. Other neutrophil proteases, such as cathepsin G,[20] cathepsin S,[29] and proteinase 3,[30] are also detected and active in the sputum of patients with CF. Cathepsin S has recently been found to degrade antimicrobial components such as lactoferrin and β-defensins.[29] Finally, a class of enzymes that belongs to the zinc-metalloproteinase family (eg, matrix metalloproteinase [MMP]-8, MMP, MMP-12, and prolyln endopeptidases), which are produced by neutrophils to degrade extracellular matrix, are abundantly recovered in the sputum of patients with CF.[31] The concomitant damaging activity of metalloproteinases and prolyn endopeptidase on collagen will result in accumulation of proteolytic products (for example, proline-glycine-proline [PGP]) that will exaggerate inflammation and neutrophil chemotaxis to the lungs.

Oxidative environment The CF ASL contains high levels of reactive oxygen species (ROS). Neutrophils are the major contributor of ROS, which they produce in abundance as part of their activation (respiratory burst) and with the release of myeloperoxidase (MPO). Airway epithelium also contributes to production and release of ROS. Furthermore, increased oxidative stress in this environment is exacerbated by altered antioxidant mechanisms. In fact, patients with CF have reduced glutathione metabolism and lowered intake and absorption of fat-soluble antioxidants such as vitamin E, carotenoids, and coenzyme Q-10. In addition, induction of cellular antioxidant responses (eg, nuclear translocation of the transcription factor Nrf-2) are blunted in CF bronchial epithelial cells. Oxidative stress invigorates the proinflammatory environment, such that oxidative stress correlates with inflammatory markers in patients with CF (Ref.[32] provides a comprehensive review).

Decreased nitric oxide Nitric oxide (NO) is produced from the amino acid L-arginine by the enzymatic action of NO synthase proteins (NOS). In the lungs, NO is produced by several cells, including airway epithelium, and immune and endothelial cells, and it is detected in exhaled air. NO is a versatile player in the immune system and is essential for controlling infection, inflammation, and autoimmune processes, as well as modulation of ciliary activity, vasodilatation, and bronchodilatation.[33] Low levels of NO have been observed in the exhaled breath of patients with CF, which is associated with poor pulmonary function and risk of infection with certain pathogens.[34] Reduced NO production in patients with CF may be due to low expression of NOS due to blunted Jak-STAT signaling,[35] and/or to the low availability of the NO substrate arginine. Indeed, elevated levels of

arginase activity, the enzyme that catabolizes arginine, have been detected in CF airways.[36] Importantly, treatment with ivacaftor resulted in increased NO in CF airways.[37,38] Although controlled inhalation of NO has been considered as a therapeutic intervention for CF, the precise and controlled administration of this gas may be challenging. Modulation of the cellular pathways that may stimulate production of NO in CF lungs may represent an alternative strategy. Interestingly, N91115, a novel inhibitor of S-nitrosoglutathione reductase, which will increase NO production, is in a phase 1 clinical trial for CF (NCT02275936).

Abnormal cell-cell connections
The airway barrier function is maintained by an integrated system of cell-cell contacts (eg, tight and gap junctions) that regulate epithelial barrier functions. In CF, loss of CFTR will result in altered levels and positioning of airway epithelial junction proteins that will lead to weak tight[39] and adherent junctions,[40,41] compromising epithelial paracellular permeability to ions and small molecules.[42] Tight junction abnormalities have also been described in CF pancreatic epithelial cells[39] and small intestine.[43] From an immunologic point of view these structural abnormalities may alter the following:

- The paracellular permeability to bacterial products that lead to infection and inflammation.[44]
- Altered signaling of the pathogen associated molecular pattern receptors (PRR) inducing the TLRs.[45,46]
- Structural changes which may interfere with tissue repair in response to inflammatory/infectious insults, thus augmenting CF lung scaring.[47]

More studies are needed to assess whether these changes in CF experimental models contribute to human disease, and therefore should be targeted for future therapies. Interestingly, the macrolide antibiotic azithromycin, which has anti-inflammatory proprieties and improves lung function in patients with CF, augments airway epithelial tight junctions and integrity.[48]

Altered Innate Immune Responses Contribute to a Proinflammatory Environment in Cystic Fibrosis

Pattern recognition receptor signaling
The innate immune system senses microorganisms by recognizing pathogen-associated molecules (eg, LPS, dsRNA, flagellin) through a repertoire of receptors called PRRs. PRRs are

expressed on immune and structural cells, including airway epithelium. PRRs are divided into several families, which will recognize specific pathogen-associated molecules.[49] Once activated, PRRs, through a tightly regulated signal transduction mechanism, initiate the inflammatory response by producing inflammatory mediators that lead to pathogen elimination, and eventually, reestablishment of tissue homeostasis. Abundance, location, turnover, and signal transduction regulation of PRRs will determine the quality, intensity, and duration of the immune response.[49] In CF, uncontrolled regulation of these receptors results in a robust and unresolved activation of proinflammatory pathways.

In CF, it was hypothesized that hyperinflammation may solely result from chronic infection. However, several studies show that CF tissues may be predisposed to hyperinflammation independently from infection.[50–52] This may be a result of the CF lung environment, which is rich in inflammatory mediators (for example, ROS,[32] PGP,[53] and mobility group box 1 [HMGB1][54]) that activate PRRs to stimulate proinflammatory pathways. In addition to the CF lung environment, CFTR protein itself directly modulates receptor signaling involved in immune responses.[45,46] Taken together, the initiation and resolution of inflammatory response through PRRs are compromised in CF.

Dysregulated immune pathways

At the cellular level, CF bronchial epithelial cells have several signaling pathways that are dysregulated and tightly associated with exaggerated inflammation. In contrast, pathways that are normally activated to regulate inflammation and to fight infections are downregulated. Several of these pathways are summarized as follows, and depicted in **Fig. 1**.

- Increased activation of the nuclear factor–kappa B (NFκB) and mitogen-activated protein kinase pathways contribute to increased secretion of proinflammatory cytokines (eg, IL-8, tumor necrosis factor-α, IL-6, and IL-1β[52,55]), which ultimately will increase lung neutrophilia.
- Abnormal basal lipid metabolism.[56] Fatty acid metabolism is skewed toward higher production of arachidonic acid (AA) and leukotriene B4 (LTB4) with decreased docosahexaenoic acid (DHA) and lipoxin A4 (LXA4).[57,58] Interestingly, dietary supplementation of DHA reduces lung inflammation in CF.[59] Cellular level and distribution of sphingolipids and cholesterol[56] are also altered, with potential consequences on inflammatory response regulation.
- Expression of proteins that favor ROS production are increased (eg, tissue transglutaminase 2[60]), whereas antioxidant proteins are downregulated (eg, PPAR-γ[61] and Nrf2[62]).
- Endoplasmic reticulum stress, the unfolded protein response, is elevated in CF airway epithelium, which promotes hyperinflammation.[63]
- Interferon (INF) signaling is blunted, which interferes with eradication of bacteria,[64] and increases susceptibility to viral infection.[65]

Altered Phagocyte Function Contributes to Dysregulated Host Defense in Cystic Fibrosis

Phagocytes (such as neutrophils and monocyte/macrophages) are fundamental effector cells that

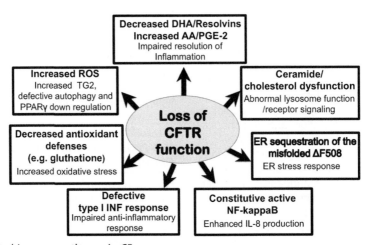

Fig. 1. Dysregulated immune pathways in CF.

are required for immune responses, pathogen killing, dead cell and debris removal, and to reestablish immune homeostasis. In CF, phagocytes do not function properly due to inherited and acquired deficiencies.

Neutrophils

Neutrophils are the most abundant immune cells recovered from the bronchoalveolar (BAL) fluid (**Fig. 2**) and sputum of patients with CF, and, as discussed previously, they play a central role in the development of CF lung disease. Migration of neutrophils into CF lung is primarily attributed to a massive increase in chemokines (eg, IL-8, LTB4, PGP, and IL-17), which promote their extravasation from the circulation. Although high in number, neutrophils fail to efficiently eradicate bacteria in CF lung. Several mechanisms may contribute to this defect:

- Bacteria, such as *P aeruginosa*, stick to mucus and form biofilms in CF airways, which prevents recognition and phagocytosis by neutrophils.
- Loss of CFTR in neutrophils impairs neutrophils' microbial killing by decreasing their ability to generate intraphagosomal hypochlorous acid.[66]
- CF neutrophils have impaired degranulation of secondary and tertiary granules, which contain several antimicrobial molecules (eg, lysozyme, lactoferrin, and cathepsins[17]).

The elevated number of neutrophils in the CF lungs can also contribute to amplifying hyperinflammation and lung damage. Some specific contributions that have been described include:

- Neutrophils contribute to the production of proinflammatory cytokines.[67]

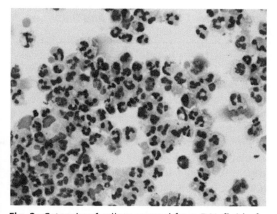

Fig. 2. Cytospin of cells recovered from BAL fluid of a patient with CF.

- Neutrophils release proteases and other inflammatory/damaging mediators into CF airways as discussed previously.
- Neutrophils are a major contributor of ROS, which they produce in abundance as part of their activation.
- Although CF neutrophils produce functional neutrophil extracellular traps (NETs), extruded chromatin that traps bacteria to improve killing,[68] the high content of DNA expelled with NETs augments viscosity of airway secretions in CF lungs.
- Neutrophils in CF airways may undergo metabolic adaptations that impact their function and that may negatively impact lymphocyte cell function.[69]

Macrophages/Monocytes

MΦs and blood-recruited monocytes are central mediators of inflammatory responses, which act by responding to external cues and contribute to the initiation and resolution of inflammation. In addition, MΦs are instrumental for maintaining tissue homeostasis, and their dysfunction leads to several human diseases.[70] Significant evidence has accumulated to prove that MΦs contribute to CF pathology.

- There are increased MΦs numbers in CF airways in the later stages of fetal development[51] and in young children with CF who are not yet chronically infected.[71] Several MΦ subsets are present within the lungs, which, in a temporal fashion, coordinate the initiation, intensity, and resolution of the inflammatory response, as well as participate in tissue repair. The 2 major characterized subsets of MΦs are classically activated (M1), which produce high levels of proinflammatory cytokines, and are involved in eliciting Th1 and Th17 responses. The alternatively activated (M2) MΦs favor resolution of inflammation; however, M2 MΦs may participate in airway remodeling in chronic diseases.[72] In CF, several studies suggest that BAL MΦs from patients with CF infected with *P aeruginosa* are skewed toward M2.[36,73] However, studies in CF models suggest a contribution of M1 MΦs to CF lung disease,[74] which suggest that further investigation is required.
- As with neutrophils, MΦ function is altered by the CF environment (eg, mucus obstruction, increased proteases, ROS), which ultimately affects their ability to properly regulate inflammatory responses and to clear bacteria. Of particular interest is the negative effect that proteases have on airway clearance of

apoptotic cells (a mechanism called efferocytosis), which are increased in sputum from patients with CF.[24] Proteases, in fact, cleave MΦ phosphatidylserine receptors, which impairs the capability of MΦs to recognize and phagocytose apoptotic cells in CF lungs. Removal of dying apoptotic neutrophils is fundamental to suppressing the release proinflammatory mediators. Thus, reduced efferocytosis in CF may contribute to immune dysregulation and hyperinflammation.[24]

- MΦs have intrinsic defects related to functional CFTR protein. Studies suggest that MΦs/monocytes from patients with CF have altered regulation of receptors (eg, TLR4, TLR5, CD11b, and major histocompatibility complex [MHC] class II molecules[75]) involved in immune regulation. Ex vivo culture of MΦs isolated from the lungs[76] or peripheral blood[46,77–79] of patients with CF have exaggerated inflammatory responses with impaired bacterial killing due to defective phagolysosomal acidification, impaired autophagy and accumulation of ceramide (Ref.[80] provides a comprehensive review).

ADAPTIVE IMMUNITY
Communication Between the Innate and Adaptive Immune Systems

The immune system is composed of multiple cell types, which together control the host response to infection. This involves the collaborative interaction between antigen-presenting innate immune cells, messenger T cells and subsequent activation of B cells, epithelial cells, MΦs, dendritic cells (DC), and neutrophils. This complex communication is driven through cell interactions at the membrane surface through the MHC. Studies from a CF genome-wide association project have shown a significant association between MHC class II polymorphisms in the HLA-DR regions and overall disease severity in CF.[81] The association between HLA-DR single nucleotide polymorphisms and CF lung disease severity was the most significant region in the genome. These results are consistent with previous studies demonstrating polymorphisms in HLA-DR4 and HLA-DR7 and CF phenotypes.[82] MHC class II polymorphisms and disease is not unique to CF, having been associated with other chronic diseases, highlighting the impact this genomic region has on host immunity.[83–86] Furthermore, antigen presentation can become altered during chronic inflammation and infection due to persistent antigen exposure,[87] also implicated in CF.[88,89]

The host response to bacterial infection requires communication between antigen-presenting cells

(APCs; eg, DC and MΦ and T cells), which is relayed through MHC class II antigen presentation to the cells of the immune system.[90] DCs are central to the integration of innate and adaptive immunity and are located throughout the respiratory mucosa and alveolar epithelium where they sense and process antigens. Peripheral blood DCs from patients with CF have lower levels of MHC class II receptors when compared with healthy controls,[75] which is also observed in CF mouse models,[91] suggesting that in CF, DCs may be inefficient at antigen presentation capability. In addition, DC maturation and function may be compromised by neutrophil elastase in CF airway fluids, which cleaves the CD86 receptor.[92] It has also become increasingly evident that B cells not only respond to T cells, but also actively participate in programming CD4 T-cell responses, including priming and induction of T-cell memory. This process occurs via the efficient uptake, processing, and presentation of antigens recognized by individual B cells and the unique B-cell receptor. In CF, there is significant evidence supporting inefficient immune resolution of infection and inflammation as well as hypergammaglobulinemia and continuous immune reactivity.[87–89]

The antigen-presentation process requires effective gene expression of transcriptional regulators, such as NFκB, which is controlled by epigenic modifications.[93,94] Importantly, there are therapies available, which are approved by the Food and Drug Administration, that target NFκB and histone modification in pulmonary inflammation.[95,96] There have also been studies that focus on improving antigen presentation to enhance the immune response to pathogen exposure.[97,98] Interestingly, epigenetic modifications have been implicated in CF,[99,100] and NFκB dysregulation has been documented in epithelial cells[101,102] and MΦ.[46]

Lymphocytes, Cystic Fibrosis, and Immune Dysfunction

Exaggerated lymphocyte responses, specifically Th17 and Th2, have been implicated in CF,[103–105] which may be related to defective activity of anti-inflammatory regulatory T cells (Tregs).[106] Some studies have suggested a lower percentage of Tregs during infection with pathogens such as Aspergillus fumigatus, with Treg concentration correlating to disease severity.[107,108] Decreased Tregs are thought to move the lung environment away from anti-inflammatory IL-10, and toward proinflammatory IL-17 and IL-8.

An association with defective tryptophan catabolism and T-cell phenotype and disease also has been implicated, suggesting nutritional contribution to T-cell activity.[109] Using T-cell–specific CFTR knockout, studies have shown aberrant cytokine secretion and hyperinflammatory adaptive immune responses.[110] In these studies, CFTR null animals demonstrated an exaggerated immunoglobulin E response toward *A fumigatus*, with higher levels of IL-13 and IL-4, which mimic responses observed in patients with CF. These studies also showed that lymphocyte CFTR expression regulated Ca^{2+} influx, which drives inflammation. In earlier studies, T cells obtained from patients with CF were found to produce less IL-10 compared with controls,[111] which was also recapitulated in CFTR knockout mice.[112]

There also has been interest in Th17 T-cells in CF because of the potential to promote neutrophil recruitment into the lungs. Although many cytokines and small molecules have been shown to recruit neutrophils into the airway[113,114](discussed previously), IL-17 participates in this process in the CF lung because it is critically important in the host response to gram negative infection.[115–117] IL-17 has also been shown to upregulate epithelial mucin-producing genes, which contributes to the pathophysiology of CF.[118,119] IL-17 is increased in CF sputum of patients with *P aeruginosa*, and decreases after antibiotic therapy.[120,121] In CF mice stimulated with *P aeruginosa*, IL-17 is elevated in BAL fluid with recent studies demonstrating a unique population of IL-17 positive neutrophils. Neutralizing IL-17, which also has been performed in other inflammatory mouse models,[116,122,123] markedly reduced neutrophil recruitment into lungs of CF mice challenged with *P aeruginosa*, implicating IL-17 as a potential therapeutic target.

Finally, another T-cell population, the invariant natural killer T cells (iNKT), has also been shown to be dysregulated in CF. In elegant studies, Siegmann and Doring show that iNKT cells are upregulated by the absence of CFTR.[124] Further, the accumulation of iNKT cells triggered cell death in CF organs and contributed to MO and neutrophil recruitment to the lung. Deleting the iNKT cells removed the effect, suggesting a direct pathophysiologic role of iNKT cells in CF.

Regulating the Immune Response Preserves Lung Function in Cystic Fibrosis

A therapeutic anti-inflammatory approach has reinforced the concept that inflammation dysregulates the CF immune response. In fact, chronic treatment with the nonsteroidal anti-inflammatory drug (NSAID) ibuprofen slows lung function decline, and increases life expectancy in patients with CF.[125] Ibuprofen is the only anti-inflammatory drug currently recommended for CF.[126] However, the high doses needed to achieve a beneficial outcome are associated with side effects, which limits its use to fewer than 10% of patients with CF. Other NSAIDs may reduce hyperinflammation in CF using a lower dose than that required for ibuprofen.[127] Additional anti-inflammatory drugs have been tested in CF, but with unsatisfactory or inconclusive results. Among these are oral[128] or inhaled corticosteroids,[129] PPAR pathway modulators (eg, thiazolidinediones and glitazones),[130] inhaled interferon-gamma,[131] antioxidant therapies (inhaled glutathione),[132,133] and N-acetyl cysteine. Of note, N-acetyl cysteine treatment, although it did not have effects on inflammatory markers, stabilized lung function.[134]

Because neutrophils have an enormous negative impact on CF lung disease progression, several therapeutic strategies have attempted to block their migration into the lung. With this goal, a potent LTB4 antagonist (amelubant) was tested in a clinical trial for CF, but was suspended because of adverse effects. In fact, blocking lung neutrophil migration was associated with impaired antimicrobial defense, which resulted in increased pulmonary exacerbations.[114] Alternative strategies that are more balanced, such as chemokine receptor antagonists (eg, CXCR2)[135] and IL-17 inhibitors, are still under consideration. The LTB4 antagonist trial has highlighted the fact that a successful anti-inflammatory therapy for CF, while halting inflammation, should not impair host defense. Promising approaches that are currently being tested in clinical trials aim to control harmful neutrophil products rather than neutrophil migration. Examples of these are inhalation of alpha 1-antitrypsin[73] and alpha1-proteinase inhibitor,[136] which target neutralizing proteases, and modulation of redox balance with pharmacologic supplementation of thiocyanate.[137,138]

In addition, approaches that boost anti-inflammatory responses, rather than interfering with the proinflammatory cascade, are being considered. These include stimulation of NO production via L-arginine administration,[139] increasing Nrf2 expression,[140] and administration of fatty acid derivatives with anti-inflammatory proprieties (eg, lipoxin and resolvins[141]). Finally, antibacterial therapies that also have anti-inflammatory properties represent an excellent CF therapeutic approach. Tobramycin[142] and azithromycin[143–145] have these characteristics, and are currently approved for CF treatment because they improve lung function, weight gain, and decrease pulmonary exacerbations in patients with CF. A comprehensive review on planned, ongoing, and completed clinical trials that ameliorate immune dysfunction in CF is available.[146] Further, even with the advent of approved CFTR potentiator and corrector therapies, which improve mutation specific functions, in many patients the smoldering inflammation is sustained. There observations suggest that combining novel anti-inflammatory strategies with these therapies will be critical to preserve long-term outcomes.[28,147,148]

SUMMARY

In summary, evidence suggests that patients with CF have inherited and acquired factors that contribute to abnormal immune regulation, which contribute to tissue hyperinflammation, defective bacterial clearance, and impaired function of the adaptive immune response. Years of research studies suggest that an effective, long-term therapy for CF also will need to target and restore these inefficiencies of the immune response. Because there remains a large knowledge gap about the mechanism(s) causing immune dysregulation in CF, future studies to better understand this aspect of CF lung disease may help to identify novel therapeutic targets that will contribute to improved clinical outcomes.

REFERENCES

1. Knowles MR, Boucher RC. Mucus clearance as a primary innate defense mechanism for mammalian airways. J Clin Invest 2002;109(5):571–7.
2. Bals R, Hiemstra PS. Innate immunity in the lung: how epithelial cells fight against respiratory pathogens. Eur Respir J 2004;23(2):327–33.
3. Pohl C, Hermanns MI, Uboldi C, et al. Barrier functions and paracellular integrity in human cell culture models of the proximal respiratory unit. Eur J Pharm Biopharm 2009;72(2):339–49.
4. Kreda SM, Davis CW, Rose MC. CFTR, mucins, and mucus obstruction in cystic fibrosis. Cold Spring Harb Perspect Med 2012;2(9):a009589.
5. Hoegger MJ, Fischer AJ, McMenimen JD, et al. Impaired mucus detachment disrupts mucociliary transport in a piglet model of cystic fibrosis. Science 2014;345(6198):818–22.
6. Quinton PM. Role of epithelial HCO3(-) transport in mucin secretion: lessons from cystic fibrosis. Am J Physiol Cell Physiol 2010;299(6):C1222–33.
7. Schutte A, Ermund A, Becker-Pauly C, et al. Microbial-induced meprin beta cleavage in MUC2 mucin and a functional CFTR channel are required to release anchored small intestinal mucus. Proc Natl Acad Sci U S A 2014;111(34):12396–401.
8. Boucher RC. Airway surface dehydration in cystic fibrosis: pathogenesis and therapy. Annu Rev Med 2007;58:157–70.
9. Lazarowski ER, Tarran R, Grubb BR, et al. Nucleotide release provides a mechanism for airway surface liquid homeostasis. J Biol Chem 2004;279(35):36855–64.
10. Yuan S, Hollinger M, Lachowicz-Scroggins ME, et al. Oxidation increases mucin polymer cross-links to stiffen airway mucus gels. Sci Transl Med 2015;7(276):276ra27.
11. Worlitzsch D, Tarran R, Ulrich M, et al. Effects of reduced mucus oxygen concentration in airway Pseudomonas infections of cystic fibrosis patients. J Clin Invest 2002;109(3):317–25.
12. Saini Y, Dang H, Livraghi-Butrico A, et al. Gene expression in whole lung and pulmonary macrophages reflects the dynamic pathology associated with airway surface dehydration. BMC Genomics 2014;15:726.
13. Abou Alaiwa MH, Reznikov LR, Gansemer ND, et al. pH modulates the activity and synergism of the airway surface liquid antimicrobials beta-defensin-3 and LL-37. Proc Natl Acad Sci U S A 2014;111(52):18703–8.
14. Rogan MP, Taggart CC, Greene CM, et al. Loss of microbicidal activity and increased formation of biofilm due to decreased lactoferrin activity in patients with cystic fibrosis. J Infect Dis 2004;190(7):1245–53.
15. Ghio AJ, Roggli VL, Soukup JM, et al. Iron accumulates in the lavage and explanted lungs of cystic fibrosis patients. J Cyst Fibros 2013;12(4):390–8.
16. Moreau-Marquis S, Coutermarsh B, Stanton BA. Combination of hypothiocyanite and lactoferrin (ALX-109) enhances the ability of tobramycin and aztreonam to eliminate Pseudomonas aeruginosa biofilms growing on cystic fibrosis airway epithelial cells. J Antimicrob Chemother 2015;70(1):160–6.
17. Pohl K, Hayes E, Keenan J, et al. A neutrophil intrinsic impairment affecting Rab27a and degranulation in cystic fibrosis is corrected by CFTR potentiator therapy. Blood 2014;124(7):999–1009.
18. Britto CJ, Cohn L. Bactericidal/Permeability-increasing protein fold-containing family member A1 in airway host protection and respiratory disease. Am J Respir Cell Mol Biol 2015;52(5):525–34.
19. Tarran R, Redinbo MR. Mammalian short palate lung and nasal epithelial clone 1 (SPLUNC1) in pH-dependent airway hydration. Int J Biochem Cell Biol 2014;52:130–5.
20. Goldstein W, Doring G. Lysosomal-enzymes from polymorphonuclear leukocytes and proteinase-inhibitors in patients with cystic-fibrosis. Am Rev Respir Dis 1986;134(1):49–56.
21. Sagel SD, Wagner BD, Anthony MM, et al. Sputum biomarkers of inflammation and lung function

decline in children with cystic fibrosis. Am J Respir Crit Care Med 2012;186(9):857–65.

22. Bruce MC, Poncz L, Klinger JD, et al. Biochemical and pathologic evidence for proteolytic destruction of lung connective tissue in cystic fibrosis. Am Rev Respir Dis 1985;132(3):529–35.

23. Hartl D, Latzin P, Hordijk P, et al. Cleavage of CXCR1 on neutrophils disables bacterial killing in cystic fibrosis lung disease. Nat Med 2007; 13(12):1423–30.

24. Vandivier RW, Fadok VA, Hoffmann PR, et al. Elastase-mediated phosphatidylserine receptor cleavage impairs apoptotic cell clearance in cystic fibrosis and bronchiectasis. J Clin Invest 2002; 109(5):661–70.

25. Doring G. The role of neutrophil elastase in chronic inflammation. Am J Respir Crit Care Med 1994; 150(6 Pt 2):S114–7.

26. Voynow JA, Young LR, Wang Y, et al. Neutrophil elastase increases MUC5AC mRNA and protein expression in respiratory epithelial cells. Am J Physiol 1999;276(5 Pt 1):L835–43.

27. Devaney JM, Greene CM, Taggart CC, et al. Neutrophil elastase up-regulates interleukin-8 via toll-like receptor 4. FEBS Lett 2003;544(1–3): 129–32.

28. Rowe SM, Heltshe SL, Gonska T, et al. Network GlotCFFTD. Clinical mechanism of the cystic fibrosis transmembrane conductance regulator potentiator ivacaftor in G551D-mediated cystic fibrosis. Am J Respir Crit Care Med 2014;190(2):175–84.

29. Weldon S, McNally P, McAuley DF, et al. miR-31 dysregulation in cystic fibrosis airways contributes to increased pulmonary cathepsin S production. Am J Respir Crit Care Med 2014;190(2):165–74.

30. Witko-Sarsat V, Halbwachs-Mecarelli L, Schuster A, et al. Proteinase 3, a potent secretagogue in airways, is present in cystic fibrosis sputum. Am J Respir Cell Mol Biol 1999;20(4):729–36.

31. Gaggar A, Hector A, Bratcher PE, et al. The role of matrix metalloproteinases in cystic fibrosis lung disease. Eur Respir J 2011;38(3):721–7.

32. Galli F, Battistoni A, Gambari R, et al. Oxidative stress and antioxidant therapy in cystic fibrosis. Biochim Biophys Acta 2012;1822(5):690–713.

33. Bogdan C. Nitric oxide and the immune response. Nat Immunol 2001;2(10):907–16.

34. Grasemann H, Michler E, Wallot M, et al. Decreased concentration of exhaled nitric oxide (NO) in patients with cystic fibrosis. Pediatr Pulmonol 1997;24(3):173–7.

35. Kelley TJ, Drumm ML. Inducible nitric oxide synthase expression is reduced in cystic fibrosis murine and human airway epithelial cells. J Clin Invest 1998;102(6):1200–7.

36. Grasemann H, Schwiertz R, Matthiesen S, et al. Increased arginase activity in cystic fibrosis airways. Am J Respir Crit Care Med 2005; 172(12):1523–8.

37. Grasemann H, Gonska T, Avolio J, et al. Effect of ivacaftor therapy on exhaled nitric oxide in patients with cystic fibrosis. J Cyst Fibros 2015; 14(6):727–32.

38. Kotha K, Szczesniak RD, Naren AP, et al. Concentration of fractional excretion of nitric oxide (FENO): a potential airway biomarker of restored CFTR function. J Cyst Fibros 2015;14(6):733–40.

39. Coyne CB, Vanhook MK, Gambling TM, et al. Regulation of airway tight junctions by proinflammatory cytokines. Mol Biol Cell 2002;13(9):3218–34.

40. Huang S, Jornot L, Wiszniewski L, et al. Src signaling links mediators of inflammation to Cx43 gap junction channels in primary and transformed CFTR-expressing airway cells. Cell Commun Adhes 2003;10(4–6):279–85.

41. Molina SA, Stauffer B, Moriarty HK, et al. Junctional abnormalities in human airway epithelial cells expressing F508del CFTR. Am J Physiol Lung Cell Mol Physiol 2015;309(5):L475–87.

42. Weiser N, Molenda N, Urbanova K, et al. Paracellular permeability of bronchial epithelium is controlled by CFTR. Cell Physiol Biochem 2011; 28(2):289–96.

43. De Lisle RC. Disrupted tight junctions in the small intestine of cystic fibrosis mice. Cell Tissue Res 2014;355(1):131–42.

44. Losa D, Kohler T, Bacchetta M, et al. Airway epithelial cell integrity protects from cytotoxicity of Pseudomonas aeruginosa quorum-sensing signals. Am J Respir Cell Mol Biol 2015;53(2):265–75.

45. Dudez T, Borot F, Huang S, et al. CFTR in a lipid raft-TNFR1 complex modulates gap junctional intercellular communication and IL-8 secretion. Biochim Biophys Acta 2008;1783(5):779–88.

46. Bruscia EM, Zhang P-X, Satoh A, et al. Abnormal trafficking and degradation of TLR4 underlie the elevated inflammatory response in cystic fibrosis. J Immunol 2011;186(12):6990–8.

47. Chanson M, Derouette JP, Roth I, et al. Gap junctional communication in tissue inflammation and repair. Biochim Biophys Acta 2005;1711(2):197–207.

48. Asgrimsson V, Gudjonsson T, Gudmundsson GH, et al. Novel effects of azithromycin on tight junction proteins in human airway epithelia. Antimicrob Agents Chemother 2006;50(5):1805–12.

49. Akira S, Uematsu S, Takeuchi O. Pathogen recognition and innate immunity. Cell 2006; 124(4):783–801.

50. Tirouvanziam R, de Bentzmann S, Hubeau C, et al. Inflammation and infection in naive human cystic fibrosis airway grafts. Am J Respir Cell Mol Biol 2000;23(2):121–7.

51. Hubeau C, Puchelle E, Gaillard D. Distinct pattern of immune cell population in the lung of human

fetuses with cystic fibrosis. J Allergy Clin Immunol 2001;108(4):524–9.

52. Bonfield TL, Panuska JR, Konstan MW, et al. Inflammatory cytokines in cystic fibrosis lungs. Am J Respir Crit Care Med 1995;152(6 Pt 1):2111–8.

53. Gaggar A, Rowe SM, Matthew H, et al. Proline-Glycine-Proline (PGP) and High Mobility Group Box Protein-1 (HMGB1): potential mediators of cystic fibrosis airway inflammation. Open Respir Med J 2010;4:32–8.

54. Rowe SM, Jackson PL, Liu G, et al. Potential role of high-mobility group box 1 in cystic fibrosis airway disease. Am J Respir Crit Care Med 2008;178(8): 822–31.

55. Khan TZ, Wagener JS, Bost T, et al. Early pulmonary inflammation in infants with cystic fibrosis. Am J Respir Crit Care Med 1995; 151(4):1075–82.

56. Worgall TS. Lipid metabolism in cystic fibrosis. Curr Opin Clin Nutr Metab Care 2009;12(2):105–9.

57. Karp CL, Flick LM, Park KW, et al. Defective lipoxin-mediated anti-inflammatory activity in the cystic fibrosis airway. Nat Immunol 2004;5(4):388–92.

58. Ringholz FC, Buchanan PJ, Clarke DT, et al. Reduced 15-lipoxygenase 2 and lipoxin A4/leukotriene B4 ratio in children with cystic fibrosis. Eur Respir J 2014;44(2):394–404.

59. Leggieri E, De Biase RV, Savi D, et al. Clinical effects of diet supplementation with DHA in pediatric patients suffering from cystic fibrosis. Minerva Pediatr 2013;65(4):389–98.

60. Maiuri L, Luciani A, Giardino I, et al. Tissue transglutaminase activation modulates inflammation in cystic fibrosis via PPARgamma down-regulation. J Immunol 2008;180(11):7697–705.

61. Ollero M, Junaidi O, Zaman MM, et al. Decreased expression of peroxisome proliferator activated receptor gamma in cftr-/- mice. J Cell Physiol 2004; 200(2):235–44.

62. Chen J, Kinter M, Shank S, et al. Dysfunction of Nrf-2 in CF epithelia leads to excess intracellular H2O2 and inflammatory cytokine production. PLoS One 2008;3(10):e3367.

63. Ribeiro CM, Boucher RC. Role of endoplasmic reticulum stress in cystic fibrosis-related airway inflammatory responses. Proc Am Thorac Soc 2010;7(6):387–94.

64. Parker D, Cohen TS, Alhede M, et al. Induction of type I interferon signaling by Pseudomonas aeruginosa is diminished in cystic fibrosis epithelial cells. Am J Respir Cell Mol Biol 2012;46(1):6–13.

65. Zheng S, De BP, Choudhary S, et al. Impaired innate host defense causes susceptibility to respiratory virus infections in cystic fibrosis. Immunity 2003;18(5):619–30.

66. Zhou Y, Song K, Painter RG, et al. Cystic fibrosis transmembrane conductance regulator recruitment to phagosomes in neutrophils. J Innate Immun 2013;5(3):219–30.

67. Su X, Looney M, Su H, et al. Role of CFTR expressed by neutrophils in modulating acute lung inflammation and injury in mice. Inflamm Res 2011;60(7):619–32.

68. Nauseef WM, Borregaard N. Neutrophils at work. Nat Immunol 2014;15(7):602–11.

69. Ingersoll SA, Laval J, Forrest OA, et al. Mature cystic fibrosis airway neutrophils suppress T cell function: evidence for a role of arginase 1 but not programmed death-ligand 1. J Immunol 2015; 194(11):5520–8.

70. Murray PJ, Wynn TA. Protective and pathogenic functions of macrophage subsets. Nat Rev Immunol 2011;11(11):723–37.

71. Brennan S, Sly PD, Gangell CL, et al. Alveolar macrophages and CC chemokines are increased in children with cystic fibrosis. Eur Respir J 2009; 34(3):655–61.

72. Locati M, Mantovani A, Sica A. Macrophage activation and polarization as an adaptive component of innate immunity. Adv Immunol 2013;120:163–84.

73. Griese M, Latzin P, Kappler M, et al. alpha1-Antitrypsin inhalation reduces airway inflammation in cystic fibrosis patients. Eur Respir J 2007;29(2): 240–50.

74. Meyer M, Huaux F, Gavilanes X, et al. Azithromycin reduces exaggerated cytokine production by M1 alveolar macrophages in cystic fibrosis. Am J Respir Cell Mol Biol 2009;41(5):590–602.

75. Hofer TP, Frankenberger M, Heimbeck I, et al. Decreased expression of HLA-DQ and HLA-DR on cells of the monocytic lineage in cystic fibrosis. J Mol Med (Berl) 2014;92(12):1293–304.

76. Lubamba BA, Jones LC, O'Neal WK, et al. X-Box binding protein 1 modulates innate immune responses of cystic fibrosis alveolar macrophages. Am J Respir Crit Care Med 2015. [Epub ahead of print].

77. Zaman MM, Gelrud A, Junaidi O, et al. Interleukin 8 secretion from monocytes of subjects heterozygous for the deltaF508 cystic fibrosis transmembrane conductance regulator gene mutation is altered. Clin Diagn Lab Immunol 2004;11(5):819–24.

78. Andersson C, Zaman MM, Jones AB, et al. Alterations in immune response and PPAR/LXR regulation in cystic fibrosis macrophages. J Cyst Fibros 2008;7(1):68–78.

79. Bonfield TL, Hodges CA, Cotton CU, et al. Absence of the cystic fibrosis transmembrane regulator (Cftr) from myeloid-derived cells slows resolution of inflammation and infection. J Leukoc Biol 2012;92(5):1111–22.

80. Hartl D, Gaggar A, Bruscia E, et al. Innate immunity in cystic fibrosis lung disease. J Cyst Fibros 2012; 11(5):363–82.

81. Wright FA, Strug LJ, Doshi VK, et al. Genome-wide association and linkage identify modifier loci of lung disease severity in cystic fibrosis at 11p13 and 20q13.2. Nat Genet 2011;43(6):539–46.

82. Aron Y, Polla BS, Bienvenu T, et al. HLA class II polymorphism in cystic fibrosis. A possible modifier of pulmonary phenotype. Am J Respir Crit Care Med 1999;159(5 Pt 1):1464–8.

83. Ramagopalan SV, Maugeri NJ, Handunnetthi L, et al. Expression of the multiple sclerosis-associated MHC class II Allele HLA-DRB1*1501 is regulated by vitamin D. PLoS Genet 2009;5(2): e1000369.

84. Knutsen AP. Immunopathology and immunogenetics of allergic bronchopulmonary aspergillosis. J Allergy (Cairo) 2011;2011:785983.

85. Koehm S, Slavin RG, Hutcheson PS, et al. HLA-DRB1 alleles control allergic bronchopulmonary aspergillosis-like pulmonary responses in humanized transgenic mice. J Allergy Clin Immunol 2007;120(3):570–7.

86. Abdulrahman BA, Khweek AA, Akhter A, et al. Autophagy stimulation by rapamycin suppresses lung inflammation and infection by Burkholderia cenocepacia in a model of cystic fibrosis. Autophagy 2011;7(11):1359–70.

87. Bunting MM, Shadie AM, Flesher RP, et al. Interleukin-33 drives activation of alveolar macrophages and airway inflammation in a mouse model of acute exacerbation of chronic asthma. Biomed Res Int 2013;2013:250938.

88. Knight RA, Kollnberger S, Madden B, et al. Defective antigen presentation by lavage cells from terminal patients with cystic fibrosis. Clin Exp Immunol 1997;107(3):542–7.

89. Hampton TH, Stanton BA. A novel approach to analyze gene expression data demonstrates that the DeltaF508 mutation in CFTR downregulates the antigen presentation pathway. Am J Physiol Lung Cell Mol Physiol 2010;298(4):L473–82.

90. Aalaei-Andabili SH, Rezaei N. Toll like receptor (TLR)-induced differential expression of microRNAs (MiRs) promotes proper immune response against infections: a systematic review. J Infect 2013;67(4):251–64.

91. Xu Y, Krause A, Limberis M, et al. Low sphingosine-1-phosphate impairs lung dendritic cells in cystic fibrosis. Am J Respir Cell Mol Biol 2013;48(2): 250–7.

92. Bhattacharya S, Ray RM, Johnson LR. Decreased apoptosis in polyamine depleted IEC-6 cells depends on Akt-mediated NF-kappaB activation but not GSK3beta activity. Apoptosis 2005;10(4): 759–76.

93. Ku CS, Pham TX, Park Y, et al. Edible blue-green algae reduce the production of pro-inflammatory cytokines by inhibiting NF-kappaB pathway in macrophages and splenocytes. Biochim Biophys Acta 2013;1830(4):2981–8.

94. Barnes PJ. Corticosteroid resistance in patients with asthma and chronic obstructive pulmonary disease. J Allergy Clin Immunol 2013;131(3):636–45.

95. Amaru Calzada A, Todoerti K, Donadoni L, et al. The HDAC inhibitor Givinostat modulates the hematopoietic transcription factors NFE2 and C-MYB in JAK2(V617F) myeloproliferative neoplasm cells. Exp Hematol 2012;40(8):634–45.e10.

96. Durham AL, Wiegman C, Adcock IM. Epigenetics of asthma. Biochim Biophys Acta 2011;1810(11): 1103–9.

97. Halili MA, Andrews MR, Labzin LI, et al. Differential effects of selective HDAC inhibitors on macrophage inflammatory responses to the Toll-like receptor 4 agonist LPS. J Leukoc Biol 2010;87(6): 1103–14.

98. Serrador JM, Cabrero JR, Sancho D, et al. HDAC6 deacetylase activity links the tubulin cytoskeleton with immune synapse organization. Immunity 2004;20(4):417–28.

99. Bartling TR, Drumm ML. Oxidative stress causes IL8 promoter hyperacetylation in cystic fibrosis airway cell models. Am J Respir Cell Mol Biol 2009;40(1):58–65.

100. Bartling TR, Drumm ML. Loss of CFTR results in reduction of histone deacetylase 2 in airway epithelial cells. Am J Physiol Lung Cell Mol Physiol 2009; 297(1):L35–43.

101. Saadane A, Soltys J, Berger M. Role of IL-10 deficiency in excessive nuclear factor-kappaB activation and lung inflammation in cystic fibrosis transmembrane conductance regulator knockout mice. J Allergy Clin Immunol 2005;115(2):405–11.

102. Perez A, Issler AC, Cotton CU, et al. CFTR inhibition mimics the cystic fibrosis inflammatory profile. Am J Physiol Lung Cell Mol Physiol 2007;292(2): L383–95.

103. Regamey N, Tsartsali L, Hilliard TN, et al. Distinct patterns of inflammation in the airway lumen and bronchial mucosa of children with cystic fibrosis. Thorax 2012;67(2):164–70.

104. Tan HL, Regamey N, Brown S, et al. The Th17 pathway in cystic fibrosis lung disease. Am J Respir Crit Care Med 2011;184(2):252–8.

105. Hartl D, Griese M, Kappler M, et al. Pulmonary T(H) 2 response in Pseudomonas aeruginosa-infected patients with cystic fibrosis. J Allergy Clin Immunol 2006;117(1):204–11.

106. Hector A, Schafer H, Poschel S, et al. Regulatory T cell impairment in cystic fibrosis patients with chronic Pseudomonas infection. Am J Respir Crit Care Med 2015;191(8):914–23.

107. Kreindler JL, Steele C, Nguyen N, et al. Vitamin D3 attenuates Th2 responses to Aspergillus fumigatus mounted by CD4+ T cells from cystic fibrosis

patients with allergic bronchopulmonary aspergillosis. J Clin Invest 2010;120(9):3242–54.

108. McGuire JK. Regulatory T cells in cystic fibrosis lung disease. More answers, more questions. Am J Respir Crit Care Med 2015;191(8):866–8.

109. Iannitti RG, Carvalho A, Cunha C, et al. Th17/Treg imbalance in murine cystic fibrosis is linked to indoleamine 2,3-dioxygenase deficiency but corrected by kynurenines. Am J Respir Crit Care Med 2013; 187(6):609–20.

110. Mueller C, Braag SA, Keeler A, et al. Lack of cystic fibrosis transmembrane conductance regulator in CD3+ lymphocytes leads to aberrant cytokine secretion and hyperinflammatory adaptive immune responses. Am J Respir Cell Mol Biol 2011;44(6):922–9.

111. Moss RB, Bocian RC, Hsu YP, et al. Reduced IL-10 secretion by CD4+ T lymphocytes expressing mutant cystic fibrosis transmembrane conductance regulator (CFTR). Clin Exp Immunol 1996; 106(2):374–88.

112. Soltys J, Bonfield T, Chmiel J, et al. Functional IL-10 deficiency in the lung of cystic fibrosis (cftr(-/-)) and IL-10 knockout mice causes increased expression and function of B7 costimulatory molecules on alveolar macrophages. J Immunol 2002;168(4): 1903–10.

113. Mayer-Hamblett N, Aitken ML, Accurso FJ, et al. Association between pulmonary function and sputum biomarkers in cystic fibrosis. Am J Respir Crit Care Med 2007;175(8):822–8.

114. Konstan MW, Doring G, Heltshe SL, et al, Investigators and Coordinators of BI Trial 543.45. A randomized double blind, placebo controlled phase 2 trial of BIIL 284 BS (an LTB4 receptor antagonist) for the treatment of lung disease in children and adults with cystic fibrosis. J Cyst Fibros 2014;13(2):148–55.

115. Ling Y, Puel A. IL-17 and infections. Actas Dermosifiliogr 2014;105(Suppl 1):34–40.

116. Nembrini C, Marsland BJ, Kopf M. IL-17-producing T cells in lung immunity and inflammation. J Allergy Clin Immunol 2009;123(5):986–94 [quiz: 995–6].

117. Ye P, Garvey PB, Zhang P, et al. Interleukin-17 and lung host defense against Klebsiella pneumoniae infection. Am J Respir Cell Mol Biol 2001;25(3): 335–40.

118. Lubberts E, van den Bersselaar L, Oppers-Walgreen B, et al. IL-17 promotes bone erosion in murine collagen-induced arthritis through loss of the receptor activator of NF-kappa B ligand/osteoprotegerin balance. J Immunol 2003;170(5): 2655–62.

119. Decraene A, Willems-Widyastuti A, Kasran A, et al. Elevated expression of both mRNA and protein levels of IL-17A in sputum of stable cystic fibrosis patients. Respir Res 2010;11:177.

120. Tan HL, Rosenthal M. IL-17 in lung disease: friend or foe? Thorax 2013;68(8):788–90.

121. Chan YR, Chen K, Duncan SR, et al. Patients with cystic fibrosis have inducible IL-17+IL-22+ memory cells in lung draining lymph nodes. J Allergy Clin Immunol 2013;131(4):1117–29, 1129.e1–5.

122. Newcomb DC, Boswell MG, Huckabee MM, et al. IL-13 regulates Th17 secretion of IL-17A in an IL-10-dependent manner. J Immunol 2012;188(3): 1027–35.

123. Cho JS, Pietras EM, Garcia NC, et al. IL-17 is essential for host defense against cutaneous Staphylococcus aureus infection in mice. J Clin Invest 2010;120(5):1762–73.

124. Siegmann N, Worbs D, Effinger F, et al. Invariant natural killer T (iNKT) cells prevent autoimmunity, but induce pulmonary inflammation in cystic fibrosis. Cell Physiol Biochem 2014;34(1):56–70.

125. Konstan MW, Schluchter MD, Xue W, et al. Clinical use of ibuprofen is associated with slower FEV1 decline in children with cystic fibrosis. Am J Respir Crit Care Med 2007;176(11):1084–9.

126. Mogayzel PJ Jr, Naureckas ET, Robinson KA, et al, Pulmonary Clinical Practice Guidelines Committee. Cystic fibrosis pulmonary guidelines. Chronic medications for maintenance of lung health. Am J Respir Crit Care Med 2013;187(7):680–9.

127. Zhang PX, Cheng J, Zou S, et al. Pharmacological modulation of the AKT/microRNA-199a-5p/CAV1 pathway ameliorates cystic fibrosis lung hyperinflammation. Nat Commun 2015;6:6221.

128. Eigen H, Rosenstein BJ, FitzSimmons S, et al. A multicenter study of alternate-day prednisone therapy in patients with cystic fibrosis. Cystic Fibrosis Foundation Prednisone Trial Group. J Pediatr 1995;126(4):515–23.

129. Ross KR, Chmiel JF, Konstan MW. The role of inhaled corticosteroids in the management of cystic fibrosis. Paediatr Drugs 2009;11(2):101–13.

130. Konstan M, Krenicky J, Hilliard K, et al. A pilot study evaluating the effect of pioglitazone, simvastatin and ibuprofen on neutrophil migration in vivo in healthy subjects. Pediatr Pulmonol 2009;289–90.

131. Moss RB, Mayer-Hamblett N, Wagener J, et al. Randomized, double-blind, placebo-controlled, dose-escalating study of aerosolized interferon gamma-1b in patients with mild to moderate cystic fibrosis lung disease. Pediatr Pulmonol 2005;39(3): 209–18.

132. Bishop C, Hudson VM, Hilton SC, et al. A pilot study of the effect of inhaled buffered reduced glutathione on the clinical status of patients with cystic fibrosis. Chest 2005;127(1):308–17.

133. Hartl D, Starosta V, Maier K, et al. Inhaled glutathione decreases PGE2 and increases lymphocytes in cystic fibrosis lungs. Free Radic Biol Med 2005;39(4):463–72.

134. Conrad C, Lymp J, Thompson V, et al. Long-term treatment with oral N-acetylcysteine: affects lung function but not sputum inflammation in cystic fibrosis subjects. A phase II randomized placebo-controlled trial. J Cyst Fibros 2015;14(2):219–27.

135. Moss RB, Mistry SJ, Konstan MW, et al. Safety and early treatment effects of the CXCR2 antagonist SB-656933 in patients with cystic fibrosis. J Cyst Fibros 2013;12(3):241–8.

136. Gaggar A, Chen J, Chmiel JF, et al. Inhaled alpha-proteinase inhibitor therapy in patients with cystic fibrosis. J Cyst Fibros 2015. [Epub ahead of print].

137. Gould NS, Gauthier S, Kariya CT, et al. Hypertonic saline increases lung epithelial lining fluid glutathione and thiocyanate: two protective CFTR-dependent thiols against oxidative injury. Respir Res 2010;11:119.

138. Chandler JD, Min E, Huang J, et al. Antiinflammatory and antimicrobial effects of thiocyanate in a cystic fibrosis mouse model. Am J Respir Cell Mol Biol 2015;53(2):193–205.

139. Grasemann H, Grasemann C, Kurtz F, et al. Oral L-arginine supplementation in cystic fibrosis patients: a placebo-controlled study. Eur Respir J 2005; 25(1):62–8.

140. Nichols DP, Ziady AG, Shank SL, et al. The triterpenoid CDDO limits inflammation in preclinical models of cystic fibrosis lung disease. Am J Physiol Lung Cell Mol Physiol 2009;297(5):L828–36.

141. Serhan CN, Chiang N, Dalli J, et al. Lipid mediators in the resolution of inflammation. Cold Spring Harb Perspect Biol 2015;7(2):a016311.

142. Ramsey BW, Dorkin HL, Eisenberg JD, et al. Efficacy of aerosolized tobramycin in patients with cystic fibrosis. N Engl J Med 1993;328(24):1740–6.

143. Ratjen F, Saiman L, Mayer-Hamblett N, et al. Effect of azithromycin on systemic markers of inflammation in patients with cystic fibrosis uninfected with *Pseudomonas aeruginosa*. Chest 2012;142(5): 1259–66.

144. Saiman L, Mayer-Hamblett N, Anstead M, et al, AZ0004 Macrolide Study Team. Open-label, follow-on study of azithromycin in pediatric patients with CF uninfected with *Pseudomonas aeruginosa*. Pediatr Pulmonol 2012;47(7):641–8.

145. Saiman L, Anstead M, Mayer-Hamblett N, et al, AZ0004 Azithromycin Study Group. Effect of azithromycin on pulmonary function in patients with cystic fibrosis uninfected with *Pseudomonas aeruginosa*: a randomized controlled trial. JAMA 2010; 303(17):1707–15.

146. Cantin AM, Hartl D, Konstan MW, et al. Inflammation in cystic fibrosis lung disease: pathogenesis and therapy. J Cyst Fibros 2015;14(4):419–30.

147. Accurso FJ, Rowe SM, Clancy JP, et al. Effect of VX-770 in persons with cystic fibrosis and the G551D-CFTR mutation. N Engl J Med 2010; 363(21):1991–2003.

148. Wainwright CE, Elborn JS, Ramsey BW, et al, TRAFFIC Study Group, TRANSPORT Study Group. Lumacaftor-ivacaftor in patients with cystic fibrosis homozygous for Phe508del CFTR. N Engl J Med 2015;373(3):220–31.

Diagnostic Testing in Cystic Fibrosis

John Brewington, MD, J.P. Clancy, MD*

KEYWORDS

- Cystic fibrosis • Diagnosis • Sweat chloride • Newborn screening • CRMS

KEY POINTS

- Cystic fibrosis (CF), caused by mutations in the cystic fibrosis transmembrane conductance regulator (CFTR) gene, leads to defects in ion and fluid balance at the epithelial surface.
- Newborn screening tests using the immunoreactive trypsinogen assay followed by a secondary test are both sensitive for identifying those at risk for CF and cost-effective.
- Sweat chloride concentration is the first-line diagnostic test for CF. Intermediate or abnormal testing should be followed with genetic evaluation for CFTR mutations.
- Fecal elastase and non–sweat ion transport testing such as nasal potential difference or intestinal current measurement can support the diagnosis of CF.
- Patients not meeting criteria for CF may be diagnosed with CFTR-related metabolic syndrome or another CFTR-related disorder, and should be followed at a CF center for progression of disease.

INTRODUCTION

Cystic fibrosis (CF) is a rare disorder affecting more than 70,000 people worldwide and approximately 30,000 people in the United States.[1–3] Patient life expectancy varies considerably across different countries, with median survival of approximately 41 years in the United States.[3] Pulmonary disease is the primary source of morbidity and mortality, with variable symptoms seen in the exocrine and endocrine pancreas, sinuses, gastrointestinal tract, hepatobiliary tree, bones, male reproductive tract, and sweat glands. CF is caused by autosomal recessive mutations in the gene encoding the cystic fibrosis transmembrane conductance regulator protein (CFTR). Nearly 2000 mutations have been described; these are summarized in 2 readily accessible databases that are inclusive of nearly all described mutations and link relatively common mutations to phenotypic information (www.genetsickkids.on.ca and www.cftr2.org, respectively).[4] CFTR is a traffic adenosine triphosphatase protein, with 2 membrane-anchored transmembrane domains, 2 cytoplasmic nucleotide binding domains (NBD-1 and -2) and a unique regulatory (R) domain. CFTR is a bicarbonate and chloride channel that regulates the transport of several ions, including additional chloride channels, thiocyanate and glutathione transport, and the epithelial sodium channel.[1,5–9] CFTR can be detected in numerous tissues, but its expression in the airways, small and large intestines, pancreatic ducts, bile ducts, vas deferens, and sweat glands are all linked directly to disease pathogenesis.[10–16] CF airway disease relates directly to CFTR defects in ion transport in submucosal glands and surface airway epithelia, governing airway surface liquid volume and pH, as well as mucus hydration and release.[17–24] Loss of CFTR

Disclosures: Dr J. Brewington has nothing to disclose. Dr J.P. Clancy has received contracted research support from Vertex Pharmaceuticals (VX12-770-115, VX12-809-105), ProQR (PQ010-002), the CFFT (Clancy14Y0, Clancy11CS0, Clancy14K1, Clancy14XX1, Clancy14XX0, Clancy14Y4, eICE-ID-10, CFFC-OB-11, AquaADEKs-2-IP-12, SHIP14K0), and the NIH (R01HL116226), none of which directly conflicts with the information presented.
Division of Pulmonary Medicine, Department of Pediatrics, Cincinnati Children's Hospital Medical Center, MLC 2021, 3333 Burnet Avenue, Cincinnati, OH 45229, USA
* Corresponding author.
E-mail address: john.clancy@cchmc.org

function decreases mucus clearance, leading to mucus stagnation, infection, inflammation, and subsequent symptoms of the disease.[25–27]

Diagnostic testing in CF has traditionally centered on the sweat chloride (SC) test in the context of appropriate signs and symptoms of disease. After the discovery of the gene encoding CFTR in 1989, diagnostic tests based on genetic techniques have become increasingly common and applied, particularly in challenging cases with equivocal symptoms and functional testing. These have been augmented by additional in vivo or ex vivo tests of CFTR function, including the nasal potential difference (NPD) and intestinal current measurement (ICM). Historically, treatment of CF has been supportive, addressing the downstream manifestations that result from the loss of CFTR activity. Recent therapeutic advancements have emerged that target the underlying cause of CF, including treatment with drugs that restore function to disease-causing CFTR mutations. These new therapies have the potential to be transformative, and highlight the value of early CF diagnosis and treatment assignment that is tailored to specific CFTR mutation defects.

SCREENING PROTOCOLS FOR CYSTIC FIBROSIS
Prenatal Screening

Prenatal CFTR screening is available both for parental carrier status and for fetal confirmation (through invasive testing such as amniocentesis). It is recommended that all pregnant women in the United States be offered genetic screening, although counseling for positive screening results is variable and often carried out by the obstetrician.[28,29] Parent/couple responses to carrier screening are also variable, often including changes in reproductive patterns.[30] In those already pregnant, prenatal diagnosis may result in termination of pregnancy, which has broad ethical implications.[31] Nonetheless, in 1 survey, the majority of adult CF patients/parents support prenatal or preconception screening for CFTR mutations.[32] In addition to screening diagnoses, a minority of CF patients are diagnosed prenatally owing to the detection of bowel abnormalities by prenatal ultrasonography.

Newborn Screening

Universal newborn screening (NBS) for CF was implemented in all 50 states within the United States as of 2010, as well as in several European countries.[33,34] In the United States, it is part of the standard newborn screen for other congenital genetic abnormalities, with some variance in the nature of testing that is state specific. The benefits of NBS and early CF diagnosis are clear, including improved lung function and growth in childhood, decreased rates of hospitalization, earlier family access to genetic counseling, and improved cognitive performance.[35–40] The reasons for these benefits produced by neonatal diagnosis compared with diagnosing CF secondary to disease manifestations likely include improved growth and nutrition in the neonatal and infant periods, avoidance of fat-soluble vitamin deficiencies, and the initiation of pulmonary therapies that prevent early lung damage.[40,41] Approximately 10% of CF patients are diagnosed soon after birth owing to meconium ileus, in which thick and poorly hydrated bowel secretions produce bowel obstruction and, in extreme cases, bowel perforation and/or microcolon; these patients are typically excluded from analyses of NBS protocols.

Risks of NBS are similar to those associated with other early screens, including parental depression and anxiety (in both patients with true disease and in false positives), altered parent–child bonding, and a misunderstanding of carrier status.[42,43] Diagnosis of CF through NBS was associated with early detection of *Pseudomonas aeruginosa* in 1 study, which may have been related to common CF clinic visits of older CF patients (enriched for this CF pathogen), and infants identified through NBS.[44] Although any screening protocol introduces new costs to a health care system, cost analysis of NBS for CF compared with late diagnosis and its downstream complications suggest significant system-level savings using an early screening model.[45] For example, NBS may provide earlier identification of the approximately 10% of CF patients who are diagnosed in adulthood.

NBS methodology typically includes a 2-tiered combination of functional and/or genetic testing. As the first tier, all current NBS protocols initially use a functional measurement of immunoreactive trypsinogen (IRT), a pancreatic exocrine biomarker that is increased in the blood of the vast majority of patients with either partial or nonfunctional CFTR mutations.[46] An increased IRT at 48 to 72 hours of life is sensitive but not specific for a diagnosis of CF, with genetic carriers also often testing positive. Other causes of increased IRT include perinatal stress, critical illness, and several trisomies.[47–49] A notable cause of falsely low IRT values is meconium ileus, which should clinically prompt evaluation for CF regardless of NBS results.[50] Values that exceed a specific threshold or that are in the highest percentile of a given day of testing at a state screening laboratory are considered positive, triggering a second-tier test, with regional variability in the subsequent testing algorithm. Examples of NBS protocols currently in use and their test characteristics can be found in **Fig. 1** and **Table 1**.

One option for second-tier testing is a repeat IRT at 2 to 4 weeks of age when this assay becomes more specific (the so-called IRT/IRT screening methodology).[51,52] This strategy has been shown to have reasonable test characteristics, but does require a second blood draw, which may lead to additional parental anxiety.[42] Alternatively, after a positive initial IRT screen, many protocols then use genetic testing as a second-tier evaluation (the IRT/DNA methodology). This can include a limited or expanded panel of CF-associated mutations, which varies from state to state and country to country. Although attractive given the recent discovery of genotype-directed therapies, genetic screening for CFTR mutations does not confirm disease. For one, many screens are of limited scope, and previously unidentified or rare mutations may be missed. Even identification of 2 CFTR mutations may not necessarily indicate disease, because both mutations can occur in cis, on the same chromosome. Moreover, this methodology likely identifies many carriers, leading to additional testing. A third evolving option for functional testing includes following a positive IRT with a test of pancreatitis-associated protein (the IRT/pancreatitis-associated protein methodology). Early evidence suggests that this method yields a sensitivity and specificity similar to genetic testing as a second-line test, and may be more cost effective.[53–56] Regardless of the algorithm, patients with a positive IRT and secondary test are considered to have a positive NBS. Some algorithms also use a "fail-safe" protocol, flagging an "ultrahigh" initial IRT (typically the top 0.1% of values for the population) as a positive NBS regardless of the secondary test. All patients with a positive NBS should be referred for SC testing as the gold standard confirmatory test (discussed elsewhere in this paper).

DIAGNOSTIC TESTING FOR CYSTIC FIBROSIS TRANSMEMBRANE CONDUCTANCE REGULATOR PROTEIN DEFECTS

In 1996, the CF Foundation convened a panel of experts to develop criteria for the diagnosis of CF. The consensus from this panel was that the diagnosis of CF should be based on the presence of 1 or more characteristic clinical features, a history of CF in a sibling, or a positive NBS test, plus laboratory evidence of an abnormality in the CFTR gene or protein. Acceptable evidence of a CFTR abnormality included biological evidence of channel dysfunction (ie, abnormal SC concentration or NPD) or identification of a CF disease-causing mutation in each copy of the CFTR gene (ie, on each chromosome).[57,58]

The diagnosis of CF is typically made in the context of CF-associated organ symptoms, functional testing (SC), and genetic identification of CFTR mutations. In newborns, the diagnosis can often be made before the detection of CF-associated symptoms by relying on screening (IRT and genetic testing) that is confirmed by SC testing. In patients with SC values above the normal range without identification of 2 CF-associated mutations in CFTR, further testing of CFTR function (NPD, ICM) and assessment for organ-specific symptoms (pulmonary pathogens, obstructive lung disease, bronchiectasis, pancreatic insufficiency, and liver disease) can generally provide a complete picture that helps to clarify whether CF is the underlying diagnosis.

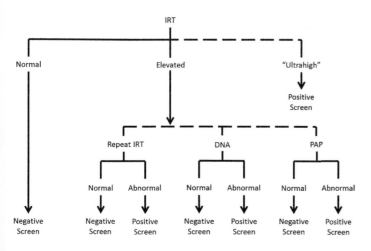

Fig. 1. Current newborn screening algorithms for cystic fibrosis. IRT and PAP cutoffs for normal, elevated, and "ultrahigh" depend on specific testing algorithms. Dotted lines represent variable components of screening algorithms. CFTR mutation-based secondary screening protocols also vary by algorithm. CFTR, cystic fibrosis transmembrane conductance regulator protein; DNA, CFTR mutation-based screening; IRT, immunoreactive trypsinogen; PAP, pancreatitis-associated protein.

Table 1
Testing characteristics of selected newborn screening algorithms

Screening Strategy	Region	Number Screened	Initial IRT Cutoff	Secondary Test	Direct Referral for Ultrahigh IRT	Sensitivity (%)	Specificity (%)
IRT/IRT	Colorado[120]	279,399	≥140 µg/L	IRT ≥80 µg/L	No	93.0	NR
	Northern Ireland[121]	108,424	≥98th percentile	IRT ≥120 µg/L	No	73.0	99.9
IRT/DNA	Wisconsin[122]	509,794	≥94th percentile	F508del screen	Yes	94.0	99.0
		90,142	≥96th percentile	25-mutation screen	Yes	95.0	99.0
	New York[123]	1,480,000	≥95th percentile	23-mutation screen	No	96.5	99.6
	Massachusetts[124]	265,610	≥95th percentile	27-mutation screen	≥99.9th percentile	97.8	99.7
	France[125]	5,947,148	≥65 µg/L	30-mutation screen or repeat IRT	≥100 µg/L (99.9th percentile)	95.1	99.9
IRT/PAP	Germany[56]	328,176	≥99th percentile	PAP ≥1.6 µg/L	≥99.9th percentile	96	99.80

All data exclude patients with meconium ileus from consideration.
Abbreviations: IRT, immunoreactive trypsinogen; NR, not reported; PAP, pancreatitis-associated protein.

Sweat Chloride Testing

The SC test is a well-established functional assessment of CFTR that has been available for decades to diagnose CF.[59] In the sweat gland, CFTR activity drives sodium reabsorption. When CFTR functions normally, sodium and chloride are absorbed in the ductal portion of the sweat gland, resulting in a low level of sodium and chloride at the skin surface.[1] Sweating is stimulated by pilocarpine iontophoresis, with a standardized time of collection.[57] The sodium and chloride concentrations in the collected sweat are then quantified, and reported for 2 simultaneous collections. In the 2005 CF Foundation Patient Registry, only 3.5% of patients with a diagnosis of CF had an SC value of less than 60 mmol/L, and only 1.2% had a value of less than 40 mmol/L.[57,60] Although the SC is a sensitive and specific test for CFTR dysfunction, there are a number of other disorders or conditions that can lead to false-positive values (summarized in **Box 1**).

Box 1
Conditions associated with falsely increased sweat chloride levels

Anorexia nervosa

Atopic dermatitis

Autonomic dysfunction

Ectodermal dysplasia

Environmental deprivation

Familial cholestasis

Fucosidosis

Glucose-6-phosphate deficiency

Hypogammaglobulinemia

Klinefelter syndrome

Long-term prostaglandin E1 infusion

Mauriac's syndrome

Mucopolysaccharidosis type 1

Nephrogenic diabetes insipidus

Nephrosis

Protein calorie malnutrition

Psuedohypoaldosteronism

Psychosocial failure to thrive

Untreated adrenal insufficiency

Untreated hypothyroidism

Data from CLSI. Sweat testing: sample collection and quantitative chloride analysis; approved guideline—third edition. CLSI document C34-A3. Wayne, PA: Clinical and Laboratory Standards Institute; 2009.

Normative values for SC concentrations currently in use were developed in the early 1960s, defining normal (<39 mmol/L), intermediate (40–59 mmol/L), and abnormal (>60 mmol/L) ranges. These ranges carry several important caveats.[61] First, no healthy controls were studied, potentially introducing a bias toward higher "normal" values. Second, the methodology used in these tests is no longer identical to modern testing, raising the possibility of systematic bias. Finally, these references were generated in patients with classic clinical signs of CF, likely missing many patients with mild disease, and were generally obtained in older pediatric patients. This may have implications for the diagnosis of adult patients with milder CF phenotypes. Nonetheless, these reference values appear to be appropriate based on registry data, with the great majority of patients with a clinical diagnosis of CF having an abnormal SC concentration.[3]

After the introduction of NBS, many infants at risk for CF are being identified and referred for SC testing. The interpretation testing in this age group is complex, because many non-CF infants have a slightly elevated SC concentration and many infants ultimately diagnosed with CF have lower values compared with the adult norms.[62,63] As such, separate normal (<29 mmol/L), intermediate (30–59 mmol/L), and abnormal (>60 mmol/L) reference ranges have been validated in infants.[64] The CF Foundation recommends use of these ranges up to age 6 months, followed by the adult reference ranges, whereas the European Cystic Fibrosis Society uses the adult reference values for all patients.[34,57]

Fecal Elastase

In cases of possible CF, evaluation of fecal elastase (FE) can be performed to examine for evidence of pancreatic dysfunction. Although this is a simple and noninvasive test, it can give false-positive results, and its sensitivity in patients with mild pancreatic insufficiency is low.[65] In addition, the FE value can vary throughout the first year of life, complicating conclusions made on a single sample. Infants with FE values that are intermediate (50–200 μg/g of stool) should have repeat testing at 1 year of age to ensure that those with falsely low levels do not continue pancreatic enzyme replacement unnecessarily. Importantly, those with initial FE values of greater than 200 μg/g can become pancreatic insufficient over time, and thus should be reevaluated periodically based on their clinical course.[66]

Nasal Potential Difference

The NPD measurement is a functional bioelectric test that is capable of isolating CFTR function. It was first described by Knowles and colleagues[67] in 1981, and over the past several years has undergone significant refinements to standardize its performance across different CF care centers.[68–74] Most of these efforts have been geared toward optimizing the assay to detect restored function for gene therapy or CFTR modulator clinical trials. However, this standardization has benefited the use of this test for diagnostic purposes. The assay includes the perfusion of different solutions in standardized concentrations across the nasal mucosa and monitoring the transepithelial potential difference by a probe electrode.[75] The solutions used include Ringers, Ringers plus amiloride (to block epithelial sodium channel and sodium resorption), zero chloride solution and amiloride (with gluconate replacing chloride to produce a chloride secretory gradient), the addition of isoproterenol (to stimulate CFTR) and adenosine triphosphate (to activate CFTR-independent chloride transport and serve as a positive control of epithelial integrity). The assay demonstrates excellent sensitivity and specificity in experienced hands, but currently does not have specific regulatory approval as a diagnostic test (eg, CLIA-approved test). Refinements to optimize this test include standardized times of perfusion of the different solutions, the use of standardized catheters and nasal mucosal placement, the use of a probe electrode made of agar (to reduce noise and breaks in PD detection), and data analysis (single vs averaged NPD values for both nostrils). Thresholds of PD values and changes have been defined that exclude CF, including the baseline value and the change in PD after amiloride perfusion (reflective of sodium absorption), and the change in PD following zero chloride plus amiloride and zero chloride plus amiloride plus isoproterenol (reflective of CFTR activity). **Table 2** includes the NPD values of non-CF controls and CF patients collected by the CF Foundation Therapeutic Development Network during the process of NPD operator qualification for use in CF clinical trials. By measuring the change in PD after 3 minutes of perfusion with zero chloride plus amiloride (100 µmol/L) and 3 minutes with zero chloride plus amiloride (100 µmol/L) plus isoproterenol (10 µmol/L), a cutoff PD change of -6.62 mV provides 94.8% sensitivity and 96.5% specificity to distinguish CF from non-CF.

Intestinal Current Measurement

ICM was developed in Europe, and provides a direct measurement of CFTR activity in rectal tissue derived from patients.[76] In this assay, intestinal tissue obtained from rectal biopsies is dissected (to remove the muscularis mucosa and retain the intact epithelial layer) and mounted in Ussing chambers to monitor either transepithelial potential (open circuit) or transepithelial short circuit current (voltage clamp conditions). Tissues are treated with reagents that isolate and quantify CFTR function by monitoring responses to various CFTR stimuli. There have been several efforts to standardize the test for use in clinical trials, and this has driven standardization for diagnostic use.[77–82] Similar to NPD, ICM is not currently a CLIA-approved test in the United States, but is applied to diagnose CF when other diagnostic tests provide unclear information (most commonly in several European countries). Several studies

---

Table 2
NPD values of CF and non-CF controls, from the CFF-TDN center for CFTR detection (University of Alabama at Birmingham)

NPD Values (mV)	Non-CF Controls (n = 135) (SD)	CF Controls (n = 144) (SD)
Ringers	−16.1 (9.32)	−35.2 (12.53)
Change amiloride	8.78 (5.2)	18.65 (9.0)
Change 0 [chloride] plus amiloride (A)	−12.0 (6.41)	1.41 (2.81)
Change 0 [chloride] plus amiloride plus isoproterenol (B)	−10.4 (6.4)	−0.23 (3.0)
Total change (A and B)	−22.41 (13.1)	1.18 (3.9)
Change ATP	−2.84 (11.8)	−7.83 (14.02)

Abbreviations: ATP, adenosine triphosphate; CF, cystic fibrosis; CFTR, cystic fibrosis transmembrane conductance regulator protein; NPD, nasal potential difference.

Adapted from Liu B, Hathorne H, Hill A, et al. Normative values and receiver operating characteristics of NPD for diagnostic measurements. Pediatr Pulmonol 2010;303(S33):307.

have demonstrated that the ICM assay can segregate CF patients with nonfunctional CFTR mutations from patients with partial function CFTR mutations and healthy non-CF controls. This is attractive because it provides a greater dynamic range than NPD, and provides the flexibility to use reagents that help to isolate CFTR that are not appropriate for in vivo use. Performance of ICM requires special expertise that is not available uniformly, including specialized expertise to dissect and study the biopsy tissue ex vivo, as well as the necessary equipment to measure ion transport. The European and US CF communities have developed standard operating procedures that have been generally harmonized for CFTR detection, allowing comparison of results between centers.[76,77,83] These efforts have also led to the development of standard operating procedures for ICM use in clinical trials of CFTR restorative therapies. The specificity of the assay for CFTR potentially allows for its use in small clinical trials,

and future efforts will likely help to establish a uniform protocol for diagnostic application. **Fig. 2** summarizes ICM differences between CF and non-CF subjects. The short circuit response to cyclic adenosine monophosphate (forskolin 10 μmol/L and IBMX 100 μmol/L) and carbachol (100 μmol/L) demonstrates excellent sensitivity and specificity to separate CF from non-CF in multicenter ICM performance.

DIAGNOSTIC CRITERIA FOR CYSTIC FIBROSIS

Diagnostic criteria for CF have been developed by the CF Foundation and the European CF care community. These include the demonstration of defects in CFTR function coupled with the identification of CF-associated mutations and organ-specific disease manifestations associated with CF. **Figs. 3** and **4** depict these guideline-based diagnostic algorithms for patients identified by

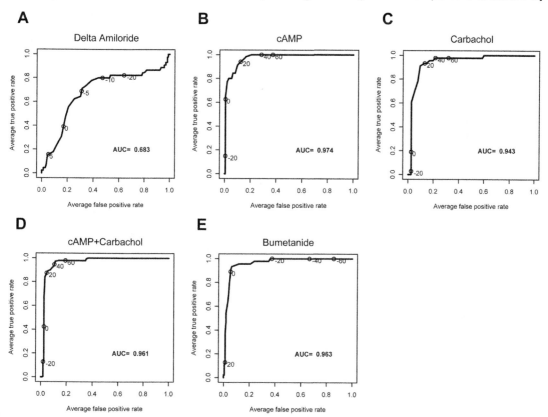

Fig. 2. Comparison of receiver operating characteristic curves of intestinal current measurement (ICM) parameters in cystic fibrosis (CF) and non-CF subjects from 4 centers. (*A-E*) Receiver operating curves for diagnosing CF based on intestinal current measurement changes with the addition of amiloride, cAMP (forskolin/IBMX), carbachol, cAMP combined with carbachol, and bumetanide (respectively). Response to cAMP and carbachol (*D*) demonstrates excellent sensitivity and specificity to separate CF From non-CF. AUC, area under the curve; cAMP, cyclic adenosine monophosphate. (*From* Clancy JP, Szczesniak RD, Ashlock MA, et al. Multicenter intestinal current measurements in rectal biopsies from CF and non-CF subjects to monitor CFTR function. PLoS One 2013;8(9):e73905.)

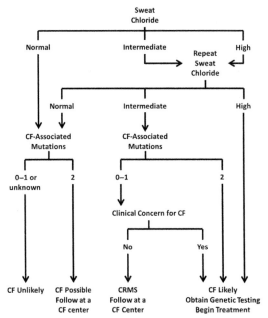

Fig. 3. Diagnostic algorithm for evaluation of an asymptomatic infant with a positive newborn screen. Different cutoff values for normal and intermediate sweat chloride are used for infants younger than 6 months of age in the Cystic Fibrosis Foundation (CFF; normal, ≤29 mmol/L; intermediate, 30–59 mmol/L) and European Cystic Fibrosis Society (ECFS; normal, ≤39 mmol/L; intermediate, 40–59 mmol/L) guidelines. For those older than 6 months of age, the same cutoff values are used (normal, ≤39 mmol/L; intermediate, 40–59 mmol/L). The ECFS guidelines also recommend consideration of nasal potential difference testing for those with "CF possible" or "CRMS" diagnoses. CF, cystic fibrosis; CFTR, cystic fibrosis transmembrane conductance regulator protein; CRMS, CFTR-related metabolic syndrome.

NBS and by clinical concern. Simplified criteria are provided in **Box 2**.

North American Cystic Fibrosis Foundation Guidelines for Diagnosis of Cystic Fibrosis

The CF Foundation criteria, last updated in 2008, recommend diagnostic testing for persons with suspected CF as defined by positive NBS, clinical concern based on classic symptoms, or a sibling with CF.[57]

Newborns with a positive NBS should be referred for SC testing. An abnormal SC value (≥60 mmol/L) is diagnostic of CF in these patients, although repeat SC and/or genetic testing for CF-associated mutations are recommended for further confirmation. A normal SC value (≤29 mmol/L) makes CF unlikely. Patients identified by a positive IRT/DNA screen with 2 known CF-associated mutations and a normal SC

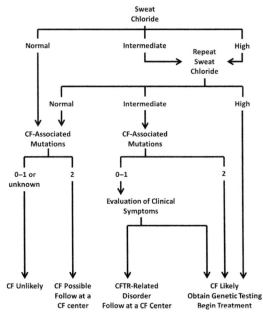

Fig. 4. Cystic Fibrosis Foundation (CFF) diagnostic algorithm for evaluation of a symptomatic patient with concern for cystic fibrosis (CF). Different cutoff values for normal and intermediate sweat chloride are used for infants younger than 6 months of age (normal, ≤29 mmol/L; intermediate, 30–59 mmol/L) and those older than 6 months of age (normal, ≤39 mmol/L; intermediate; 40–59 mmol/L).

Box 2
Diagnostic criteria for CF in children

Positive newborn screen -or- family history -or- clinical concern for CF plus one of the below

- Confirmed positive sweat chloride concentration

- Two CF-associated mutations identified

- Confirmed intermediate sweat chloride concentration with 0 to 1 identified mutations and additional evidence of CF, including:

  ○ Respiratory tract colonization with *Pseudomonas aeruginosa*;

  ○ Pancreatic insufficiency based on fecal elastase testing;

  ○ Chronic respiratory complaints and/or bronchiectasis; and

  ○ NPD testing consistent with CF (if available).

Abbreviations: CF, cystic fibrosis; NPD, nasal potential difference.

Adapted from Farrell PM, Rosenstein BJ, White TB, et al. Guidelines for diagnosis of cystic fibrosis in newborns through older adults: Cystic Fibrosis Foundation Consensus Report. J Pediatr 2008;153(2):S4-14.

concentration may, in rare circumstances, have CF, and should be followed in a CF center. In these cases, maternal genetic testing should be considered to clarify if the mutations are in cis or in trans. Infants with a SC value in the intermediate range (30–59 mmol/L) should undergo genetic testing, which is considered confirmatory of CF if 2 CF-associated mutations are present. Infants with 0 or 1 identified mutations, a positive newborn screen, and an intermediate SC fall under the CFTR related metabolic syndrome classification, and should be followed routinely at a CF center, with ongoing evaluation for clinical evidence of CF (see Cystic Fibrosis Transmembrane Conductance Regulator Protein-Related Metabolic Syndrome). This longitudinal follow-up should continue in a routine fashion until the patient is confirmed to have CF (positive sweat test or clinical evidence of disease) or ruled unlikely to have disease by negative sweat test.

Individuals with concern for CF owing to symptoms or a family history should also be referred for SC measurement. As stated, an abnormal SC value ($\geq$60 mmol/L) is diagnostic of CF in these patients, with repeat SC and/or genetic testing for CFTR mutations recommended for further confirmation. A normal SC value ($\leq$29–39 mmol/L, depending on age) makes CF unlikely, although patients with 2 identified CF-associated mutations in this group may have CF and should continue to follow at a CF center. Those with intermediate SC values (between 30–40 and 59 mmol/L, depending on age) should undergo genetic testing, confirming CF whether 2 CF-associated mutations are identified. Similar to the algorithm presented, patients with intermediate SC levels and 0 or 1 identified mutations should be followed routinely in a CF center until either CF disease is confirmed, a negative SC is obtained (making CF unlikely), or a CFTR-related disorder is diagnosed.

European Cystic Fibrosis Society Diagnostic Guidelines

The most recent European CF Society diagnostic guidelines, updated in 2009, are similar to the North American guidelines with 2 notable differences.[34,84] First, there is no recommendation to use separate infant SC cutoff values; instead, adult values are used for all patients regardless of age. Second, in cases of equivocal diagnoses, the European guidelines also suggest use of other electrophysiological diagnostic techniques (such as NPD or ICM) to aid in diagnosis CF. No specific choice of testing method or reference range is provided.

CYSTIC FIBROSIS TRANSMEMBRANE CONDUCTANCE REGULATOR PROTEIN-RELATED METABOLIC SYNDROME

One side effect of universal NBS has been the identification of children with CFTR abnormalities that do not meet the full diagnostic criteria for CF, leading to clinical uncertainty. These are typically asymptomatic patients with elevated IRT on testing, 1 or no CF-associated mutations in CFTR, and sweat tests that are intermediate but fail to meet CF diagnostic criteria. These features have been termed the CFTR-related metabolic syndrome (CRMS). Counseling and management of these patients is a significant challenge for the CF care community, and have been the topic of deliberation among experts in CF. These issues can be particularly challenging in states with a diverse ethnic populations (such as California) where common CF-associated mutations characterized in the Caucasian population are reduced, and less well-described CFTR mutations from Hispanic (or other) ethnicities are enriched. This can also be a diagnostic dilemma for patients with a combination of CFTR mutations with known phenotypic variability (such as R117H-T7).

Diagnosis and Management of Cystic Fibrosis Transmembrane Conductance Regulator Protein-Related Metabolic Syndrome

Published in 2009, the North American CFF guidelines for management of infants with CRMS provide recommendations for these patients.[85] Here, CRMS is defined as an asymptomatic infant with a positive NBS (either by IRT/IRT or IRT/DNA methods), 0 or 1 identified disease-causing CFTR mutations, and an intermediate SC concentration. For initial evaluation, these patients should undergo in-depth genetic analysis (if not already performed as part of their NBS) and have a repeat SC before the age of 2 months. At that time, they should be seen by a CF care provider including a full history and physical examination, with special note paid to growth and nutrition. Genetic counseling services should be made available to patients and their families to discuss both CF and CRMS. Exocrine pancreatic function evaluation via FE is recommended, and further testing (including chest or abdominal radiograph, fat-soluble vitamin levels, complete blood count, and liver function testing) can be considered based on the presence of any symptoms. Finally, an oropharyngeal culture should be obtained and processed as a "CF culture" sample. In the absence of concerning findings and persistence of an intermediate SC value, patients should be seen again with a repeat SC after the age of

6 months. Thereafter, CRMS patients should be seen by a CF care provider at least yearly with repeat oropharyngeal culture and reassessment for clinical evidence of disease at each visit. Consideration should be made for salt supplementation in patients with higher SC values (who by definition have increased salt losses compared with the population average).

Patients with CRMS may be changed to a formal diagnosis of CF if at any time they have a positive SC measurement ($\geq$60 mmol/L), if they have other significant clinical disease consistent with CF (chronic respiratory disease, failure to thrive, evidence of pancreatic insufficiency), or if *Pseudomonas aeruginosa* is persistently cultured from their respiratory tract. Alternatively, patients with subsequent normal SC measurements ($\leq$29 mmol/L) are "cleared" of their CRMS diagnosis.

Similar guidelines are available from the European CF Society for diagnosis and management of CRMS.[86] Common to the European Cystic Fibrosis Society CF diagnostic guidelines, infant SC reference values are not used, instead using the adult reference values for all individuals. Alternative ion transport testing (eg, NPD and ICM) is again suggested in asymptomatic patients with 1 or no CF-associated mutations and persistently equivocal SC measurements. Further ion transport testing is also suggested for those with 2 known in trans CF-associated mutations and persistently normal measurements (considered diagnostic of CF by CF Foundation guidelines). The guidelines do not specify which alternative ion transport testing method to use, nor do they provide normative data for evaluation.

Simplified diagnostic criteria for CRMS are presented in **Box 3**, and the annual evaluation of patients with CRMS is presented in **Box 4**.

Box 3
Diagnostic criteria for CFTR-related metabolic syndrome

- Positive newborn screen
- Confirmed intermediate sweat chloride concentration
- Zero or one identified CF-associated mutations
- Absence of CF-related symptoms

Abbreviations: CF, cystic fibrosis; CFTR, cystic fibrosis transmembrane conductance regulator protein.
Adapted from Borowitz D, Parad RB, Sharp JK, et al. Cystic Fibrosis Foundation practice guidelines for the management of infants with cystic fibrosis transmembrane conductance regulator-related metabolic syndrome during the first two years of life and beyond. J Pediatr 2009;155(6 Suppl):S106-16.

Box 4
Annual evaluation of CFTR-related metabolic syndrome

- Weight/growth parameters
- History/physical
- Spirometry (once able)
- Consider additional testing based on symptoms
  - GI: abdominal radiograph, repeat fecal elastase
  - Pulmonary: chest radiograph
  - ID: bronchoscopy with BAL
  - Nutrition: fat-soluble vitamin levels
- Oropharyngeal culture

Abbreviations: BAL, bronchoalveolar lavage; CFTR, cystic fibrosis transmembrane conductance regulator protein; GI, gastrointestinal; ID, infectious disease.
Adapted from Borowitz D, Parad RB, Sharp JK, et al. Cystic Fibrosis Foundation practice guidelines for the management of infants with cystic fibrosis transmembrane conductance regulator-related metabolic syndrome during the first two years of life and beyond. J Pediatr 2009;155(6 Suppl):S106-16.

Outcomes in Cystic Fibrosis Transmembrane Conductance Regulator Protein-Related Metabolic Syndrome

A recent case series evaluated outcomes in patients with CRMS.[87] Although it was published after the release of the CF Foundation guidelines, this retrospective review describes patients cared for before the guideline availability, and therefore does not adhere entirely to the current definition of CRMS. Twelve patients diagnosed with CRMS were followed for an average of 36 months and compared with a similar-aged cohort of patients diagnosed with CF. All patients had 1 or more CF-associated mutation, although many included variable-phenotype mutations such as R334W and R117H-7T. All 12 patients were pancreatic sufficient by FE. Only 1 CRMS patient was hospitalized over the first 4 years of life (for bronchiolitis owing to respiratory syncytial virus), whereas almost 50% of the patients with CF were hospitalized during that age. Three patients had positive oropharyngeal cultures for *P aeruginosa*, which the authors did not use as automatic criteria for a CF diagnosis. All 3 such patients had 2 CF-associated mutations, and in all 3 cases 1 mutation was R117H-7T. One of these 3 patients ultimately was diagnosed with CF owing to an increased repeat SC concentration; this was the only CRMS patient in the cohort to convert to a diagnosis of CF. Interestingly, if positive oropharyngeal cultures for *P aeruginosa* had been used as criteria for conversion to a diagnosis of CF (as is suggested in the CFF guidelines), than the 25% (3/12) conversion rate would be very similar to an older Australian cohort following patients with intermediate SC values.[88] This further highlights the importance of close follow-up for patients with CRMS, especially those with variable-phenotype mutations in CFTR.

CYSTIC FIBROSIS TRANSMEMBRANE CONDUCTANCE REGULATOR PROTEIN-RELATED DISORDERS

CFTR dysfunction is a spectrum, and CFTR mutations can contribute to disorders that do not meet the diagnostic criteria for CF. These are categorized as CFTR-related disorders, and are well-described for subgroups of patients with congenital bilateral absence of the vas deferens (CBAVD), recurrent acute or chronic pancreatitis, and respiratory disorders, including disseminated bronchiectasis.[89] A current definition of CFTR-related disorders is "a clinical entity associated with CFTR dysfunction that does not fulfill the diagnostic criteria for CF." An algorithm to guide the evaluation of these patients has been published recently, providing caregivers a roadmap for patient examination and management. It should be stressed that CFTR-related disorders is still being identified and defined, and that long-term prognostic information is currently limited.

Congenital Bilateral Absence of the Vas Deferens

CBAVD accounts for approximately 3% of male infertility, producing azoospermia that is clearly related to the detection of CFTR mutations.[90–92] CFTR is expressed in the vas deferens, which is very sensitive to loss of CFTR function. In several studies, cohorts of male patients with CBAVD have been described to have a high incidence of CF-associated mutations in CFTR.[93] This can include patients who are carriers for nonfunctional CFTR mutations and patients with 2 CFTR mutations (with at least 1 with partial function, such as the common IVS8-5T allele that is found in approximately 5% of CFTR alleles and reduces splicing efficiency of CFTR).[89] It has been estimated that 70% to 90% of CBAVD cases are caused by mutations in the CFTR gene depending on ethnic and population contributions.[94,95] The distribution of CFTR mutations in CBAVD patients differs from patients with CF. CBAVD males typically possess either a severe and a mild/variable (88%) mutation, or 2 mild/variable (12%) CFTR mutations.[96,97] In contrast, CF patients typically possess 2 severe mutations (88%), or 1 severe and 1 mild/variable CFTR mutation (12%). There are numerous other potential genetic contributors to the functional CFTR deficiency observed in CBAVD, including the penetrance of the IVS8-5T allele (approximately 50%), the polymorphic dinucleotide repeat TG lying immediately upstream of the IVS8-Tn tract that influences the efficiency of exon 9 splicing, and additional single nucleotide polymorphisms in CFTR exons that can produce complex alleles.[89,98] The majority of males with isolated CBAVD are otherwise asymptomatic, but some may have other organ symptoms reflective of CFTR dysfunction (such as nasal polyps, rhinosinusitis, recurrent bronchitis, and/or increased SC values).[99,100] Owing to this phenotypic heterogeneity, their management can be a challenge for care providers. It is generally recommended that patients with CBAVD, and identified CFTR mutations, undergo further examination for CF diagnosis, including extended genetic testing, functional tests (eg, SC, NPD, and potentially ICM if available), and assessment for CF disease manifestations in other organs (eg, sinopulmonary, liver, gastrointestinal tract, and pancreas). Management is driven by the results of these further analyses, and can range from no intervention to the initiation of established CF therapies.

Recurrent Pancreatitis

Recurrent pancreatitis is another disorder that can have contributions from CFTR mutations, often in concert with additional non-CFTR mutations associated with recurrent pancreatitis. CFTR is expressed on the ductal cell apical surface of the exocrine pancreas, where it regulates cyclic adenosine monophosphate–stimulated bicarbonate transport and alkalization of pancreatic secretions.[101,102] Studies have demonstrated an association between the detection of CFTR mutations and idiopathic chronic pancreatitis (ICP).[103,104] Up to 30% of patients with ICP or recurrent acute pancreatitis have CFTR mutations.[89] The risk of ICP has been demonstrated to increase to 6.3, 2.4, and 37 times that of healthy controls with a CF-causing allele, the IVS8-5T allele, and a CF-associated mutation plus a mild allele in trans, respectively.[105] There are additional ICP susceptibility genes involved in the pathway of protease activation and inactivation.[106,107] One of these (*SPINK1* – serine peptidase inhibitor, Kazal type 1) has been shown to have gene-gene interactions with CFTR that dramatically impacts the risk of developing ICP. Synergistic effects have been described between a CFTR compound heterozygote genotype and *SPINK1* mutations, with a pancreatitis risk increased approximately 40-fold with 2 CFTR mutations, 20-fold with a *SPINK1* mutation, and a 900-fold increased risk with both CFTR and *SPINK1* mutations.[108] There have also been suggestions of relationships between CFTR mutations and other pancreatitis syndromes (alcoholic pancreatitis, tropical chronic pancreatitis) but these relationships are less clear.[89] Again, patients with recurrent pancreatitis and CFTR mutations should be examined further for evidence of other organ manifestations of CF, and should complete further diagnostic testing to determine if CF therapies would be beneficial.

Idiopathic Bronchiectasis

Approximately one-half of patients with bronchiectasis have a primary underlying diagnosis, such as CF, primary ciliary dyskinesia, or immune deficiency, that is felt to be causative.[89] Recent evidence suggests that some patients with idiopathic bronchiectasis also have CFTR mutations or CFTR dysfunction. At least 1 CFTR mutation has been reported in 10% to 50% of patients with idiopathic bronchiectasis, and a minority has been reported to harbor 2 mutations.[89,109–111] The contribution of CFTR dysfunction may be more difficult to assign in these subjects, and the evaluation for CF is part of a broader workup for the numerous potential causes of bronchiectasis. This is complicated by additional factors, such as concurrent chronic pulmonary infections that frequently contribute to their clinical manifestations. In addition, cigarette smoke (a common confounding factor in adults with lung disease) has also been shown to reduce CFTR function, potentially contributing to smoking-related lung disease in some patients with chronic obstructive pulmonary disease.[112–116] CF pulmonary therapies such as chronic azithromycin have been shown to be beneficial to patients with chronic obstructive pulmonary disease and idiopathic bronchiectasis, and other therapies may be valuable to manage chronic bronchitis and mucus obstruction.[117–119] Further evaluation for CFTR deficits can be helpful, clarifying what other established CF treatments may provide benefit to these patients.

SUMMARY

Over the last 60 years, the process of diagnosing CF has evolved from sole use of SC to complex screening, functional, and genetic analyses. As our diagnostic finesse has improved, we are now able to identify a spectrum of CFTR dysfunction, ranging from minimal clinical disease to classic CF. Currently, clinicians have access to consensus-based algorithms for the use of various testing methods in the diagnosis of CF and CFTR-related disorders. With further understanding of CFTR dysfunction we will need further refinement of these testing modalities and diagnostic algorithms, and may ultimately require novel methods of evaluation.

REFERENCES

1. Rowe SM, Miller S, Sorscher EJ. Cystic fibrosis. N Engl J Med 2005;352(19):1992–2001.
2. Pilewski JM, Frizzell RA. Role of CFTR in airway disease. Physiol Rev 1999;79(1 Suppl):S215–55.
3. North American Cystic Fibrosis Foundation (NACF). 2013 North American CFF annual data report to center directors. 2013. Available at: https://www.cff.org/2013_CFF_Annual_Data_Report_to_the_Center_Directors.pdf. Accessed October 16, 2015.
4. CFF JHM. CFTR2 database. 2015. Available at: www.cftr2.org. Accessed July 28, 2015.
5. Schweibert EM, Benos DJ, Egan ME, et al. *CFTR* is a conductance regulator as well as a chloride Channel. Physiol Rev 1999;79(1 Suppl):S145–66.
6. Hudson VM. Rethinking cystic fibrosis pathology: the critical role of abnormal reduced glutathione (GSH) transport caused by *CFTR* mutation. Free Radic Biol Med 2001;30(12):1440–61.
7. Moskwa P, Lorentzen D, Excoffon KJ, et al. A novel host defense system of airways is defective in cystic fibrosis. Am J Respir Crit Care Med 2007; 175(2):174–83.
8. Park M, Ko SB, Choi JY, et al. The cystic fibrosis transmembrane conductance regulator interacts with and regulates the activity of the HCO_3-salvage transporter human Na+-HCO_3- cotransport isoform 3. J Biol Chem 2002;277(52):50503–9.
9. Anderson MP, Gregory RJ, Thompson S, et al. Demonstration that CFTR is a chloride channel by alteration of its anion selectivity. Science 1991; 253(5016):202–5.
10. Cohn JA, Strong TV, Picciotto MR, et al. Localization of the cystic fibrosis transmembrane conductance regulator in human bile duct epithelial cells. Gastroenterology 1993;105(6):1857–64.
11. Grubb BR, Gabriel SE. Intestinal physiology and pathology in gene-targeted mouse models of cystic fibrosis. Am J Physiol 1997;273(2 Pt 1): G258–66.
12. Marino CR, Matovcik LM, Gorelick FS, et al. Localization of the cystic fibrosis transmembrane conductance regulator in pancreas. J Clin Invest 1991;88(2):712–6.
13. Meyerholz DK, Stoltz DA, Namati E, et al. Loss of cystic fibrosis transmembrane conductance regulator function produces abnormalities in tracheal development in neonatal pigs and young children. Am J Respir Crit Care Med 2010;182(10):1251–61.

14. Patrizio P, Asch RH, Handelin B, et al. Aetiology of congenital absence of vas deferens: genetic study of three generations. Hum Reprod (Oxford, England) 1993;8(2):215–20.

15. Reddy MM, Bell CL, Quinton PM. Cystic fibrosis affects specific cell type in sweat gland secretory coil. Am J Physiol 1997;273(2 Pt 1):C426–33.

16. Stoltz DA, Rokhlina T, Ernst SE, et al. Intestinal CFTR expression alleviates meconium ileus in cystic fibrosis pigs. J Clin Invest 2013;123(6):2685–93.

17. Joo NS, Irokawa T, Wu JV, et al. Absent secretion to vasoactive intestinal peptide in cystic fibrosis airway glands. J Biol Chem 2002;277(52):50710–5.

18. Wu JV, Krouse ME, Wine JJ. Acinar origin of CFTR-dependent airway submucosal gland fluid secretion. Am J Physiol Lung Cell Mol Physiol 2007; 292(1):L304–11.

19. Joo NS, Irokawa T, Robbins RC, et al. Hyposecretion, not hyperabsorption, is the basic defect of cystic fibrosis airway glands. J Biol Chem 2006; 281(11):7392–8.

20. Joo NS, Lee DJ, Winges KM, et al. Regulation of antiprotease and antimicrobial protein secretion by airway submucosal gland serous cells. J Biol Chem 2004;279(37):38854–60.

21. Choi JY, Joo NS, Krouse ME, et al. Synergistic airway gland mucus secretion in response to vasoactive intestinal peptide and carbachol is lost in cystic fibrosis. J Clin Invest 2007;117(10):3118–27.

22. Wine JJ, Joo NS. Submucosal glands and airway defense. Proc Am Thorac Soc 2004;1(1):47–53.

23. Chen JH, Stoltz DA, Karp PH, et al. Loss of anion transport without increased sodium absorption characterizes newborn porcine cystic fibrosis airway epithelia. Cell 2010;143(6):911–23.

24. Hoegger MJ, Fischer AJ, McMenimen JD, et al. Impaired mucus detachment disrupts mucociliary transport in a piglet model of cystic fibrosis. Science (New York, NY) 2014;345(6198):818–22.

25. Konstan MW, Berger M. Current understanding of the inflammatory process in cystic fibrosis: onset and etiology. Pediatr Pulmonol 1997;24(2):137–42 [discussion: 159–61].

26. Chmiel JF, Konstan MW. Inflammation and anti-inflammatory therapies for cystic fibrosis. Clin Chest Med 2007;28(2):331–46.

27. Cohen-Cymberknoh M, Kerem E, Ferkol T, et al. Airway inflammation in cystic fibrosis: molecular mechanisms and clinical implications. Thorax 2013;68(12):1157–62.

28. Jelin AC, Anderson B, Wilkins-Haug L, et al. Obstetrician and gynecologists' population-based screening practices. J Matern Fetal Neonatal Med 2015. [Epub ahead of print].

29. American College of Obstetricians and Gynecologists Committee on Genetics. ACOG Committee Opinion No. 486: Update on carrier screening for cystic fibrosis. Obstet Gynecol 2011;117(4): 1028–31.

30. Ioannou L, Delatycki MB, Massie J, et al. "Suddenly having two positive people who are carriers is a whole new thing"- experiences of couples both identified as carriers of cystic fibrosis through a population-based carrier screening program in Australia. J Genet Couns 2015;24:987–1000.

31. Hadj Fredj S, Ouali F, Siala H, et al. Prenatal diagnosis of cystic fibrosis: 10-years experience. Pathol Biol 2015;63(3):126–9.

32. Janssens S, Chokoshvili D, Binst C, et al. Attitudes of cystic fibrosis patients and parents toward carrier screening and related reproductive issues. Eur J Hum Genet 2015. [Epub ahead of print].

33. Wagener JS, Zemanick ET, Sontag MK. Newborn screening for cystic fibrosis. Curr Opin Pediatr 2012;24(3):329–35.

34. Castellani C, Southern KW, Brownlee K, et al. European best practice guidelines for cystic fibrosis neonatal screening. J Cyst Fibros 2009; 8(3):153–73.

35. Waters DL, Wilcken B, Irwing L, et al. Clinical outcomes of newborn screening for cystic fibrosis. Arch Dis Child Fetal Neonatal Ed 1999;80(1):F1–7.

36. Accurso FJ, Sontag MK, Wagener JS. Complications associated with symptomatic diagnosis in infants with cystic fibrosis. J Pediatr 2005;147(3 Suppl):S37–41.

37. Farrell PM, Kosorok MR, Laxova A, et al. Nutritional benefits of neonatal screening for cystic fibrosis. Wisconsin cystic fibrosis neonatal screening study group. N Engl J Med 1997;337(14):963–9.

38. Collins MS, Abbott MA, Wakefield DB, et al. Improved pulmonary and growth outcomes in cystic fibrosis by newborn screening. Pediatr Pulmonol 2008;43(7):648–55.

39. Sims EJ, McCormick J, Mehta G, et al. Neonatal screening for cystic fibrosis is beneficial even in the context of modern treatment. J Pediatr 2005; 147(3 Suppl):S42–6.

40. Koscik RL, Farrell PM, Kosorok MR, et al. Cognitive function of children with cystic fibrosis: deleterious effect of early malnutrition. Pediatrics 2004;113(6): 1549–58.

41. Lai HJ, Cheng Y, Farrell PM. The survival advantage of patients with cystic fibrosis diagnosed through neonatal screening: evidence from the United States Cystic Fibrosis Foundation registry data. J Pediatr 2005;147(3 Suppl):S57–63.

42. Tluczek A, Mischler EH, Farrell PM, et al. Parents' knowledge of neonatal screening and response to false-positive cystic fibrosis testing. J Dev Behav Pediatr 1992;13(3):181–6.

43. Mischler EH, Wilfond BS, Fost N, et al. Cystic fibrosis newborn screening: impact on

reproductive behavior and implications for genetic counseling. Pediatrics 1998;102(1 Pt 1):44–52.

44. Hayes D Jr, West SE, Rock MJ, et al. Pseudomonas aeruginosa in children with cystic fibrosis diagnosed through newborn screening: assessment of clinic exposures and microbial genotypes. Pediatr Pulmonol 2010;45(7):708–16.

45. Sims EJ, Mugford M, Clark A, et al. Economic implications of newborn screening for cystic fibrosis: a cost of illness retrospective cohort study. Lancet 2007;369(9568):1187–95.

46. Crossley JR, Elliott RB, Smith PA. Dried-blood spot screening for cystic fibrosis in the newborn. Lancet 1979 3;1(8114):472–4.

47. Heeley AF, Fagan DG. Trisomy 18, cystic fibrosis, and blood immunoreactive trypsin. Lancet 1984; 1(8369):169–70.

48. Priest FJ, Nevin NC. False positive results with immunoreactive trypsinogen screening for cystic fibrosis owing to trisomy 13. J Med Genet 1991; 28(8):575–6.

49. Ravine D, Francis RI, Danks DM. Non-specific elevation of immunoreactive trypsinogen in sick infants. Eur J Pediatr 1993;152(4):348–9.

50. Docherty JG, Coutts JA, Evans TJ, et al. Immunoreactive trypsinogen concentrations in infants with meconium ileus. BMJ (Clinical research ed) 1991; 303(6793):56.

51. Southern KW, Munck A, Pollitt R, et al. A survey of newborn screening for cystic fibrosis in Europe. J Cyst Fibros 2007;6(1):57–65.

52. Wilcken B, Brown AR, Urwin R, et al. Cystic fibrosis screening by dried blood spot trypsin assay: results in 75,000 newborn infants. J Pediatr 1983; 102(3):383–7.

53. Sommerburg O, Lindner M, Muckenthaler M, et al. Initial evaluation of a biochemical cystic fibrosis newborn screening by sequential analysis of immunoreactive trypsinogen and pancreatitis-associated protein (IRT/PAP) as a strategy that does not involve DNA testing in a Northern European population. J Inherit Metab Dis 2010;33(Suppl 2):S263–71.

54. Sarles J, Giorgi R, Berthezene P, et al. Neonatal screening for cystic fibrosis: comparing the performances of IRT/DNA and IRT/PAP. J Cyst Fibros 2014;13(4):384–90.

55. Nshimyumukiza L, Bois A, Daigneault P, et al. Cost effectiveness of newborn screening for cystic fibrosis: a simulation study. J Cyst Fibros 2014;13(3):267–74.

56. Sommerburg O, Hammermann J, Lindner M, et al. Five years of experience with biochemical cystic fibrosis newborn screening based on IRT/PAP in Germany. Pediatr Pulmonol 2015;50(7):655–64.

57. Farrell PM, Rosenstein BJ, White TB, et al. Guidelines for diagnosis of cystic fibrosis in newborns through older adults: cystic fibrosis foundation consensus Report. J Pediatr 2008;153(2):S4–14.

58. Rosenstein BJ, Cutting GR. The diagnosis of cystic fibrosis: a consensus statement. Cystic Fibrosis Foundation Consensus Panel. J Pediatr 1998; 132(4):589–95.

59. Gibson LE, Cooke RE. A test for concentration of electrolytes in sweat in cystic fibrosis of the pancreas utilizing pilocarpine by iontophoresis. Pediatrics 1959;23(3):545–9.

60. Cystic Fibrosis Foundation (CFF). 2005 Annual Report to the Center Directors. CFF Patient Registry Report 2005. Available at: www.cff.org. Accessed October 16, 2015.

61. Shwachman H, Mahmoodian A. Pilocarpine iontophoresis sweat testing results of seven years' experience. Bibl Paediatr 1967;86:158–82.

62. Eng W, LeGrys VA, Schechter MS, et al. Sweat-testing in preterm and full-term infants less than 6 weeks of age. Pediatr Pulmonol 2005;40(1):64–7.

63. Parad RB, Comeau AM, Dorkin HL, et al. Sweat testing infants detected by cystic fibrosis newborn screening. J Pediatr 2005;147(3 Suppl):S69–72.

64. Farrell PM, Koscik RE. Sweat chloride concentrations in infants homozygous or heterozygous for F508 cystic fibrosis. Pediatrics 1996;97(4):524–8.

65. Wali PD, Loveridge-Lenza B, He Z, et al. Comparison of fecal elastase-1 and pancreatic function testing in children. J Pediatr Gastroenterol Nutr 2012;54(2):277–80.

66. O'Sullivan BP, Baker D, Leung KG, et al. Evolution of pancreatic function during the first year in infants with cystic fibrosis. J Pediatr 2013;162(4):808–12. e1.

67. Knowles MR, Carson JL, Collier AM, et al. Measurements of nasal transepithelial electric potential differences in normal human subjects in vivo. Am Rev Respir Dis 1981;124(4):484–90.

68. Boyle MP, Diener-West M, Milgram L, et al. A multicenter study of the effect of solution temperature on nasal potential difference measurements. Chest 2003;124(2):482–9.

69. Bronsveld I, Vermeulen F, Sands D, et al. Influence of perfusate temperature on nasal potential difference. Eur Respir J 2013;42(2):389–93.

70. Keenan K, Avolio J, Rueckes-Nilges C, et al. Nasal potential difference: best or average result for CFTR function as diagnostic criteria for cystic fibrosis? J Cyst Fibros 2015;14(3):310–6.

71. Naehrlich L, Ballmann M, Davies J, et al. Nasal potential difference measurements in diagnosis of cystic fibrosis: an international survey. J Cyst Fibros 2014;13(1):24–8.

72. Solomon GM, Konstan MW, Wilschanski M, et al. An international randomized multicenter comparison of nasal potential difference techniques. Chest 2010;138(4):919–28.

73. Vermeulen F, Proesmans M, Feyaerts N, et al. Nasal potential measurements on the nasal floor

and under the inferior turbinate: does it matter? Pediatr Pulmonol 2011;46(2):145–52.

74. Yaakov Y, Kerem E, Yahav Y, et al. Reproducibility of nasal potential difference measurements in cystic fibrosis. Chest 2007;132(4):1219–26.

75. Rowe SM, Clancy JP, Wilschanski M. Nasal potential difference measurements to assess CFTR ion channel activity. Methods Mol Biol 2011;741:09–80.

76. Hug MJ, Derichs N, Bronsveld I, et al. Measurement of ion transport function in rectal biopsies. Methods Mol Biol 2011;741:87–107.

77. Clancy JP, Szczesniak RD, Ashlock MA, et al. Multicenter intestinal current measurements in rectal biopsies from CF and non-CF subjects to monitor CFTR function. PLoS One 2013;8(9):e73905.

78. van Barneveld A, Stanke F, Tamm S, et al. Functional analysis of F508del CFTR in native human colon. Biochim Biophys Acta 2010;1802(11):1062–9.

79. Hirtz S, Gonska T, Seydewitz HH, et al. CFTR Cl-channel function in native human colon correlates with the genotype and phenotype in cystic fibrosis. Gastroenterology 2004;127(4):1085–95.

80. Cohen-Cymberknoh M, Yaakov Y, Shoseyov D, et al. Evaluation of the intestinal current measurement method as a diagnostic test for cystic fibrosis. Pediatr Pulmonol 2013;48(3):229–35.

81. Derichs N, Sanz J, Von Kanel T, et al. Intestinal current measurement for diagnostic classification of patients with questionable cystic fibrosis: validation and reference data. Thorax 2010;65(7):594–9.

82. Hug MJ, Tummler B. Intestinal current measurements to diagnose cystic fibrosis. J Cyst Fibros 2004;3(Suppl 2):157–8.

83. De Boeck K, Kent L, Davies J, et al. CFTR biomarkers: time for promotion to surrogate end-point. Eur Respir J 2013;41(1):203–16.

84. De Boeck K, Wilschanski M, Castellani C, et al. Cystic fibrosis: terminology and diagnostic algorithms. Thorax 2006;61(7):627–35.

85. Borowitz D, Parad RB, Sharp JK, et al. Cystic Fibrosis Foundation practice guidelines for the management of infants with cystic fibrosis transmembrane conductance regulator-related metabolic syndrome during the first two years of life and beyond. J Pediatr 2009;155(6 Suppl):S106–16.

86. Mayell SJ, Munck A, Craig JV, et al. A European consensus for the evaluation and management of infants with an equivocal diagnosis following newborn screening for cystic fibrosis. J Cyst Fibros 2009;8(1):71–8.

87. Ren CL, Desai H, Platt M, et al. Clinical outcomes in infants with cystic fibrosis transmembrane conductance regulator (CFTR) related metabolic syndrome. Pediatr Pulmonol 2011;46(11):1079–84.

88. Massie J, Clements B. Diagnosis of cystic fibrosis after newborn screening: the Australasian experience–twenty years and five million babies later: a consensus statement from the Australasian Paediatric Respiratory Group. Pediatr Pulmonol 2005;39(5):440–6.

89. Bombieri C, Claustres M, De Boeck K, et al. Recommendations for the classification of diseases as CFTR-related disorders. J Cyst Fibros 2011;10(Suppl 2):S86–102.

90. Holsclaw DS, Perlmutter AD, Jockin H, et al. Genital abnormalities in male patients with cystic fibrosis. J Urol 1971;106(4):568–74.

91. Oates RD, Amos JA. The genetic basis of congenital bilateral absence of the vas deferens and cystic fibrosis. J Androl 1994;15(1):1–8.

92. Mak V, Jarvi KA. The genetics of male infertility. J Urol 1996;156(4):1245–56 [discussion: 1256–7].

93. Wilschanski M, Dupuis A, Ellis L, et al. Mutations in the cystic fibrosis transmembrane regulator gene and in vivo transepithelial potentials. Am J Respir Crit Care Med 2006;174(7):787–94.

94. Chillon M, Casals T, Mercier B, et al. Mutations in the cystic fibrosis gene in patients with congenital absence of the vas deferens. N Engl J Med 1995;332(22):1475–80.

95. Costes B, Girodon E, Ghanem N, et al. Frequent occurrence of the CFTR intron 8 (TG)n 5T allele in men with congenital bilateral absence of the vas deferens. Eur J Hum Genet 1995;3(5):285–93.

96. Dork T, Dworniczak B, Aulehla-Scholz C, et al. Distinct spectrum of CFTR gene mutations in congenital absence of vas deferens. Hum Genet 1997;100(3–4):365–77.

97. Claustres M, Guittard C, Bozon D, et al. Spectrum of CFTR mutations in cystic fibrosis and in congenital absence of the vas deferens in France. Hum Mutat 2000;16(2):143–56.

98. Cuppens H, Lin W, Jaspers M, et al. Polyvariant mutant cystic fibrosis transmembrane conductance regulator genes. The polymorphic (Tg)m locus explains the partial penetrance of the T5 polymorphism as a disease mutation. J Clin Invest 1998;101(2):487–96.

99. Casals T, Bassas L, Egozcue S, et al. Heterogeneity for mutations in the CFTR gene and clinical correlations in patients with congenital absence of the vas deferens. Hum Reprod (Oxford, England) 2000;15(7):1476–83.

100. Josserand RN, Bey-Omar F, Rollet J, et al. Cystic fibrosis phenotype evaluation and paternity outcome in 50 males with congenital bilateral absence of vas deferens. Hum Reprod (Oxford, England) 2001;16(10):2093–7.

101. Ko SB, Zeng W, Dorwart MR, et al. Gating of CFTR by the STAS domain of SLC26 transporters. Nat Cell Biol 2004;6(4):343–50.

102. Poulsen JH, Fischer H, Illek B, et al. Bicarbonate conductance and pH regulatory capability of cystic fibrosis transmembrane conductance regulator. Proc Natl Acad Sci U S A 1994;91(12):5340–4.

103. Cohn JA, Friedman KJ, Noone PG, et al. Relation between mutations of the cystic fibrosis gene and idiopathic pancreatitis. N Engl J Med 1998; 339(10):653–8.

104. Sharer N, Schwarz M, Malone G, et al. Mutations of the cystic fibrosis gene in patients with chronic pancreatitis. N Engl J Med 1998;339(10):645–52.

105. Cohn JA. Reduced CFTR function and the pathobiology of idiopathic pancreatitis. J Clin Gastroenterol 2005;39(4 Suppl 2):S70–7.

106. Audrezet MP, Chen JM, Le Marechal C, et al. Determination of the relative contribution of three genes-the cystic fibrosis transmembrane conductance regulator gene, the cationic trypsinogen gene, and the pancreatic secretory trypsin inhibitor gene-to the etiology of idiopathic chronic pancreatitis. Eur J Hum Genet 2002;10(2):100–6.

107. Chen JM, Ferec C. Chronic pancreatitis: genetics and pathogenesis. Annu Rev Genomics Hum Genet 2009;10:63–87.

108. Noone PG, Zhou Z, Silverman LM, et al. Cystic fibrosis gene mutations and pancreatitis risk: relation to epithelial ion transport and trypsin inhibitor gene mutations. Gastroenterology 2001;121(6): 1310–9.

109. Casals T, De-Gracia J, Gallego M, et al. Bronchiectasis in adult patients: an expression of heterozygosity for CFTR gene mutations? Clin Genet 2004;65(6):490–5.

110. Divac A, Nikolic A, Mitic-Milikic M, et al. CFTR mutations and polymorphisms in adults with disseminated bronchiectasis: a controversial issue. Thorax 2005;60(1):85.

111. Girodon E, Cazeneuve C, Lebargy F, et al. CFTR gene mutations in adults with disseminated bronchiectasis. Eur J Hum Genet 1997;5(3):149–55.

112. Dransfield MT, Wilhelm AM, Flanagan B, et al. Acquired cystic fibrosis transmembrane conductance regulator dysfunction in the lower airways in COPD. Chest 2013;144(2):498–506.

113. Hassan F, Xu X, Nuovo G, et al. Accumulation of metals in GOLD4 COPD lungs is associated with decreased CFTR levels. Respir Res 2014;15:69.

114. Raju SV, Jackson PL, Courville CA, et al. Cigarette smoke induces systemic defects in cystic fibrosis transmembrane conductance regulator function. Am J Respir Crit Care Med 2013;188(11):1321–30.

115. Rasmussen JE, Sheridan JT, Polk W, et al. Cigarette smoke-induced Ca2+ release leads to cystic fibrosis transmembrane conductance regulator (CFTR) dysfunction. J Biol Chem 2014;289(11): 7671–81.

116. Xu X, Balsiger R, Tyrrell J, et al. Cigarette smoke exposure reveals a novel role for the MEK/ERK1/2 MAPK pathway in regulation of CFTR. Biochim Biophys Acta 2015;1850(6):1224–32.

117. Haworth CS, Bilton D, Elborn JS. Long-term macrolide maintenance therapy in non-CF bronchiectasis: evidence and questions. Respir Med 2014; 108(10):1397–408.

118. Ni W, Shao X, Cai X, et al. Prophylactic use of macrolide antibiotics for the prevention of chronic obstructive pulmonary disease exacerbation: a meta-analysis. PLoS One 2015;10(3):e0121257.

119. Lourdesamy Anthony AI, Muthukumaru U. Efficacy of azithromycin in the treatment of bronchiectasis. Respirology (Carlton, Vic) 2014;19(8):1178–82.

120. Hammond KB, Abman SH, Sokol RJ, et al. Efficacy of statewide neonatal screening for cystic fibrosis by assay of trypsinogen concentrations. N Engl J Med 1991;325(11):769–74.

121. Roberts G, Stanfield M, Black A, et al. Screening for cystic fibrosis: a four year regional experience. Arch Dis Child 1988;63(12):1438–43.

122. Rock MJ, Hoffman G, Laessig RH, et al. Newborn screening for cystic fibrosis in Wisconsin: nine-year experience with routine trypsinogen/DNA testing. J Pediatr 2005;147(3 Suppl):S73–7.

123. Kay DM, Maloney B, Hamel R, et al. Screening for cystic fibrosis in New York State: considerations for algorithm improvements. Eur J Pediatr 2015. [Epub ahead of print].

124. Comeau AM, Parad RB, Dorkin HL, et al. Population-based newborn screening for genetic disorders when multiple mutation DNA testing is incorporated: a cystic fibrosis newborn screening model demonstrating increased sensitivity but more carrier detections. Pediatrics 2004;113(6): 1573–81.

125. Audrézet MP, Munck A, Scotet V, et al. Comprehensive CFTR gene analysis of the French cystic fibrosis screened newborn cohort: implications for diagnosis, genetic counseling, and mutation-specific therapy. Genet Med 2015;17(2):108–16.

Diagnosis of Adult Patients with Cystic Fibrosis

Jerry A. Nick, MD[a,b,*], David P. Nichols, MD[b,c]

KEYWORDS

- Cystic fibrosis • Diagnosis • Adult • Bronchiectasis • Genotype

KEY POINTS

- Cystic fibrosis (CF) diagnosed in adulthood typically occurs because of the presence of a residual function (milder) mutation combined with a more severe mutation.
- The phenotype associated with an adult diagnosis is usually milder and limited to fewer organs at the time of presentation.
- The diagnosis is based on identification of CF transmembrane receptor (the gene responsible for CF) dysfunction in the presence of characteristic clinical features of the disease.
- Often the diagnosis is inconclusive at the time of initial evaluation, and may depend on clinical judgment supported by ancillary testing.
- With age, adult diagnosed patients can develop severe bronchiectasis and all features of the classic disease.

NATURE OF THE PROBLEM

Cystic fibrosis (CF) is a disease that is nearly always diagnosed in early childhood.[1] As newborn screening (NBS) has gradually been adopted by all 50 states, the 2013 Cystic Fibrosis Foundation (CFF) Patient Registry reports that 62% of patients are now diagnosed at birth, and 72.4% within the first year of life.[1] However, since the discovery of the genetic basis for CF in 1989, major advances have been made in understanding the potential for variability in the clinical phenotype and onset of symptoms. Thus, although diagnosis by NBS is becoming more common, the diagnosis of CF in adults has also increased.[2] Adults constituted 7.7% of new diagnoses between 1995 and 2000, and 9.0% between 2001 and 2005.[2] As a result, the subpopulation of patients enrolled in the CFF registry diagnosed after the age of 18 years has increased from only 2.8% in 1982 to 4.1% in 2002, and to 7% in 2013.[1,3] This value almost certainly underestimates the number of adult-diagnosed patients with CF in the United States, because less than half attend CF care centers.[4] This increase in incidence is likely caused by a combination of factors, including greater awareness by physicians and the public, widespread availability of CF transmembrane receptor (*CFTR*) mutation testing, and more straightforward diagnostic criteria.[5] Although previously the adult diagnosis was often viewed as a medical curiosity or a missed diagnosis of a childhood disease, it is now understood that it often results from *CFTR* mutations with residual function, resulting in both delayed onset and lesser disease severity.

Disclosures: The Cystic Fibrosis Foundation (NICK14G0), and the Rebecca Runyon Bryan Chair for Cystic Fibrosis.
[a] Department of Medicine, National Jewish Health, 1400 Jackson, Denver, CO 80206, USA; [b] Department of Medicine, University of Colorado Denver School of Medicine, 13001 East 17th Pl, Aurora, CO 80045, USA; [c] Department of Pediatrics, National Jewish Health, Denver, CO 80206, USA
* Corresponding author.
E-mail address: nickj@njhealth.org

Clin Chest Med 37 (2016) 47–57
http://dx.doi.org/10.1016/j.ccm.2015.11.006
0272-5231/16/$ – see front matter © 2016 Elsevier Inc. All rights reserved.

Although both scenarios can be challenging, the diagnosis of CF in adults differs fundamentally from the diagnosis prompted by NBS. Most newborns are asymptomatic,[1] and physicians must reconcile the abnormal test result with the apparent lack of a clinical phenotype. In contrast, adult patients present with a clinical phenotype, and the role of the physician is to guide diagnostic testing to prove or disprove the presence of CF. Nearly always the newborn diagnosis is extremely distressing to the family. In contrast, the adult diagnosis is often sought by the patient and is met with a sense of relief, because it may come following years of medical consultations for a variety of symptoms, and allows access to a unified and evidence-based approach to care. However, knowledge of the pathophysiology of CF is incomplete and frequently the adult CF diagnosis remains challenging and inconclusive. This article reviews the criteria used to establish the diagnosis of CF in adults and highlights unique aspects of the genotype and phenotype, with special emphasis on clinical features that lead to diagnosis in these patients.

DIAGNOSTIC CRITERIA

Current diagnostic criteria for CF in the United States follows consensus guidelines developed by the CFF in 2008 (**Box 1**).[5] When applied to adults, all patients must have 1 or more symptoms of CF (**Box 2**) combined with evidence of CFTR dysfunction, through sweat testing and/or genotype analysis. Despite its apparent simplicity, application of the criteria is sometimes difficult in the clinical care setting. Available tests for CFTR dysfunction are imperfect, and the list of phenotypic features consistent with the disease is broad and nonspecific (discussed later).

Sweat Chloride Testing

Evidence of CFTR dysfunction is derived primarily through sweat chloride testing. Acceptable methods and techniques for this test have been reviewed elsewhere,[6] and it is recommended that it is performed by laboratories associated with CF care centers. Sweat chloride analysis was developed primarily for infants, and is less sensitive and specific in adults.[5] It is now well recognized that patients with sweat chloride levels less than the diagnostic threshold of 60 mmol/L can develop CF,[5,7–9] and this is most commonly seen when the age of diagnosis is less than 18 years.[2] In our experience, a diagnosis of CF is unlikely with a chloride level less than 30 mmol/L, which is the lower limit of the established indeterminate range. When collecting sweat for testing from older individuals, clinicians should be careful to determine whether an adequate volume of sweat was collected to help ensure the reliability of the chloride level.

Cystic Fibrosis Transmembrane Receptor Genotype Analysis

CFTR is the gene responsible for CF. As with sweat chloride testing, analysis of the *CFTR* genotype can be inconclusive for a variety of reasons. In the CFF registry, 86.4% of the population has at least 1 copy of F508del and 46.5% are F508del homozygotes.[1] However, a vast array of molecular abnormalities have been detected within *CFTR*, and often the less common mutations are those that afford residual CFTR function, which are linked to the less severe phenotype typical of the adult diagnosis.[10] Although F508del is the most common allele in adult-diagnosed cohorts,[2,11–13] these patients often have a genotype that includes 1 or more class IV to VI mutations or an unidentified genetic abnormality.[2,12–18] In rare cases, a severe genotype, including homozygote F508del, is identified in a patient diagnosed as an adult,[10,12,13,19] which likely reflects the contribution of a growing list of genetic modifiers of CF.[20–24] Other genetic abnormalities of *CFTR* may contribute to the presentation of the milder

---

Box 1
Diagnostic criteria for CF in adulthood

Presence of symptoms of CF (see Box 2) or a family history

And 1 of the following:

- Sweat chloride value greater than or equal to 60 mmol/L
- Two identified CF-causing mutations
- Sweat chloride value 40 to 59 mmol/L with no or 1 CF-causing mutation, but with family history and/or ancillary testing and clinical presentation strongly suggestive of CF.

Adapted from Farrell PM, Rosenstein BJ, White TB, et al. Guidelines for diagnosis of cystic fibrosis in newborns through older adults: Cystic Fibrosis Foundation consensus report. J Pediatr 2008;153:S10.

Box 2
Phenotypic features consistent with a diagnosis of CF

Chronic sinopulmonary disease, manifested by:

Persistent colonization/infection with typical CF pathogens[a]

Chronic cough and sputum production

Persistent chest radiograph abnormalities[b]

Airway obstruction by examination or spirometry testing

Sinus disease[c]

Digital clubbing

Gastrointestinal and nutritional abnormalities, including:

Intestinal:

  Meconium ileus

  Distal intestinal obstruction syndrome

  Rectal prolapse

Pancreatic:

  Pancreatic insufficiency

  Recurrent acute or chronic pancreatitis

  Pancreatic abnormalities on imaging

Hepatic:

  Prolonged neonatal jaundice

  Chronic hepatic disease[d]

Nutritional:

  Failure to thrive (protein-calorie malnutrition)

  Hypoproteinemia and edema

  Clinical or laboratory evidence of fat-soluble vitamin deficiencies

Salt loss syndromes

Acute salt depletion

Chronic metabolic alkalosis

Genital abnormalities in male patients

Obstructive azoospermia

[a] *Staphylococcus aureus*, nontypable *Haemophilus influenzae*, mucoid and nonmucoid *Pseudomonas aeruginosa*, *Stenotrophomonas maltophilia*, and *Burkholderia cepacia*.
[b] May include bronchiectasis, atelectasis, infiltrates, and hyperinflation.
[c] Radiographic or computed tomography (CT) abnormalities of the paranasal sinuses, presence of nasal polyps.
[d] Clinical or histologic evidence of focal biliary cirrhosis or multilobular cirrhosis.
Adapted from Farrell PM, Rosenstein BJ, White TB, et al. Guidelines for diagnosis of cystic fibrosis in newborns through older adults: Cystic Fibrosis Foundation consensus report. J Pediatr 2008;153:S4–14; with permission.

---

phenotype, include the noncoding 5T allele of the polythymidine tract in intron 8 (IVS8),[10,25] as well as large sequence deletions, duplications, and in-cis distribution of benign polymorphisms.[26–28] Even with extensive sequencing of all exons and intron/exon junctions, only a single mutation is identified in more than a quarter of individuals with the diagnosis of mild or atypical CF.[28] Even if 2 *CFTR* abnormalities have been identified, only a small percentage of the more than 1800 identified genetic changes have been rigorously confirmed as CF-causing mutations.[29] In many cases, available reports linking phenotypic characteristics to a rare mutation are very limited and may describe a patient of a much younger age. Some CFTR mutations that are thought not to cause disease based on studies in young patients or in vitro models have later been reported in adult-diagnosed patients with CF with disease phenotype, further complicating the interpretation of genetic testing in the adult population.

Other Considerations

If sweat chloride testing and genotype analysis are not conclusive in adults with features consistent with CF, clinical judgment plays a role in making the diagnosis, and ancillary testing can often prove invaluable in this regard (discussed later).[5] Comprehensive investigation for other potential causes of disease, and close follow-up to determine the individual response to CF-directed therapies, are additional and important considerations to help inform clinical judgment. Difficulties in reconciling laboratory testing and clinical manifestations in newborns and infants have led to several new terms and proposed classifications, including CFTR-related metabolic syndrome, CFTR-related disease, CF screen positive, inconclusive diagnosis, and delayed CF.[30] However, there is little consensus surrounding these classifications, and they are rarely applied to adults. A new consensus conference will be convened in October 2015 under the sponsorship of the CFF to review this rapidly evolving field.[30]

CLINICAL MANIFESTATIONS

Adults diagnosed with CF can eventually develop all of the clinical features associated with the classic childhood disease, although usually at the time of diagnosis clinically relevant involvement is more limited (see **Box 2**). The most important features are discussed here.

Pulmonary Manifestations

Respiratory symptoms are the most common feature leading to the adult CF diagnosis.[2,11,13,31–33] Bronchiectasis is usually present and is easily detected by high-resolution computed tomography (CT) scanning. When young, these patients are often given the diagnosis of either asthma or chronic obstructive pulmonary disease based on obstructive physiology, bronchodilator response, and chronic sputum production. Cohorts of adult-diagnosed patients with CF show less severe lung disease compared with childhood-diagnosed cohorts, despite being significantly older.[4,11,32,34] However, for patients who survive past 40 years, 85% of patients with the adult diagnosis died of respiratory-related complications or transplant-related complications, which was similar to the

87% of childhood-diagnosed patients surviving past 40 years.[4]

Airway Infections

Recurrent or chronic airway infection is often the finding that leads to the consideration of CF in adults. Although patients with CF diagnosed as adults have a lower frequency of *Pseudomonas aeruginosa* infection (both mucoid and nonmucoid) than childhood-diagnosed patients,[11,12,31,32] it is still the most common airway infection in most reports.[2,11,12,31,34] Some investigators have reported a greater prevalence of *Staphylococcus aureus*, which is another common respiratory pathogen in CF.[33] Other typical CF pathogens, such as *Burkholderia cepacia*, can also be recovered, as well as pathogens not usually seen in the general CF population. Detection of nontuberculous mycobacteria (NTM) in the sputum correlates strongly with increasing age in patients with CF,[35–39] and is especially common in adult-diagnosed patients with CF.[2] We detected NTM 3 times more often in the adult diagnosis group ($P<006$), with *Mycobacterium avium* complex representing the most commonly detected species.[12] In a national epidemiologic study of NTM in CF, the age of mycobacteria-positive individuals was greater (26 vs 22 years), and subjects tended to have milder abnormalities in lung function (forced expiratory volume in 1 second [FEV_1], percentage predicted, 60% vs 54%).[35] Although age of diagnosis was not analyzed in that study, those data support the observation made by many investigators that older patients with milder disease are predisposed to infection with NTM, which may be the presenting feature at the time of diagnosis.[35,37,39,40]

Chronic Sinusitis

Chronic or recurrent sinusitis and nasal polyps are also common in patients with CF diagnosed as adults.[31,33] In a cohort of patients with CF with residual function mutations, mild lung disease, and an average age of diagnosis of 42.6 ± 17.2 years, we found that sinus CT findings were markedly worse than in a control group of patients without CF with chronic rhinosinusitis.[41]

Gastrointestinal Manifestations

The absence of pancreatic insufficiency (PI) is a major distinction between adult-diagnosed patients and those with the classic disease,[2,4,11,12,31–34] and is likely the primary reason for the diagnosis of CF not being made earlier in these patients. Accordingly, these patients have less CF-related diabetes,[4,12,32,34] and better overall nutrition.[11,12,32] Some adults present with PI at time of diagnosis and have adopted an extremely low-fat diet in order to reduce the symptoms of bloating and steatorrhea. However, patients with unrecognized, severe PI are usually markedly malnourished and deficient in fat-soluble vitamins. More commonly, adult patients report nonspecific symptoms of intermittent constipations and diarrhea, and often ascribe a beneficial response to low-dose pancreatic enzyme replacement even in the absence of overt PI. Many adults do not initially recognize the connection between these symptoms and their respiratory complaints, and are frequently assigned the diagnosis of irritable bowel syndrome. Over time, progression toward worsening PI can occur, even in the absence of clinically evident pancreatitis.[42–44] Our experience is consistent with that of multiple other groups reporting pancreatic enzyme supplementation in approximately half of patients diagnosed at the age of 18 years or greater.[2,12,32,45]

Pancreatitis

Idiopathic and recurrent pancreatitis is well recognized as a presenting manifestation of CF in adults,[34,46] frequently in the absence of apparent respiratory disease. These episodes can occur episodically over a series of years, with significant associated morbidity. In the original reports, many individuals were identified as having only a single CFTR mutation, based on limited genetic screening.[46,47] However, sequencing analysis of CFTR confirms that increased risk of pancreatitis requires 2 CFTR mutations (or a 5T allele) when other hereditary forms of pancreatitis are excluded.[48] Adults diagnosed with CF based on the clinical presentation of pancreatitis with the confirmed presence of 2 CFTR mutations are often considered to represent a single-organ manifestation of CF. However, with more extensive testing, many of these individuals have additional findings consistent with CF, including abnormal sweat testing, congenital bilateral absence of the vas deferens (CBAVD), sinusitis, and chronic bronchial infection with CF-typical pathogens.[48]

Congenital Bilateral Absence of the Vas Deferens

Absence of the vas deferens is nearly universal in male patients with CF, and is one of the most sensitive predictors for the presence of 2 clinically significant CFTR mutations in male patients.[49] Detection of CBAVD or other forms of obstructive azoospermia usually occurs in young men undergoing infertility evaluation, in the absence of clinically relevant respiratory complaints.[34] However, these men often have some degree of pulmonary or sinus disease,[50–52] and bronchoalveolar lavage studies of the airways of men with CBAVD and 1 or 2 identified CFTR mutations showed bacterial infection and inflammation in the absence of respiratory symptoms.[34] These results support the conclusion that young men presenting with CBAVD as a single-organ manifestation of CF are at risk to develop CF lung disease over time. Very rarely, normal reproductive function is present in men with mild mutations associated with the diagnosis of CF in adults.[49]

Female Gender

The diagnosis of CF in adulthood is made most frequently in women. In a cohort of 109 adult-diagnosed patients more than age 40 years at our center, 72.5% were women ($P = .0038$), and in a comparable cohort from the CFF registry 54.1% were women ($P<.0001$).[4] This finding has been reported by other centers worldwide.[11–13,33] Several factors could contribute to an increased frequency of adult diagnosis in women, including greater persistence in seeking the diagnosis and overall greater use of the health care system. In addition, a bias may exist against referral of men presenting with CBAVD to CF centers, resulting in an underrepresentation of men in databases of patients with adult-diagnosed CF. However, it is also possible that female predominance is based on molecular mechanisms and differences in phenotype.[53–55] Before widespread use of NBS, the CF diagnosis in female infants occurred later than in male infants.[56–58] This delay in diagnosis is also seen in adult-diagnosed patients in the CFF registry, in which the median age of diagnosis for men was 35.7 years compared with 39.2 for women ($P = .0014$).[4]

CLINICAL FINDINGS
Physical Examination

Findings on examination are usually nonspecific. Unlike patients diagnosed in childhood with the classic disease phenotype, adult-diagnosed patients may not be thin or have short stature. because respiratory symptoms are the most common presentation, patients often have a respiratory examination consistent with obstructive lung disease, with a prolonged expiratory phase or wheezing with forced expiration, and occasionally with scattered rhonchi. Nasal mucosa may be inflamed and polyps may be visible. Recurrent middle ear infections and subsequent deafness are not typical features of CF, and if present are more consistent with primary ciliary dyskinesia.[59] The abdominal examination is typically benign. Digital clubbing sometimes occurs.

Ancillary Testing

A variety of tests beyond sweat chloride analysis and *CFTR* genotyping may be helpful in establishing the CF diagnosis (**Table 1**). The nasal potential difference (NPD) test can be useful in assessment of patients with inconclusive sweat chloride values. However, access to NPD testing is not widely available beyond large research centers. The test requires a high level of operator training and expertise, and the usefulness of results are limited by a shortage of reference values and validation studies. Current guidelines state that the test should be used only to provide contributory evidence in a diagnostic evaluation.[5]

In adult patients, a high-resolution CT scan can detect even mild bronchiectasis and other early features of the disease.[60] Also valuable is an assessment of pancreatic exocrine function, which, if present, strongly argues in favor of CF, and helps guide treatment as well. A wide range of tests for assessing pancreatic function are available. The fecal elastase assay is usually preferred, but, depending on the setting of care and available resources, other testing could include a 72-hour stool collection, assays of fecal trypsin and chymotrypsin, and serum trypsinogen. Measurement of the fat-soluble vitamins A, D, and E, as well as indirect assessment of vitamin K through measurement of the prothrombin time and International Normalized Ratio (INR), can provide evidence of malabsorption, supporting the presence of PI. As discussed earlier, assessment of pancreatic function may need to be repeated over time, because PI develops gradually in some patients

Table 1
Ancillary testing for the assessment of the CF diagnosis in adults

Tests	Indications and Comments
Respiratory tract cultures	CF-associated pathogens, especially *P aeruginosa* but also *S aureus*, nontypable *Haemophilus influenzae*, *Stenotrophomonas maltophilia*, *Burkholderia cepacia*, and NTM
Exocrine pancreatic function tests	Presence of PI strongly supports CF diagnosis. Available tests include fecal elastase assay, 72-h stool collection, fecal trypsin or chymotrypsin, and serum trypsinogen
Fat-soluble vitamins	Deficiency in vitamins A, D, or E, as well as a prolonged INR (vitamin K), support the presence of fat malabsorption, a symptom of untreated PI
Genital evaluation in men	Genital examination, rectal ultrasonography for detection of vas deferens, semen analysis. Presence of sperm makes the CF diagnosis unlikely
Pancreatic imaging	CT and/or ultrasonography findings of pancreatic atrophy, fatty replacement, or lipomatous pseudohypertrophy are supportive of the CF diagnosis[64]
High-resolution chest CT	Capable of detecting very early radiographic features of CF, and in some cases can suggest alternative causes of bronchiectasis[60]
Bronchoalveolar lavage	Including microbiology assessment
Pulmonary function testing	Spirometry may be normal even with clinically and radiographically significant disease. With more advanced disease, an obstructive pattern of airflow limitation is expected
NPD testing	Useful in the setting of inconclusive sweat chloride values, but not universally available and limited by a lack of reference values and validation studies
Exclusionary testing for ciliary dyskinesia	Measurement of nasal nitric oxide, analysis of ciliary beat or ciliary composition, genetic testing[59]
Exclusionary testing for immunodeficiencies	Immunoglobulin levels, complement levels, leukocyte functional assays
Exclusionary testing for acute recurrent pancreatitis	Evaluation for gallstone disease, sphincter of Oddi dysfunction, anatomic variant of pancreatic ductal anatomy, genotype for *PRSS1* and *SPINK1* mutations[65]

Box 3
Disease associated with the development of diffuse bronchiectasis

Infection (primary)

    Bacteria: *Klebsiella pneumoniae, S aureus, H influenzae, Bordetella pertussis*

    Mycobacteria: *Mycobacterium tuberculosis*, NTM

    Mycoplasma

    Viruses: influenza, adenoviruses, measles, human immunodeficiency virus

    Fungus

Allergic bronchopulmonary aspergillosis

Mucoid impaction

Bronchocentric granulomatosis

Primary ciliary dyskinesia

    Kartagener syndrome

Young syndrome

Immunodeficiency states

    Immunoglobulin (Ig) G deficiency

    IgG subclass deficiency

    IgA deficiency

    Leukocyte dysfunction

    Lymphocyte dysfunction

    Complement deficiencies

Alpha1-antitrypsin deficiency

Autoimmune or hyperimmune disorders

    Rheumatoid arthritis

    Ulcerative colitis

    Cutaneous vasculitis

    Hashimoto thyroiditis

    Pernicious anemia

    Primary biliary cirrhosis

    Relapsing polychondritis

    Celiac disease

Yellow nail syndrome

Diseases of tracheal or bronchial cartilage

    Williams-Campbell syndrome

    Tracheobronchomegaly (Mounier-Kuhn)

Inhalation of noxious fumes and dust

    Anhydrous ammonia, silica, sulfur dioxide, talc, cork, Bakelite, cooking fumes

Heroin

Chronic fibrosing diseases

Chronic gastric aspiration

Marfan syndrome

Heart-lung transplant

Idiopathic (without known cause)

with CF of all ages who were initially determined to be pancreatic sufficient.[42–44]

Also of high value are respiratory tract cultures, which may include induced sputum and bronchoalveolar lavage. In our experience, patients presenting for evaluation of CF as adults may not have had frequent respiratory cultures during the course of their care, despite a high prevalence of productive cough. The presence of typical CF pathogens, in particular mucoid *P aeruginosa*, is supportive of the CF diagnosis.

Ancillary testing is also valuable for the purpose of eliminating other diagnostic considerations, as discussed later; in particular, the common causes of diffuse bronchiectasis, such as primary ciliary dyskinesia, and immunoglobulin deficiencies. When sweat chloride testing and CFTR genotype analysis remain inconclusive, the elimination of many other plausible causes of bronchiectasis can be an important consideration in deciding to assign the CF diagnosis to an adult.

DIAGNOSTIC DILEMMAS

The CF phenotype includes several signs and symptoms that overlap with a wide variety of obstructive lung diseases, various immunodeficiencies, and a broad range of gastrointestinal disorders. Because the most common presentation is with respiratory complaints, the most frequent consideration is other causes of diffuse bronchiectasis. The differential diagnosis of bronchiectasis is complicated and challenging, and often remains labeled as idiopathic despite exhaustive evaluation. The most relevant causes are listed in **Box 3**. The involvement of an organ outside the respiratory tract is the most important clinical feature in many cases. The same processes that result in bronchiectasis often also involve the sinuses to varying degrees; however, clinically significant involvement of the pancreas, bowel, or vas deferens is not expected in most of the disease processes that result in the common causes of bronchiectasis.

OUTCOMES FOR PATIENTS WITH CYSTIC FIBROSIS DIAGNOSED AS ADULTS

There is a paucity of data concerning response to treatment and outcomes in patients with CF diagnosed in adulthood. We have found that newly diagnosed adult patients with CF receiving multidisciplinary, guideline-based care at a CF center achieve a significant and sustained improvement in FEV_1 from baseline (time of diagnosis) over a period of 4 years.[4] This finding is particularly notable because there is no evidence-based treatment approach specific to adult-diagnosed patients, and available therapies were generally developed for children and adolescents with the classic phenotype, who typically have different *CFTR* mutations, different absorption of nutrition and medications, and different patterns of airway infection. Unexpectedly, we found that, following diagnosis, less than half of adult-diagnosed patients received their care at a CF center.[4] A general lack of familiarity with the adult diagnosis, even within the CF care community, may contribute to a reluctance of these patients to continue long-term follow-up at CF care centers. However, the significant and sustained benefit to lung function observed after initiating typical CF therapy within our center argues in support of both incorporating and aggressively treating patients diagnosed with CF later in life. As expected, adult-diagnosed patients have substantially better survival than the CF population as a whole, with a median survival of 76.9 years for adult-diagnosed patients in our Colorado database, and 68.2 years for patients followed in the CFF Patient Registry.[4] Note that women who were diagnosed as adults enjoyed a distinct survival advantage of 13.5 years in the Colorado database and 9.2 years in the CFF registry database compared with their male counterparts.[4] To our knowledge, this reverse gender gap is the first example of a clinical advantage of women with CF compared with men. However, despite a much longer lifespan, most adult-diagnosed patients followed in the CFF Patient Registry died of respiratory failure (76%) or transplant-related complications (9%), with an almost identical frequency to long-term survivors of the childhood diagnosis.[4]

SUMMARY

Clinical manifestations of adult-diagnosed CF include an extremely diverse spectrum of disease, ranging from mild single-organ involvement to the classic phenotype. As a result of greater CFTR activity associated with residual function mutations, these patients generally have less severe lung and gastrointestinal involvement despite achieving a greater age than patients diagnosed in childhood. Adult-diagnosed patients can be expected to have a lower prevalence of PI and *P aeruginosa* infections, but over time have a higher frequency of pancreatitis, are at greater risk for NTM infection, and historically have primarily died of respiratory complications.

We believe that CF remains undiagnosed in a significant number of adults, and, when diagnosed, most individuals do not receive care at CF centers. Thus, these patients are under-represented in the

CF patient registries. Physicians encountering patients with bronchiectasis of unknown cause, especially when associated with chronic infection with *P aeruginosa*, *S aureus*, or NTM, should consider CF regardless of the age and associated symptoms. Clearly, CF must be included in the differential diagnosis of recurrent idiopathic pancreatitis or CBAVD, but other symptoms that may be diagnosed as irritable bowel syndrome should also be considered as possible manifestations of CF. When CF is suspected, the work-up typically requires both a sweat chloride test and *CFTR* genotyping, associated with ancillary testing as clinically indicated. Physicians need to be mindful that their understanding of the genetic basis of CF continues to evolve, and the clinical phenotype within an individual may not be fully evident until late adulthood. Thus, follow-up is often warranted in cases in which a conclusive diagnosis is not possible at the time of presentation. If CF is diagnosed, referral to a CF care center for aggressive disease management should be encouraged.

Going forward, patients with the adult diagnosis may be well positioned to benefit from recent advances in CF care. In particular, the CFTR potentiator ivacaftor has now been approved for use in patients with the *Arg117His-CFTR* mutation,[61] which is frequently associated with the adult diagnosis.[4] This result was predicted by in vitro studies in which ivacaftor induced significant improvements in chloride transport in cell lines expressing *Arg117His* and a range of other residual function mutations that are commonly associated with the adult diagnosis.[62] Case reports have documented a favorable response to CFTR modulation treatment in individual patients with these mutations,[63] and an n-of-1 trial was recently completed to examine this effect in predominantly adult-diagnosed patients (NCT01685801), with a trial of ivacaftor in combination with VX-661 for patients with residual function mutations underway (NCT02392234). Regardless of the results of these trials, the adult diagnosis of CF should be pursued aggressively when clinical suspicion exists, because patients have been shown to respond to conventional CF therapy.[4] The adult CF diagnosis allows a unified approach to multisystem complaints, allows the patient to alert family members who are potential carriers, and often provides a sense of relief for patients who have struggled to conceptualize progressively worsening symptoms in the absence of a diagnosis or rational treatment plan.

REFERENCES

1. 2013 annual data report; Cystic Fibrosis Foundation patient registry. 2014.

2. Keating CL, Liu X, Dimango EA. Classic respiratory disease but atypical diagnostic testing distinguishes adult presentation of cystic fibrosis. Chest 2010;137: 1157–63.

3. Nick JA, Rodman DM. Manifestations of cystic fibrosis diagnosed in adulthood. Curr Opin Pulm Med 2005;11:513–8.

4. Nick JA, Chacon CS, Brayshaw SJ, et al. Effects of gender and age at diagnosis on disease progression in long-term survivors of cystic fibrosis. Am J Respir Crit Care Med 2010;182:614–26.

5. Farrell PM, Rosenstein BJ, White TB, et al. Guidelines for diagnosis of cystic fibrosis in newborns through older adults: Cystic Fibrosis Foundation consensus report. J Pediatr 2008;153:S4–14.

6. LeGrys VA, Yankaskas JR, Quittell LM, et al, Cystic Fibrosis Foundation. Diagnostic sweat testing: the Cystic Fibrosis Foundation guidelines. J Pediatr 2007;151:85–9.

7. Groves T, Robinson P, Wiley V, et al. Long-term outcomes of children with intermediate sweat chloride values in infancy. J Pediatr 2015;166:1469–74. e1-e3.

8. Highsmith WE, Burch LH, Zhou Z, et al. A novel mutation in the cystic fibrosis gene in patients with pulmonary disease but normal sweat chloride concentrations. N Engl J Med 1994;331:974–80.

9. Stewart B, Zabner J, Shuber AP, et al. Normal sweat chloride values do not exclude the diagnosis of cystic fibrosis. Am J Respir Crit Care Med 1995; 151:899–903.

10. Noone PG, Knowles MR. 'CFTR-opathies': disease phenotypes associated with cystic fibrosis transmembrane regulator gene mutations. Respir Res 2001;2:328–32.

11. Gan KH, Geus WP, Bakker W, et al. Genetic and clinical features of patients with cystic fibrosis diagnosed after the age of 16 years. Thorax 1995;50: 1301–4.

12. Rodman DM, Polis JM, Heltshe SL, et al. Late diagnosis defines a unique population of long-term survivors of cystic fibrosis. Am J Respir Crit Care Med 2005;171:621–6.

13. Modolell I, Alvarez A, Guarner L, et al. Gastrointestinal, liver, and pancreatic involvement in adult patients with cystic fibrosis. Pancreas 2001;22:395–9.

14. Choo-Kang LR, Zeitlin PL. Type I, II, III, IV, and V cystic fibrosis transmembrane conductance regulator defects and opportunities for therapy. Curr Opin Pulm Med 2000;6:521–9.

15. Durno C, Corey M, Zielenski J, et al. Genotype and phenotype correlations in patients with CF and pancreatitis. Gastroenterology 2002;123:1857–64.

16. Hubert D, Bienvenu T, Desmazes-Dufeu N, et al. Genotype-phenotype relationships in a cohort of adult cystic fibrosis patients. Eur Respir J 1996;9: 2207–14.

17. McKone EF, Emerson SS, Edwards KL, et al. Effect of genotype on phenotype and mortality in cystic fibrosis: a retrospective cohort study. Lancet 2003;361:1671–6.

18. McKone EF, Goss CH, Aitken ML. CFTR genotype as a predictor of prognosis in cystic fibrosis. Chest 2006;130:1441–7.

19. Burke W, Aitken ML, Chen SH, et al. Variable severity of pulmonary disease in adults with identical cystic fibrosis mutations. Chest 1992;102:506–9.

20. Cutting GR. Modifier genes in mendelian disorders: the example of cystic fibrosis. Ann N Y Acad Sci 2010;1214:57–69.

21. Joly P, Restier L, Bouchecareilh M, et al. DEFI-ALPHA cohort and POLYGEN DEFI-ALPHA clinical research hospital programme. A study about clinical, biological and genetics factors associated with the occurrence and the evolution of hepatic complications in children with alpha-1 antitrypsin deficiency. Rev Mal Respir 2015;32(7):759–67 [in French].

22. Coutinho CA, Marson FA, Marcelino AR, et al. TNF-alpha polymorphisms as a potential modifier gene in the cystic fibrosis. Int J Mol Epidemiol Genet 2014;5:87–99.

23. Blackman SM, Commander CW, Watson C, et al. Genetic modifiers of cystic fibrosis-related diabetes. Diabetes 2013;62:3627–35.

24. Bradley GM, Blackman SM, Watson CP, et al. Genetic modifiers of nutritional status in cystic fibrosis. Am J Clin Nutr 2012;96:1299–308.

25. Chillon M, Casals T, Mercier B, et al. Mutations in the cystic fibrosis gene in patients with congenital absence of the vas deferens. N Engl J Med 1995; 332:1475–80.

26. Taulan M, Viart V, Theze C, et al. Identification of a novel duplication CFTRdup2 and functional impact of large rearrangements identified in the CFTR gene. Gene 2012;500:194–8.

27. Ni WH, Jiang L, Fei QJ, et al. The CFTR polymorphisms poly-T, TG-repeats and M470V in Chinese males with congenital bilateral absence of the vas deferens. Asian J Androl 2012;14:687–90.

28. Strom CM, Crossley B, Buller-Buerkle A, et al. Cystic fibrosis testing 8 years on: Lessons learned from carrier screening and sequencing analysis. Genet Med 2011;13:166–72.

29. US CF Foundation JHU, The Hospital for Sick Children. The clinical and functional translation of CFTR (CFTR2). 2011. Available at: http://cftr2.Org. Accessed December 2, 2015.

30. Levy H, Farrell PM. New challenges in the diagnosis and management of cystic fibrosis. J Pediatr 2015; 166:1337–41.

31. Shwachman H, Kowalski M, Khaw KT. Cystic fibrosis: a new outlook. Medicine 1977;56:129–49.

32. McCloskey M, Redmond AO, Hill A, et al. Clinical features associated with a delayed diagnosis of cystic fibrosis. Respiration 2000;67:402–7.

33. Widerman E, Millner L, Sexauer W, et al. Health status and sociodemographic characteristics of adults receiving a CF diagnosis after age 18 years. Chest 2000;118:427–33.

34. Gilljam M, Ellis L, Corey M, et al. Clinical manifestations of cystic fibrosis among patients with diagnosis in adulthood. Chest 2004;126:1215–24.

35. Olivier KN, Weber DJ, Wallace RJ Jr, et al. Nontuberculous mycobacteria. I: Multicenter prevalence study in cystic fibrosis. Am J Respir Crit Care Med 2003;167:828–34.

36. Esther CR Jr, Esserman DA, Gilligan P, et al. Chronic mycobacterium abscessus infection and lung function decline in cystic fibrosis. J Cyst Fibros 2010;9: 117–23.

37. Aitken ML, Burke W, McDonald G, et al. Nontuberculous mycobacterial disease in adult cystic fibrosis patients. Chest 1993;103:1096–9.

38. Levy I, Grisaru-Soen G, Lerner-Geva L, et al. Multicenter cross-sectional study of nontuberculous mycobacterial infections among cystic fibrosis patients, Israel. Emerg Infect Dis 2008;14:378–84.

39. Fauroux B, Delaisi B, Clement A, et al. Mycobacterial lung disease in cystic fibrosis: a prospective study. Pediatr Infect Dis J 1997;16:354–8.

40. Olivier KN, Weber DJ, Lee JH, et al. Nontuberculous mycobacteria. II: Nested-cohort study of impact on cystic fibrosis lung disease. Am J Respir Crit Care Med 2003;167:835–40.

41. Ferril GR, Nick JA, Getz AE, et al. Comparison of radiographic and clinical characteristics of low-risk and high-risk cystic fibrosis genotypes. Int Forum Allergy Rhinol 2014;4(11):915–20.

42. Couper RT, Corey M, Durie PR, et al. Longitudinal evaluation of serum trypsinogen measurement in pancreatic-insufficient and pancreatic-sufficient patients with cystic fibrosis. J Pediatr 1995;127:408–13.

43. Couper RT, Corey M, Moore DJ, et al. Decline of exocrine pancreatic function in cystic fibrosis patients with pancreatic sufficiency. Pediatr Res 1992;32:179–82.

44. Bronstein MN, Sokol RJ, Abman SH, et al. Pancreatic insufficiency, growth, and nutrition in infants identified by newborn screening as having cystic fibrosis. J Pediatr 1992;120:533–40.

45. Simmonds NJ, Cullinan P, Hodson ME. Growing old with cystic fibrosis - the characteristics of long-term survivors of cystic fibrosis. Respir Med 2009;103: 629–35.

46. Sharer N, Schwarz M, Malone G, et al. Mutations of the cystic fibrosis gene in patients with chronic pancreatitis. N Engl J Med 1998;339:645–52.

47. Cohn JA, Friedman KJ, Noone PG, et al. Relation between mutations of the cystic fibrosis gene and idiopathic pancreatitis. N Engl J Med 1998;339:653–8.

48. Noone PG, Zhou Z, Silverman LM, et al. Cystic fibrosis gene mutations and pancreatitis risk: Relation to

epithelial ion transport and trypsin inhibitor gene mutations. Gastroenterology 2001;121:1310–9.

49. Groman JD, Karczeski B, Sheridan M, et al. Phenotypic and genetic characterization of patients with features of "nonclassic" forms of cystic fibrosis. J Pediatr 2005;146:675–80.

50. Kerem E, Rave-Harel N, Augarten A, et al. A cystic fibrosis transmembrane conductance regulator splice variant with partial penetrance associated with variable cystic fibrosis presentations. Am J Respir Crit Care Med 1997;155:1914–20.

51. Culard JF, Desgeorges M, Romey MC, et al. A novel splice site mutation in the first exon of the cystic fibrosis transmembrane regulator (CFTR) gene identified in a CBAVD patient. Hum Mol Genet 1994;3: 369–70.

52. Claustres M, Guittard C, Bozon D, et al. Spectrum of CFTR mutations in cystic fibrosis and in congenital absence of the vas deferens in France. Hum Mutat 2000;16:143–56.

53. Morea A, Cameran M, Rebuffi AG, et al. Gender-sensitive association of CFTR gene mutations and 5T allele emerging from a large survey on infertility. Mol Hum Reprod 2005;11:607–14.

54. Strom CM, Crossley B, Redman JB, et al. Cystic fibrosis screening: lessons learned from the first 320,000 patients. Genet Med 2004;6:136–40.

55. Sun W, Anderson B, Redman J, et al. CFTR 5T variant has a low penetrance in females that is partially attributable to its haplotype. Genet Med 2006;8:339–45.

56. Farrell P, Joffe S, Foley L, et al. Diagnosis of cystic fibrosis in the Republic of Ireland: epidemiology and costs. Ir Med J 2007;100:557–60.

57. McCormick J, Sims EJ, Mehta A. Delayed diagnosis of females with respiratory presentation of cystic fibrosis did not segregate with poorer clinical outcome. J Clin Epidemiol 2006;59:315–22.

58. Lai HC, Kosorok MR, Laxova A, et al. Delayed diagnosis of US females with cystic fibrosis. Am J Epidemiol 2002;156:165–73.

59. Werner C, Onnebrink JG, Omran H. Diagnosis and management of primary ciliary dyskinesia. Cilia 2015;4:2.

60. Dodd JD, Lavelle LP, Fabre A, et al. Imaging in cystic fibrosis and non-cystic fibrosis bronchiectasis. Semin Respir Crit Care Med 2015;36:194–206.

61. Moss RB, Flume PA, Elborn JS, et al. Efficacy and safety of ivacaftor in patients with cystic fibrosis who have an Arg117His-CFTR mutation: a double-blind, randomised controlled trial. Lancet Respir Med 2015;3:524–33.

62. Van Goor F, Yu H, Burton B, et al. Effect of ivacaftor on CFTR forms with missense mutations associated with defects in protein processing or function. J Cyst Fibros 2014;13:29–36.

63. Yousef S, Solomon GM, Brody A, et al. Improved clinical and radiographic outcomes after treatment with ivacaftor in a young adult with cystic fibrosis with the P67I CFTR mutation. Chest 2015;147:e79–82.

64. Lavelle LP, McEvoy SH, Ni Mhurchu E, et al. Cystic fibrosis below the diaphragm: abdominal findings in adult patients. Radiographics 2015;35:680–95.

65. Testoni PA. Acute recurrent pancreatitis: Etiopathogenesis, diagnosis and treatment. World J Gastroenterol 2014;20:16891–901.

The Microbiome in Cystic Fibrosis

Yvonne J. Huang, MD[a],*, John J. LiPuma, MD[b]

KEYWORDS

- Microbiota • Lung • Gut • Bacteria • Fungi • Virus • Culture-independent

KEY POINTS

- Culture-independent investigations have revealed a complex community of microbes, including bacteria, fungi, and viruses, harbored in the respiratory and gastrointestinal tracts of patients with cystic fibrosis (CF).
- Bacterial community composition in the respiratory and gastrointestinal tracts is heterogeneous between patients with CF, such that unique microbial signatures are generally patient specific.
- Evidence suggests that gut microbiota composition in CF may influence disease features both within and beyond the gut, but further research is needed.
- Culture-independent characterization of microbial community composition is complemented by methods that provide insight into functional features of the microbiome and mechanistic relationships to clinical outcomes.
- Multiomic analyses of airway and gut microbiota have the potential to refine current management strategies in CF.

INTRODUCTION

Recent elucidation of the richness and complexity of the microbiome in patients with cystic fibrosis (CF) has invigorated new discussions of the role of microbial infection in CF beyond pathogens classically linked to CF, like *Pseudomonas aeruginosa*. An increasing number of studies have characterized the composition of airway microbiota in patients from different CF cohorts,[1–12] and common threads have emerged across studies in the relationships observed between features of the respiratory microbiome and clinical outcomes. However, extending these observations to the clinical realm in a predictive manner remains a challenge for several reasons, including the interpatient heterogeneity in airway microbiota composition that has come to be appreciated from these studies.

Most studies to date have focused on bacterial members of the respiratory microbiome, but some recent investigations have also begun to characterize fungal and viral communities in CF.[13–16] Such efforts are important because these other microbial kingdoms have largely been ignored in the schema of lung microbiome investigation. In addition, recent studies have begun to explore the microbiome in other organs affected by CF, such as the gastrointestinal tract.[17–20] Because gut dysfunction is another prominent feature of CF, findings from these studies may have important clinical implications.[21]

This article highlights recent insights in the rapidly evolving area of CF microbiome investigation. Advances in knowledge about the nature of microbial dysbiosis (ie, altered microbial balance) in CF are reshaping the conceptual framework

Disclosures: The authors have nothing to disclose.

[a] Division of Pulmonary/Critical Care Medicine, University of Michigan Medical School, 6301 MSRB III/SPC 5642, 1150 West Medical Center Drive, Ann Arbor, MI 48109, USA; [b] Department of Pediatrics and Communicable Diseases, University of Michigan Medical School, 8323 MSRB III/SPC 5646, 1150 West Medical Center Drive, Ann Arbor, MI 48109, USA

* Corresponding author. 6301 MSRB III/SPC 5642, 1150 West Medical Center Drive, Ann Arbor, MI 48109-5642.
E-mail address: yvjhuang@umich.edu

Clin Chest Med 37 (2016) 59–67
http://dx.doi.org/10.1016/j.ccm.2015.10.003
0272-5231/16/$ – see front matter © 2016 Elsevier Inc. All rights reserved.

within which the role of infection in CF has long been considered. Select studies are discussed that have contributed to the current understanding of the structure, composition, and collective functions of CF microbiota, and their relationship to disease benchmarks. In addition, both the challenges and opportunities presented from these recent insights are discussed in terms of how such knowledge may be leveraged to inform the care of patients with CF.

OVERVIEW OF METHODS AND CONSIDERATIONS IN LUNG MICROBIOME INVESTIGATION

Advances in sequence-based analysis of microbial genomes have laid the foundation for techniques to characterize the types of microbial species present in a sample. For bacteria, the most widely used approaches are based on analysis of the 16S ribosomal RNA gene, whose conservation across species, along with polymorphisms in hypervariable regions of the gene, enables both the broad detection of bacteria present in a sample and their phylogenetic identities. For more comprehensive discussions regarding methods and tools to study the microbiome, including in the context of lung disease, readers are referred to recent articles in this area.[22–24]

The unique anatomy of the lung presents challenges to studying its microbiome. Collecting lower airway samples requires passage through the upper respiratory tract or oropharynx, which has previously raised questions about the extent of oral contamination in such samples. However, several studies now have established that microbiota identified from lower respiratory specimens are distinguishable from upper airway microbiota (especially nasopharyngeal) in measures of diversity and also in the types and relative abundance of specific bacterial groups.[25–29] Moreover, the architecture of the bronchial airways leads to regional differences in lung biology and the airway microenvironment, even in the healthy state.[30] In CF, it is likely that patterns of dysbiosis are greatly influenced by the altered airway milieu related to CF transmembrane receptor dysfunction and subsequent changes to mucus clearance.[31]

THE CYSTIC FIBROSIS RESPIRATORY MICROBIOME
Bacteria: Culture-based Investigations

Bronchiectasis and chronic infection are well-recognized clinical features of CF that contribute the most to disease morbidity and mortality. Although it is well established that P aeruginosa is an important pathogen in CF lung disease, other bacteria that also contribute to pulmonary morbidity in CF include Burkholderia cepacia complex,[32] methicillin-resistant Staphylococcus aureus,[33] and certain nontuberculous mycobacteria such as Mycobacterium abscessus complex or Mycobacterium avium complex.[34] Microbiological features of these organisms, including factors responsible for virulence and resistance to antimicrobial therapies, have been extensively studied.[35,36] Additional potential pathogens associated with CF include Stenotrophomonas maltophilia and Achromobacter spp, including Achromobacter xylosoxidans and Achromobacter ruhlandii, which can be difficult to treat.[37–41]

The role of anaerobic bacteria in CF lung disease remains uncertain, but they are frequently identifiable and prevalent by both culture-targeted and culture-independent methods.[2,42–45] Current data support an argument for anaerobes playing an important role in the CF airway microenvironment, especially given the steep oxygen gradients present.[45] In addition to contributing to the CF antibiotic resistome (ie, the collection of all antibiotic resistance genes in microorganisms), certain prevalent anaerobic species produce quorum-sensing molecules that mediate interspecies signaling pathways[46] and potentially influence virulence characteristics of pathogens like P aeruginosa.[47] More recent evidence also suggests that metabolic products associated with anaerobes,[43,48] including short-chain fatty acids detected in airway specimens, may increase the release of interleukin (IL)-8, granulocyte-macrophage colony-stimulating factor, and IL-6 and reduce inducible NOS (nitric oxide synthase) gene expression. Thus anaerobic bacteria may be a group of keystone organisms that collectively have a large influence on the CF pulmonary ecosystem.

Bacteria: Culture-independent Molecular Studies

Culture-independent investigations within the past 10 to 15 years have expanded and are reshaping traditional views of CF airway microbiology. Across both cross-sectional and longitudinal studies of CF respiratory samples, several similar observations have been made.

First, studies of respiratory samples from young children with CF have noted that several distinct bacterial groups are present in both directly sampled, CF-affected lung tissue[26] and bronchoalveolar lavage fluid.[1,11] Coupled with the knowledge that structural and physiologic function of the lung is compromised in the early life of CF-affected children,[49,50] this suggests a direct relationship between the early development of microbial dysbiosis in the lungs and these clinical outcomes.

Second, airway bacterial diversity in patients with CF is greatest in early life up to adolescence, declining thereafter into adulthood. These observations have been made from both cross-sectional and longitudinal analyses, including 1 birth cohort study that found that bacterial diversity in the first 2 years of life was influenced by feeding habit and that a decline in specific bacteria, such as *Haemophilus*, preceded colonization of *P aeruginosa*.[12] Similar trends have been observed from cross-sectional analyses across different age groups.[3,4] Selective pressure from cumulative courses of antibiotics is the predominant factor shaping this change in bacterial community structure.[7]

Third, studies in adults with CF have observed great heterogeneity among patients in the composition of bacterial communities identified from airway samples (mostly sputum).[2,6,8] That is, the types and relative abundance of different bacterial groups detected vary considerably between patients, as shown by a representative example from one study (**Fig. 1**). Another consistent finding

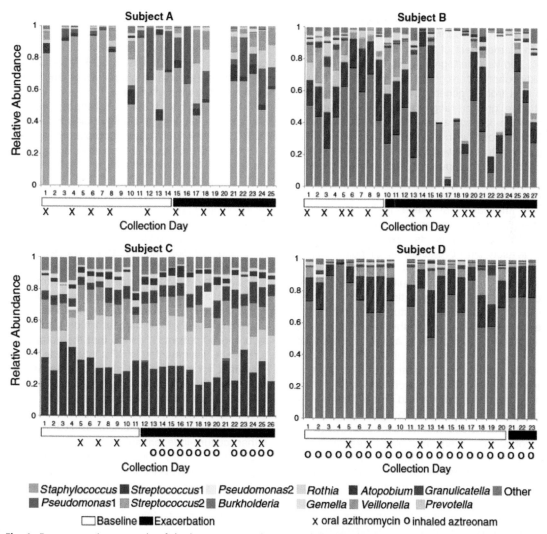

Fig. 1. Representative example of the heterogeneity between different patients with CF in bacterial community composition of sputum. The relative abundance of the top operational taxonomic units identified in daily sputum samples collected from 4 subjects during periods of clinical stability (*white horizontal bars*) and onset of exacerbation (*black horizontal bars*). Symbols below the plots indicate days when maintenance antibiotics were taken. Each plot ends on the day preceding the prescription of antibiotics for treatment of exacerbation. (*From* Carmody LA, Zhao J, Kalikin LM, et al. The daily dynamics of cystic fibrosis airway microbiota during clinical stability and at exacerbation. Microbiome 2015;3:12; with permission under Creative Commons Attribution License.)

is that bacterial groups that are most prevalent within a patient also do not tend to vary substantially in relative abundance over time. The most prevalent communities identified by culture-independent investigations mirror those species or genera detected in clinical cultures, such as *P aeruginosa*, *Burkholderia*, and *Staphylococcus*. When prevalent, these bacterial groups in essence represent core members of the CF respiratory microbiome, but results of culture-independent analyses suggest that additional bacterial groups, not usually detected by typical CF clinical culture methods, comprise this core. For example, using approaches that partition the distribution of species based on statistical variance/abundance ratios, investigators in one study reported that, in addition to *Pseudomonas*, anaerobic species, such as members of the *Porphyromonas*, *Prevotella*, and *Veillonella* genera, also contribute to their study cohort's core group of microbiota (a total of 15 taxa from 7 genera).[5] This finding contrasted with the greater range of bacterial groups (67 taxa from 33 genera) comprising a satellite group of microbiota, which did not correlate with any clinical factors. However, whether satellite species nonetheless contribute ecological interactions of importance within the CF microbiome remains an outstanding question.

An implication of these findings is that a molecular-based bacterial community signature that distinguishes patients clinically has been difficult to ascertain. For example, in CF pulmonary exacerbations, no consistent changes in airway bacterial burden or community composition have been observed among patients within a given study or compared across studies.[6,7,51] Some patients show marked shifts in their respiratory bacterial community structures at a given exacerbation, whereas others show very little change despite clinical symptoms suggestive of such events. Moreover, patients across different studies have shown exacerbation-related reductions in the abundance of baseline predominant species, suggesting that increased abundance of less prevalent microbiota members may play a greater role in certain exacerbations. In addition, antibiotic treatments for exacerbations do not cause a sustained shift in bacterial community structure following exacerbation.[6,7] The CF airway microbiome is generally resilient to these perturbations with community reassembly after recovery resembling a patient's baseline community structure.[7]

Fungal Microbiota in Cystic Fibrosis

Characterization of fungal microbial communities (mycobiome") has in general lagged behind studies of bacteria, and only recently have some advances been made in respiratory studies.[52–54] Several factors make identifying fungi and analysis of the mycobiome challenging.[52] Similar to bacteria, most fungal species are difficult, if at all possible, to culture.[55] As such, the application of high-throughput sequencing approaches has better delineated the diversity of fungal species harbored in the lungs, and in the context of respiratory disease.[53,54] However, approaches for sample preparation, from extraction of fungal DNA and choice of primers to amplify fungal sequences, are nonuniform across studies and that can influence readouts of fungal composition.[52] Moreover, existing reference databases for comparing fungal sequences are less rich and robust than those for bacteria (eg, 16S ribosomal RNA databases), further limiting analytical efforts. Investigators considering such studies should therefore be cognizant of factors that could bias or limit fungal community characterization.

Notwithstanding these challenges, several studies have explored the respiratory mycobiome in CF. In a study of sputum samples from 4 patients with CF, 60% of the identified fungal taxa were not detected by mycological cultures.[13] In addition to *Candida albicans* and *Aspergillus fumigatus*, 30 fungal species or genera identified included other species of *Candida* and *Aspergillus*, *Penicillium*, *Malassezia*, and *Kluyveromyces*. Another study of 6 subjects with CF found that a mixture of *Candida* and *Malassezia* species dominated 74% to 99% of fungal sequence reads from sputum, although the samples were collected at the time of admission, and after completion of antibacterial therapy, which could influence these findings.[14] One of the largest studies to date, involving 56 patients,[54] found that the number of fungal species detected in CF sputum was higher than that for bacteria but also fluctuated much more over time. The investigators concluded that this suggests that inhalational exposure is a greater driving factor in the detection of fungi than established fungal colonization in CF airways. Other culture-independent, nonsequencing approaches to identify fungal species, such as denaturing high-performance liquid chromatography,[15] have also been explored using CF sputa. However, the utility of this approach compared with others remains uncertain.

Viral Microbiota in Cystic Fibrosis Airways

Infections by RNA viruses (eg, rhinovirus, coronavirus, parainfluenzae) are important triggers of CF pulmonary exacerbations.[56–59] However, few studies have examined the respiratory virome in

CF, in part because of the challenges of conducting comprehensive viral sequencing studies.[60] Several studies have focused on bacteriophage populations in the airways.[16,61–63] Because these DNA viruses infect specific bacteria, specific phages have been studied as alternative therapeutic approaches to potentially target particular bacterial pathogens, like *P aeruginosa*.[62,63]

Metagenomic studies that provide a more comprehensive picture of DNA viruses in the respiratory tract of patients with CF have noted CF-associated phage communities to be highly similar to each other, in contrast with those found in patients without CF.[16] This finding likely reflects the range of bacterial species selected for in the CF lung. High phage/bacteria ratios have been described in a variety of mucosal environments, including human gingival samples, and *in vitro* studies have shown phage adherence to mucus to be mediated by binding interactions between immunoglobulinlike domains on phage capsids and glycan residues on mucin glycoproteins.[64] Further, pretreatment of mucus-producing cell lines with T4 phages led to subsequent decreased bacterial attachment (*Escherichia coli*) to the cells. These findings have led investigators to propose that bacteriophage adherence to mucus may serve as a form of antibacterial immunity along mucosal surfaces. However, the potential significance of this system extrapolated to the CF lung remains unclear. Other data also suggest that phages may be functionally synergistic with antibiotics, wherein antibiotics stimulate phage production and/or activity to aid bacterial killing.[65] Lytic activity of temperate phages may also be preserved long-term in chronic *P aeruginosa* infection and potentially contribute to controlling *P aeruginosa* density.[62]

FUNCTIONAL FEATURES OF THE CYSTIC FIBROSIS MICROBIOME

Compositional studies of the microbiota harbored within patients with CF have broadened the knowledge of microbial diversity associated with this disease. However, it is likely that the functions and metabolic features encoded for, and expressed by, a collective microbial community span species-level differences in taxonomic composition, which in itself is nonuniform across patients. Evidence for this cross-phylogeny sharing of gene functions has been found in the gut microbiome, via known mechanisms such as horizontal gene transfer between bacteria,[66] and has served as a premise for the development of in silico approaches to determine functional capacities of bacterial microbiota based on metagenome predictions.[67]

Using a combined metagenomic and metatranscriptomic approach in which sequencing of both DNA and RNA were performed, Quinn and colleagues[68] examined the functional capacities of microbiota detected from the sputa of patients with CF. Enriched functions expressed by CF-associated organisms included amino acid catabolism, folate biosynthesis, and nitrate reduction pathways, with the nitrate reduction pathways largely encoded by *Pseudomonas* and *Rothia*. Their data also suggested that ammonia may accumulate in the airway environment, because oxidative pathways involved in the nitrogen cycle were incomplete.

Artificial culture systems have also been applied in attempts to simulate and study CF microbial-related physiology in the airways.[69] One approach used glass capillary tubes instilled with artificial sputum medium intended to mimic CF physiologic conditions, which were then inoculated with bacterial strains derived from patients with CF collected serially during periods of clinical stability and exacerbation. Using a combination of techniques to evaluate the physiology of the system, the investigators observed increased gas production and a 2-unit reduction in pH before the onset of exacerbation. Parallel analysis of the microbial community noted an increase in the abundance of fermentative anaerobes, suggesting that metabolic activities of these organisms may contribute to the development of exacerbations.

THE GASTROINTESTINAL MICROBIOME IN CYSTIC FIBROSIS

Although studies of respiratory microbiota have dominated CF microbiome studies, recently investigations have also begun to characterize and analyze relationships between gastrointestinal bacterial microbiota, clinical disease markers, and profiles of airway bacterial community composition. Gastrointestinal complications of CF are a significant cause of disease morbidity, and problems beyond pancreatic insufficiency are often difficult to manage.[21] Two studies[17,18] involving a cohort of patients with CF found that numbers of Enterobacteriaceae were marginally higher in CF fecal samples, whereas there was significant underrepresentation of *Bifidobacterium* and members of *Clostridium* cluster XIVa. Two-year longitudinal analysis of 2 patients with CF and their healthy siblings observed a trend toward lower species richness and temporal stability of CF fecal microbiota.[17]

Patterns of gut and respiratory microbiome development in early life in children with CF have been reported in 2 studies from a single birth cohort.[19,20] Although the number of subjects was small, the investigators observed initial diversification in gut and respiratory microbiota composition, followed by subsequent shifts in community composition related to changes in diet, namely cessation of breastfeeding and introduction of solid foods. Although children without CF were not included as a control group for comparison in these studies, this observation is consistent with normal patterns of gut microbiome maturation in early life in healthy infants.[70,71] Changes in diet also influenced respiratory microbiota composition, indicating links to nutritional intake.[19] Decreases in specific bacterial genera, both in the gut (*Parabacteroides*) and in the respiratory tract (*Haemophilus*), preceded airway colonization with *P aeruginosa*.[20] Another interesting observation was that intestinal, but not respiratory, bacterial community structure in the first 6 months of life was associated with the occurrence of CF exacerbations during that time frame. Findings from these types of studies, as well as those from interventional trials using probiotic species,[72,73] suggest that manipulations of the gut microbiome to foster a less proinflammatory environment could be an avenue to mitigate pulmonary morbidity in CF.

FUTURE DIRECTIONS IN CYSTIC FIBROSIS MICROBIOME RESEARCH

The new insights afforded by the studies described earlier provide a foundation for addressing several important questions pertaining to the microbiology of CF. As clinicians continue to explore the long-term dynamics of airway bacterial community structure, a focus will be on better elucidating the relationship between decreasing community diversity and advancing patient age and lung disease. An intriguing question is whether maintaining more diverse communities might have a positive impact on lung health, and, if so, whether novel treatment strategies (eg, targeted species-specific antimicrobial therapy) may enable maintenance of healthier airway communities. A more complete understanding of short-term community dynamics may identify reproducible changes in community structure and/or activity that are associated with changes in patient clinical condition. If multiomic analyses identify, for example, biomarkers of impending exacerbation, it will be of great interest to determine whether these can be monitored in real time and exploited to prevent or better manage these events. Similarly, specific patterns of community change may be identified that predict exacerbation severity and/or recovery.

Moving forward, it will be important to complement the growing understanding of bacterial ecology in CF airways with attention to the broader microbial community, including viral and fungal species. Advances in the appreciation of how microbial interactions drive the activity of polymicrobial communities are expected to provide opportunities for novel therapies. In addition, continued investigation of the relationship between disordered gut microbiota and lung disorder in CF has the potential to translate to creative management strategies and to generate mechanistic hypotheses addressing CF pathobiology.

REFERENCES

1. Harris JK, De Groote MA, Sagel SD, et al. Molecular identification of bacteria in bronchoalveolar lavage fluid from children with cystic fibrosis. Proc Natl Acad Sci U S A 2007;104(51):20529–33.
2. Tunney MM, Field TR, Moriarty TF, et al. Detection of anaerobic bacteria in high numbers in sputum from patients with cystic fibrosis. Am J Respir Crit Care Med 2008;177:995–1001.
3. Cox MJ, Allgaier M, Taylor B, et al. Airway microbiota and pathogen abundance in age-stratified cystic fibrosis patients. PLoS One 2010;5(6):e11044.
4. Klepac-Ceraj V, Lemon KP, Martin TR, et al. Relationship between cystic fibrosis respiratory tract bacterial communities and age, genotype, antibiotics and *Pseudomonas aeruginosa*. Environ Microbiol 2010;12:1293–303.
5. van der Gast CJ, Walker AW, Stressmann FA, et al. Partitioning core and satellite taxa from within cystic fibrosis lung bacterial communities. ISME J 2011; 5(5):780–91.
6. Fodor AA, Klem ER, Gilpin DF, et al. The adult cystic fibrosis airway microbiota is stable over time and infection type, and highly resilient to antibiotic treatment of exacerbations. PLoS One 2012; 7(9):e45001.
7. Zhao J, Schloss PD, Kalikin LM, et al. Decade-long bacterial community dynamics in cystic fibrosis airways. Proc Natl Acad Sci U S A 2012;109(15): 5809–14.
8. Carmody LA, Zhao J, Kalikin LM, et al. The daily dynamics of cystic fibrosis airway microbiota during clinical stability and at exacerbation. Microbiome 2015;3:12.
9. Price KE, Hampton TH, Gifford AH, et al. Unique microbial communities persist in individual cystic fibrosis patients throughout a clinical exacerbation. Microbiome 2013;1(1):27.
10. Zemanick ET, Harris JK, Wagner BD, et al. Inflammation and airway microbiota during cystic fibrosis pulmonary exacerbations. PLoS One 2013;8(4): e62917.

11. Renwick J, McNally P, John B, et al. The microbial community of the cystic fibrosis airway is disrupted in early life. PLoS One 2014;9(12):e109798.

12. Coburn B, Wang PW, Diaz Caballero J, et al. Lung microbiota across age and disease stage in cystic fibrosis. Sci Rep 2015;5:10241.

13. Delhaes L, Monchy S, Fréalle E, et al. The airway microbiota in cystic fibrosis: a complex fungal and bacterial community–implications for therapeutic management. PLoS One 2012;7(4):e36313.

14. Willger SD, Grim SL, Dolben EL, et al. Characterization and quantification of the fungal microbiome in serial samples from individuals with cystic fibrosis. Microbiome 2014;2:40.

15. Mounier J, Gouëllo A, Keravec M, et al. Use of denaturing high-performance liquid chromatography (DHPLC) to characterize the bacterial and fungal airway microbiota of cystic fibrosis patients. J Microbiol 2014;52(4):307–14.

16. Willner D, Furlan M, Haynes M, et al. Metagenomic analysis of respiratory tract DNA viral communities in cystic fibrosis and non-cystic fibrosis individuals. PLoS One 2009;4(10):e7370.

17. Duytschaever G, Huys G, Bekaert M, et al. Cross-sectional and longitudinal comparisons of the predominant fecal microbiota compositions of a group of pediatric patients with cystic fibrosis and their healthy siblings. Appl Environ Microbiol 2011; 77(22):8015–24.

18. Duytschaever G, Huys G, Bekaert M, et al. Dysbiosis of bifidobacteria and Clostridium cluster XIVa in the cystic fibrosis fecal microbiota. J Cyst Fibros 2013; 12(3):206–15.

19. Madan JC, Koestler DC, Stanton BA, et al. Serial analysis of the gut and respiratory microbiome in cystic fibrosis in infancy: interaction between intestinal and respiratory tracts and impact of nutritional exposures. MBio 2012;3(4) [pii:e00251–12].

20. Hoen AG, Li J, Moulton LA, et al. Associations between gut microbial colonization in early life and respiratory outcomes in cystic fibrosis. J Pediatr 2015; 167(1):138–47.e1-3.

21. Gelfond D, Borowitz D. Gastrointestinal complications of cystic fibrosis. Clin Gastroenterol Hepatol 2013;11(4):333–42 [quiz: e30–1].

22. Han MK, Huang YJ, Lipuma JJ, et al. Significance of the microbiome in obstructive lung disease. Thorax 2012;67(5):456–63.

23. Huang YJ, Charlson ES, Collman RG, et al. The role of the lung microbiome in health and disease. A National Heart, Lung, and Blood Institute workshop report. Am J Respir Crit Care Med 2013;187(12):1382–7.

24. Dickson RP, Erb-Downward JR, Huffnagle GB. The role of the bacterial microbiome in lung disease. Expert Rev Respir Med 2013;7(3):245–57.

25. Morris A, Beck JM, Schloss PD, et al. Lung HIV microbiome project. Comparison of the respiratory microbiome in healthy nonsmokers and smokers. Am J Respir Crit Care Med 2013;187(10):1067–75.

26. Brown PS, Pope CE, Marsh RL, et al. Directly sampling the lung of a young child with cystic fibrosis reveals diverse microbiota. Ann Am Thorac Soc 2014; 11(7):1049–55.

27. Zemanick ET, Wagner BD, Robertson CE, et al. Assessment of airway microbiota and inflammation in cystic fibrosis using multiple sampling methods. Ann Am Thorac Soc 2015;12(2):221–9.

28. Boutin S, Graeber SY, Weitnauer M, et al. Comparison of microbiomes from different niches of upper and lower airways in children and adolescents with cystic fibrosis. PLoS One 2015;10(1):e0116029.

29. Venkataraman A, Bassis CM, Beck JM, et al. Application of a neutral community model to assess structuring of the human lung microbiome. MBio 2015; 6(1) [pii:e02284–14].

30. Dickson RP, Erb-Downward JR, Huffnagle GB. Towards an ecology of the lung: new conceptual models of pulmonary microbiology and pneumonia pathogenesis. Lancet Respir Med 2014;2(3):238–46.

31. Willner D, Haynes MR, Furlan M, et al. Spatial distribution of microbial communities in the cystic fibrosis lung. ISME J 2012;6(2):471–4.

32. Gilligan PH. Infections in patients with cystic fibrosis: diagnostic microbiology update [Review]. Clin Lab Med 2014;34(2):197–217.

33. Dasenbrook EC, Checkley W, Merlo CA, et al. Association between respiratory tract methicillin-resistant Staphylococcus aureus and survival in cystic fibrosis. JAMA 2010;303(23):2386–92.

34. Martiniano SL, Nick JA. Nontuberculous mycobacterial infections in cystic fibrosis [Review]. Clin Chest Med 2015;36(1):101–15.

35. Wolter DJ, Emerson JC, McNamara S, et al. Staphylococcus aureus small-colony variants are independently associated with worse lung disease in children with cystic fibrosis. Clin Infect Dis 2013; 57(3):384–91.

36. Muhlebach MS, Heltshe SL, Popowitch EB, et al, The STAR-CF Study Team. Multicenter observational study on factors and outcomes associated with different MRSA types in children with cystic fibrosis. Ann Am Thorac Soc 2015;12(6):864–71.

37. Cogen J, Emerson J, Sanders DB, et al, EPIC Study Group. Risk factors for lung function decline in a large cohort of young cystic fibrosis patients. Pediatr Pulmonol 2015;50(8):763–70.

38. Parkins MD, Floto RA. Emerging bacterial pathogens and changing concepts of bacterial pathogenesis in cystic fibrosis. J Cyst Fibros 2015; 14(3):293–304.

39. De Baets F, Schelstraete P, Van Daele S, et al. Achromobacter xylosoxidans in cystic fibrosis: prevalence and clinical relevance. J Cyst Fibros 2007; 6(1):75–8.

40. Lambiase A, Catania MR, Del Pezzo M, et al. *Achromobacter xylosoxidans* respiratory tract infection in cystic fibrosis patients. Eur J Clin Microbiol Infect Dis 2011;30(8):973–80.

41. Marzuillo C, De Giusti M, Tufi D, et al. Molecular characterization of *Stenotrophomonas maltophilia* isolates from cystic fibrosis patients and the hospital environment. Infect Control Hosp Epidemiol 2009; 30(8):753–8.

42. Tunney MM, Klem ER, Fodor AA, et al. Use of culture and molecular analysis to determine the effect of antibiotic treatment on microbial community diversity and abundance during exacerbation in patients with cystic fibrosis. Thorax 2011;66:579–84.

43. Twomey KB, Alston M, An SQ, et al. Microbiota and metabolite profiling reveal specific alterations in bacterial community structure and environment in the cystic fibrosis airway during exacerbation. PLoS One 2013;8(12):e82432.

44. Chmiel JF, Aksamit TR, Chotirmall SH, et al. Antibiotic management of lung infections in cystic fibrosis. II. Nontuberculous mycobacteria, anaerobic bacteria, and fungi. Ann Am Thorac Soc 2014;11(8): 1298–306.

45. Jones AM. Anaerobic bacteria in cystic fibrosis: pathogens or harmless commensals? Thorax 2011; 66(7):558–9.

46. Field TR, Sibley CD, Parkins MD, et al. The genus *Prevotella* in cystic fibrosis airways. Anaerobe 2010;16(4):337–44.

47. Duan K, Dammel C, Stein J, et al. Modulation of *Pseudomonas aeruginosa* gene expression by host microflora through interspecies communication. Mol Microbiol 2003;50(5):1477–91.

48. Ghorbani P, Santhakumar P, Hu Q, et al. Short-chain fatty acids affect cystic fibrosis airway inflammation and bacterial growth. Eur Respir J 2015;46(4): 1033–45.

49. Ramsey KA, Ranganathan S, Park J, et al. Early respiratory infection is associated with reduced spirometry in children with cystic fibrosis. Am J Respir Crit Care Med 2014;190(10):1111–6.

50. Wielpütz MO, Puderbach M, Kopp-Schneider A, et al. Magnetic resonance imaging detects changes in structure and perfusion, and response to therapy in early cystic fibrosis lung disease. Am J Respir Crit Care Med 2014;189(8):956–65.

51. Carmody LA, Zhao J, Schloss PD, et al. Changes in cystic fibrosis airway microbiota at pulmonary exacerbation. Ann Am Thorac Soc 2013;10(3): 179–87.

52. Cui L, Morris A, Ghedin E. The human mycobiome in health and disease [Review]. Genome Med 2013; 5(7):63.

53. Nguyen LD, Viscogliosi E, Delhaes L. The lung mycobiome: an emerging field of the human respiratory microbiome [Review]. Front Microbiol 2015;6:89.

54. Kramer R, Sauer-Heilborn A, Welte T, et al. A cohort study of the airway mycobiome in adult cystic fibrosis patients: differences in community structure of fungi compared to bacteria reveal predominance of transient fungal elements. J Clin Microbiol 2015; 53(9):2900–7.

55. Nagano Y, Elborn JS, Millar BC, et al. Comparison of techniques to examine the diversity of fungi in adult patients with cystic fibrosis. Med Mycol 2010;48: 166–76.

56. Goffard A, Lambert V, Salleron J, et al. Virus and cystic fibrosis: rhinoviruses are associated with exacerbations in adult patients. J Clin Virol 2014; 60(2):147–53.

57. Esther CR Jr, Lin FC, Kerr A, et al. Respiratory viruses are associated with common respiratory pathogens in cystic fibrosis. Pediatr Pulmonol 2014; 49(9):926–31.

58. Flight WG, Bright-Thomas RJ, Tilston P, et al. Incidence and clinical impact of respiratory viruses in adults with cystic fibrosis. Thorax 2014;69(3): 247–53.

59. Asner S, Waters V, Solomon M, et al. Role of respiratory viruses in pulmonary exacerbations in children with cystic fibrosis. J Cyst Fibros 2012;11(5):433–9.

60. Wylie KM, Weinstock GM, Storch GA. Emerging view of the human virome [Review]. Transl Res 2012;160(4):283–90.

61. Lim YW, Schmieder R, Haynes M, et al. Metagenomics and metatranscriptomics: windows on CF-associated viral and microbial communities. J Cyst Fibros 2013;12(2):154–64.

62. James CE, Davies EV, Fothergill JL, et al. Lytic activity by temperate phages of *Pseudomonas aeruginosa* in long-term cystic fibrosis chronic lung infections. ISME J 2015;9(6):1391–8.

63. Saussereau E, Vachier I, Chiron R, et al. Effectiveness of bacteriophages in the sputum of cystic fibrosis patients. Clin Microbiol Infect 2014;20(12): O983–90.

64. Barr JJ, Auro R, Furlan M, et al. Bacteriophage adhering to mucus provide a non-host-derived immunity. Proc Natl Acad Sci U S A 2013;110:10771–6.

65. Kamal F, Dennis JJ. *Burkholderia cepacia* complex phage-antibiotic synergy (PAS): antibiotics stimulate lytic phage activity. Appl Environ Microbiol 2015; 81(3):1132–8.

66. Smillie CS, Smith MB, Friedman J, et al. Ecology drives a global network of gene exchange connecting the human microbiome. Nature 2011;480: 241–4.

67. Langille MG, Zaneveld J, Caporaso JG, et al. Predictive functional profiling of microbial communities using 16S rRNA marker gene sequences. Nat Biotechnol 2013;31(9):814–21.

68. Quinn RA, Lim YW, Maughan H, et al. Biogeochemical forces shape the composition and physiology of

polymicrobial communities in the cystic fibrosis lung. MBio 2014;5(2):e00956-13.

69. Quinn RA, Whiteson K, Lim YW, et al. Winogradsky-based culture system shows an association between microbial fermentation and cystic fibrosis exacerbation. ISME J 2015;9(4):1024–38 [Erratum appears in ISME J 2015;9(4):1052].

70. Saavedra JM, Dattilo AM. Early development of intestinal microbiota: implications for future health. Gastroenterol Clin North Am 2012;41(4):717–31.

71. Bäckhed F, Roswall J, Peng Y, et al. Dynamics and stabilization of the human gut microbiome during the first year of life. Cell Host Microbe 2015;17(5): 690–703.

72. del Campo R, Garriga M, Pérez-Aragón A, et al. Improvement of digestive health and reduction in proteobacterial populations in the gut microbiota of cystic fibrosis patients using a *Lactobacillus reuteri* probiotic preparation: a double blind prospective study. J Cyst Fibros 2014;13(6):716–22.

73. Bruzzese E, Callegari ML, Raia V, et al. Disrupted intestinal microbiota and intestinal inflammation in children with cystic fibrosis and its restoration with *Lactobacillus* GG: a randomised clinical trial. PLoS One 2014;9(2):e87796.

The Approach to *Pseudomonas aeruginosa* in Cystic Fibrosis

Jaideep S. Talwalkar, MD[a,b,*], Thomas S. Murray, MD, PhD[c,d]

KEYWORDS

- Cystic fibrosis • *Pseudomonas aeruginosa* • Eradication • Inhaled antibiotics
- Pulmonary exacerbation

KEY POINTS

- There is an epidemiologic link between infection with *Pseudomonas aeruginosa* and morbidity and mortality in cystic fibrosis.
- Strict infection control is the most effective strategy to prevent *Pseudomonas aeruginosa* infection; efforts to develop vaccines are underway.
- There is consensus among cystic fibrosis professional societies that there is benefit to eradication therapy at time of newly acquired *Pseudomonas aeruginosa*.
- Maintenance therapy for chronic infection with *Pseudomonas aeruginosa* consists of inhaled antibiotics and oral azithromycin.
- Susceptibility testing poorly predicts in vivo clinical effect in acute pulmonary exacerbations, and antibiotic dosing is higher than that used in non–cystic fibrosis populations.

INTRODUCTION

Pseudomonas aeruginosa is a gram-negative non–lactose fermenting oxidase-positive bacterium that causes infection in patients with compromised immune systems and/or disrupted epithelial barriers. As a versatile opportunist, *P aeruginosa* is capable of causing acute infection, which may result in sepsis and death, and a chronic infection that can persist for years.[1] During acute infection, *P aeruginosa* secretes exotoxins into the environment that damage host tissue, and *P aeruginosa* also uses a surface-associated needle-like structure, the type III secretion system, to directly inject toxins into host cells.[1] Chronic infection is thought to be characterized by the formation of biofilms, surface-associated organized communities of bacteria residing within the thick mucus of the cystic fibrosis (CF) lung. These biofilms persist despite a robust immune response and aggressive antibiotic therapy.

Patients with CF are specifically at risk for chronic *P aeruginosa* respiratory infections because of defects in the immune response to bacterial infection, and an inability to clear thick secretions that trap microorganisms. Given the epidemiologic association between *P aeruginosa* respiratory infection and increased morbidity and mortality in the CF population, emphasis has

Disclosure Statement: The authors have nothing to disclose.
[a] Department of Internal Medicine, Yale School of Medicine, 333 Cedar Street, PO Box 208086, New Haven, CT 06520-8086, USA; [b] Department of Pediatrics, Yale School of Medicine, 333 Cedar Street, PO Box 208084, New Haven, CT 06520-8084, USA; [c] Department of Medical Sciences, Frank H Netter MD School of Medicine, Quinnipiac University, 275 Mount Carmel Avenue, Hamden, CT 06518, USA; [d] Division of Infectious Diseases and Immunology, Connecticut Children's Medical Center, 282 Washington Street, Suite 2L, Hartford, CT 06106, USA
* Corresponding author. Department of Internal Medicine, Yale School of Medicine, 333 Cedar Street, PO Box 208086, New Haven, CT 06520-8086.
E-mail address: jaideep.talwalkar@yale.edu

been placed on the prevention of acquiring *P aeruginosa* in the respiratory tract, eradication when it is first identified, therapeutic regimens for patients chronically infected with *P aeruginosa*, and appropriate treatment of acute pulmonary exacerbations (APE).

PREVENTION
Infection Control

P aeruginosa is ubiquitous in the environment surviving in water, in the soil, and in some cases on the surface of respiratory equipment.[2] If *P aeruginosa* acquisition can be prevented for patients with CF this has the potential to preserve lung function. Prevention strategies start with infection control in the home and health care setting. The Cystic Fibrosis Foundation (CFF) provides evidence-based guidelines to assist patients, families, and health care providers to prevent the spread of common CF pathogens including *P aeruginosa*.[3] Patient and health care provider education, hand hygiene with either antimicrobial soap or alcohol, and the appropriate use of personal protective equipment (eg, gowns and gloves in the health care setting) are the foundation for effective infection control.[3] Additional measures include the appropriate disinfection and cleaning of respiratory equipment, and limiting the contact of patients with CF with other patients with CF to prevent respiratory pathogen transmission between patients.[3]

Vaccination Against Pseudomonas aeruginosa

Another potential method to prevent acquisition of *P aeruginosa* is the development of a vaccine, which has been challenging despite years of work (reviewed in Ref.[4]). A variety of different bacterial surface-associated antigens have shown promise in eliciting protective immune responses, with evidence of protection in animal studies.[5] Additionally, children with CF infected with *P aeruginosa* possess higher levels of IgA, IgG, and IgM antibodies against a variety of potential vaccine antigens in bronchoalveolar lavage fluid and serum, compared with uninfected children with CF, and healthy control subjects.[6]

As an example, most strains of *P aeruginosa* possess a single unipolar flagella required for swimming motility and surface attachment that has been the focus of *P aeruginosa* vaccine development.[7] The only published randomized controlled phase III anti-*Pseudomonas* vaccine study used a bivalent flagella vaccine and compared vaccinated, uninfected children with CF (N = 239) with placebo control subjects (N = 244) over a 2-year period.[7] The results showed modest protection with the primary outcome of a

positive *P aeruginosa* culture (relative risk, 0.66; 95% confidence interval, 0.46–0.93) in patients who completed the protocol (N = 189 vaccinated group; N = 192 placebo group). Rates of chronic *P aeruginosa* infection were too low in either group to measure a statistically significant difference, and the authors hypothesized that this was caused by the institution of aggressive antibiotic-based eradication protocols.[7] Vaccine administration resulted in high levels of antiflagella antibodies, and was well tolerated. Only two severe adverse events were attributed to the vaccine: persistent pain at the injection site and atelectasis.[7] However, a second industry-sponsored randomized clinical trial was stopped early because of lack of benefit, and a recent Cochrane review concluded that vaccines against *P aeruginosa* could not be recommended, and additional studies were needed.[4,8]

Several challenges to vaccine development must be overcome to achieve an effective product. First, there is significant genotypic and phenotypic variability among *P aeruginosa* clinical isolates, reducing the effectiveness of vaccines with single antigens.[7,9] Second, antibodies against multiple *P aeruginosa* antigens present in uninfected children may interfere with the vaccine response.[6] Additionally many children with these antibodies go on to develop infection with *P aeruginosa* suggesting that the presence of antibody does not independently prevent infection.[6] Finally, patients with CF have immune dysfunction related to their underlying disease, and it is possible this also contributes to the lack of vaccine efficacy despite the presence of antipseudomonal antibodies (see Bruscia EM, Bonfield TL: Innate and Adaptive Immunity in Cystic Fibrosis, in this issue).

Given the medical need for a *P aeruginosa* vaccine, work continues with several target antigens. A recent phase I placebo-controlled trial of healthy volunteers injected with a hybrid vaccine containing the outer membrane proteins OprF and OprI found that IgG was effectively induced without safety concerns.[10] Alginate, the primary polysaccharide component of the extracellular matrix produced by mucoid *P aeruginosa*, has been studied extensively as a vaccine candidate to prevent chronic infection. A recent study conjugating alginate to the outer membrane vesicle of *Neisseria meningitides*, already used in human vaccines, elicited opsonic antibodies in mice that resulted in increased CF mouse survival when challenged with *P aeruginosa* and compared with unvaccinated control animals.[11]

In addition to active immunization, passive immunization with IgY antibodies derived from eggs inoculated with *P aeruginosa* is being studied as a gargle to prevent initial *P aeruginosa* upper airway colonization in two randomized clinical trials in Europe.[12,13] An earlier study found 17 patients on IgY prophylaxis had decreased numbers of positive *P aeruginosa* cultures over a 12-year period compared with 24 control subjects, and this was without adverse events.[14]

Prophylactic Antibiotics

Historically, the use of oral antibiotics to prevent chronic infection has been more extensively studied and reviewed in relation to *Staphylococcus aureus*[15] than with *P aeruginosa*. In a recent placebo-controlled trial, Tramper-Standers and colleagues[16] studied a combination regimen of 3-week treatments of oral and inhaled antipseudomonal antibiotics administered every 3 months for 3 years to children without *P aeruginosa* infection. No differences in rates of *P aeruginosa* infection or

forced expiratory volume in 1 second (FEV_1) % predicted were found, although higher rates of non-*Pseudomonas* gram-negative bacteria pulmonary infection were seen in the treatment group. Balancing the lack of data in support of this strategy with the potential risks (drug toxicity, impact on host microbiome) and cost (treatment time, expense), the use of prophylactic antibiotics against *P aeruginosa* is not currently a standard treatment modality in CF care.[17] Therefore, antibiotics are reserved for treating pulmonary infections. **Table 1** summarizes the antibiotics used to treat *P aeruginosa* pulmonary infections in patients with CF.

EARLY ERADICATION THERAPY

Studies support the concept of clinical decline following first isolation of *P aeruginosa* in

---

Table 1
Antibiotics for *Pseudomonas aeruginosa* infection in patients with cystic fibrosis

Antibiotic Classes	Considerations
Fluoroquinolones: ciprofloxacin, levofloxacin	• Trials of inhaled formulations ongoing[18,19] • Less data and experience with levofloxacin but has added benefit to improve spectrum against gram-positive organisms compared with ciprofloxacin[20] • Lack of data to support prophylactic or long-term use[21] • Delayed oral absorption caused by CF transmembrane conductance regulator defect[20]
Aminoglycosides: tobramycin, amikacin, gentamicin	• Inhaled tobramycin recommended for eradication therapy[22,23] and long-term use for chronic infection[24–26] • Trials of inhaled liposomal amikacin ongoing[27] • Once-daily dosing intravenously[28] • Synergy with β-lactams in vitro[29] • Cationic moieties impair ability to penetrate sputum • Increased dosing in CF because of increased renal clearance[30] • Higher rates of nephrotoxicity with gentamicin in CF[30]
Antipseudomonal β-lactams: piperacillin-tazobactam, ticarcillin-clavulanate, ceftazidime, cefepime	• Time-dependent killing has generated interest in extended-interval and continuous infusion[20] • Increased dosing in CF because of increased volume of distribution[31] • Dose-related adverse effects with piperacillin-tazobactam, although it is commonly used by CF providers[31]
Monobactam: aztreonam	• Inhaled aztreonam recommended for long-term use for chronic infection[25] • Infrequently used by CF providers in intravenous formulation[32] • Determination of optimal pharmacokinetic/pharmacodynamic parameters warrants further study[32]
Carbapenems: imipenem-cilastatin, meropenem, doripenem	• Increased *P aeruginosa* resistance to imipenem-cilastatin may limit use in patients with CF[20] • Time-dependent killing has generated interest in extended-interval and continuous infusion[20]
Polymyxin: colistin	• Inhaled form recommended for eradication therapy and long-term use for chronic infection by United Kingdom CF Trust[24] • High rates of neurotoxicity and nephrotoxicity limit its use intravenously[33] • Used for multidrug-resistant *P aeruginosa*, or when other agents are ineffective or contraindicated[33]

respiratory specimens of individuals with CF. Important clinical outcomes include worsening of respiratory symptoms and chest radiograph scores. The time of first isolation of P aeruginosa presents an opportunity for clinical intervention, because chronic infection and conversion from nonmucoid to mucoid phenotype can be delayed with early, aggressive treatment.[34] The development of chronic infection with mucoid P aeruginosa predicts more dramatic clinical deterioration, with decreases in FEV_1 and quality of life, and increases in hospitalization, need for antibiotics, and mortality.[34,35] Therefore, there has been much interest in P aeruginosa eradication on first acquisition, and a multitude of treatment protocols have been described and reviewed.[22,36]

The most commonly used strategies for P aeruginosa eradication are inhaled antibiotics (eg, colistin or tobramycin) with or without oral ciprofloxacin. Valerius and colleagues[37] administered 3 weeks of twice-daily inhaled colistin and oral ciprofloxacin to children naive to antipseudomonal antibiotics on initial growth of P aeruginosa, and with each subsequent positive culture. Over the 27-month trial, children in the treatment arm demonstrated decreased rates of chronic P aeruginosa infection (14%) relative to those receiving no treatment (58%). Gibson and colleagues[38] randomized children to a 28-day course of twice-daily tobramycin inhalation solution (TIS) or placebo. All participants had grown P aeruginosa within a year of the trial. The trial was stopped early when Day 28 bronchoalveolar lavage samples were free of P aeruginosa in 100% of the TIS-treated patients compared with 7.4% of the placebo group. A landmark comparative efficacy trial, Early Pseudomonas Infection Control (EPIC), noted no difference in microbiologic outcomes or rates of APE when oral ciprofloxacin or placebo was added to a 28-day course of TIS in children with recently acquired P aeruginosa.[39] More recently, an open-label trial of aztreonam lysine for inhalation (AZLI) demonstrated that 89.1% of children were culture negative for P aeruginosa after 4 weeks of treatment, decreasing to 47.5% at the 28-week timepoint.[40] Although the bulk of the literature pertains to children, eradication efforts in adults have also been successful.[41]

Comparing the results of these and other trials is challenging because of varying outcome measures and methods for detection of P aeruginosa. Accordingly, a 2014 Cochrane review concluded that eradication therapy is better than no treatment, but noted insufficient evidence to support a particular eradication strategy.[35] Additionally, long-term data, including impact on mortality and effects on lung microbiome, are lacking.[42] Given

that eradication is now the standard of care, it is unlikely that long-term placebo-controlled trials will be forthcoming.[17]

There is consensus among CF professional societies that there is benefit to eradication therapy at time of newly acquired P aeruginosa in children and adults with CF, and acknowledgment among these groups that no particular regimen has proven to be more beneficial than another. Nevertheless, specific recommendations vary. For example, given the methodological rigor of the EPIC study, the CFF[22] and European Cystic Fibrosis Society (ECFS)[23] suggest inhaled tobramycin, 300 mg, twice a day for 28 days, whereas the United Kingdom Cystic Fibrosis Trust (CFT) advocates twice-daily nebulized colistin and oral ciprofloxacin for at least 3 weeks.[24] Multicenter trials are currently recruiting patients to compare these and other eradication strategies.[43,44] For the time being, in the absence of definitive comparative efficacy trials other than EPIC, specific therapy should be tailored to the clinical situation, taking into account such issues as severity of illness, potential side effects, and access to medications.[22,24]

MAINTENANCE THERAPY FOR CHRONIC INFECTION

Eradication therapy can postpone chronic infection with P aeruginosa,[34] but by adulthood colonization ultimately develops in most patients with CF. Although a variety of definitions for chronic infection exist,[45] the term generally refers to persistent isolation of the organism on repeat cultures over time (eg, 6–12 months).[1,23,45] Chronic infection with P aeruginosa differs from early infection in that different virulence factors exist in strains associated with the chronic state. These virulence factors result in the formation of biofilms, organized communities of bacteria encased in respiratory secretions that often lead to the mucoid phenotype. Growth as a biofilm offers protection against phagocytosis, increased antibiotic resistance because of reduced antibiotic penetration, and altered bacterial metabolism. Mucoid P aeruginosa is a predictor of clinical deterioration,[42] and once chronic infection has been established, treatment goals switch from eradication to suppression.[17,46]

The use of inhaled antibiotics is an established standard of care in CF,[25] with supporting data accumulated over the past 70 years.[47] In theory, by delivering high concentrations of antibiotics directly into the airways, bacterial load is decreased, the host's inflammatory response is tempered, tissue destruction is reduced, and there are fewer side effects.[48]

Early studies of inhaled antibiotics used compounded versions of intravenous antibiotics. These studies showed clinical benefit despite difficulties related to bronchospasm, likely caused by preservatives in the intravenous solutions that were not designed for inhalation. Despite their shortcomings, these studies laid the groundwork for the development of formulations specifically designed for nebulization.[17]

Tobramycin

In 1997, TIS became the first inhaled antibiotic to gain Food and Drug Administration (FDA) approval. Numerous randomized trials have demonstrated its clinical benefit.[25,48] The largest study by Ramsey and colleagues[49] included 520 patients at least 6 years of age, with FEV_1 between 25% and 75% predicted. Patients were randomized to twice-daily administration of TIS, 300 mg, or taste-masked placebo for 28 days, alternating with 28 days off. Patients continued the on-off cycle for the 24-week duration of the trial. Those in the treatment group saw an 11.9% relative improvement in FEV_1 compared with the placebo group, and significant differences in forced vital capacity, sputum density of *P aeruginosa*, quality of life, and rates of hospitalization and intravenous antibiotic use.[49] Voice alteration and mild, transient tinnitus were the only statistically significant adverse effects of treatment, although bronchospasm has been described in other trials.[26] No significant differences were found in serum creatinine or audiologic testing. Clinical benefit has been demonstrated as far out as 96 weeks into treatment, although the improvement in FEV_1 declined with time on therapy.[50] Subsequent studies performed in patients with milder lung disease have also demonstrated benefit in decreasing sputum density of *P aeruginosa* and lower rates of APE.[25] An epidemiologic study based on the US CFF Patient Registry identified a mortality benefit in patients treated with TIS.[51]

Taken together, the strength of the evidence has led the CFF,[25] the ECFS,[26] and the CFT[24] to recommend the use of TIS for patients with CF. The CFF has issued the most specific recommendation, which is to use chronic inhaled tobramycin in those 6 and older with mild, moderate, and severe lung disease.[25]

A considerable downside to TIS is the treatment burden; each treatment takes 15 to 20 minutes plus additional time for nebulizer cleaning and disinfection.[52] Suboptimal adherence, presumably related to burden of treatment, led to the development of tobramycin inhalation powder (TIP). Advantages for TIP over TIS include shorter treatment time (approximately 5 vs 15–20 minutes), ease of disinfection, portability, and lack of need for electricity.[53] Two recent multicenter studies[54,55] have demonstrated the clinical benefit of TIP over placebo and one has shown its equivalence with TIS.[56] Improved adherence and patient satisfaction have been shown with TIP relative to TIS.[52,56] Cough is the most frequently reported adverse effect of TIP.[55]

Aztreonam

AZLI gained FDA approval in 2010 after two phase III trials were followed by an open-label follow-up study. In a randomized trial, Retsch-Bogart and colleagues[57] administered AZLI, 75 mg, or placebo, three times daily for 28 days to 164 patients at least 6 years of age with FEV_1 between 25% and 75% predicted, who were chronically infected with *P aeruginosa*. Patients in the treatment group had a 10.3% relative improvement in FEV_1, improved symptom scores, reduced sputum density of *P aeruginosa*, fewer hospital days, and improved weight compared with control subjects. Similar findings emerged in the second phase III trial,[58] and clinical benefit persisted in an 18-month open-label follow-up study using a 28-day on/off treatment approach.[59] In addition, the CFF identified one study demonstrating clinical benefit of AZLI in patients with mild lung disease.[25]

A recent short-term open-label comparative efficacy trial of AZLI and TIS demonstrated superiority of the former in terms of FEV_1, number of APEs, symptom scores, and weight gain.[60] Given that most patients in the study had regular use of TIS before enrollment, and that effects of TIS have been shown to diminish over time,[50] these findings were not entirely surprising.

The CFF recommends the use of AZLI for patients 6 and older with chronic *P aeruginosa* infection and mild, moderate, or severe lung disease.[25] Although AZLI is approved for use in many European countries, the ECFS[26] and the CFT[24] do not make specific recommendations about its use.

Colistin

Colistin, a polymyxin antibiotic that is bactericidal against gram-negative bacteria, is used infrequently through the intravenous route because of high rates of neurotoxicity and nephrotoxicity. However, it has been used in nebulized formulations for more than 25 years for patients with CF with *P aeruginosa* infection. Many of the studies performed over this time period have shown modest clinical benefit but have suffered from small sample sizes.[33] A larger head-to-head trial of colistin and TIS revealed reduction in sputum density of *P aeruginosa* with both agents, but only TIS demonstrated improvement in FEV_1.[61] Notably, patients were on inhaled colistin before the trial.

Cough and bronchospasm are frequently noted as adverse effects of inhaled colistin,[33,61] but the systemic effects seen with intravenous administration are not observed. Additionally, if colistin is dispensed as a dry powder for reconstitution, it should be mixed with 0.9% saline or sterile water to make 4 mL of solution for nebulization.[24] It must then be inhaled within 24 hours because the drug breaks down into polymyxin E1, which has been associated with airway damage.[62]

More recently, a dry powder inhalation (DPI) form of colistin has become available in Europe. Colistin DPI was noninferior to TIS in a 24-week comparative effectiveness trial of 373 patients. In this study, change in FEV_1 was minute (<1%) in both arms, although patients on colistin DPI reported higher quality of life scores because of reduced treatment burden.[63]

Colistin is used off-label in the United States, and the CFF concludes that the data are insufficient to recommend for or against its use.[25] The ECFS recommends colistin as an alternative to TIS,[26] and it is the CFT's first-line recommendation for chronic inhaled therapy.[24]

Fluoroquinolones

Inhaled formulations of fluoroquinolones have been recently developed. In a 28-day placebo-controlled phase 2 trial, use of levofloxacin inhalation solution resulted in decreased sputum density of *P aeruginosa*, dose-dependent increase in FEV_1, and reduction in need for other antibiotics.[64] Two phase III trials have been completed and published as conference abstracts[65] and press releases.[18] In a 28-day placebo-controlled trial that used twice-daily dosing, no difference was seen in the primary end point of time to first pulmonary exacerbation, although reduction in sputum density of *P aeruginosa* was found.[18] In a 6-month, open-label, comparative efficacy trial, alternating month therapy with levofloxacin inhalation solution was noninferior to TIS in terms of the primary end point, change in FEV_1. Patients in the levofloxacin group saw longer time to first need for antipseudomonal antibiotics and improved quality of life scores.[65] Full results of the phase III trials and FDA review are pending an ongoing open-label extension study.[18]

A DPI form of ciprofloxacin showed promise in phase I trials[66,67] but failed to meet the primary end point of change in FEV_1 in a randomized, placebo-controlled, 28-day phase IIb study.[68] It

is now being evaluated in a phase III trial for non-CF bronchiectasis.[19]

Amikacin

In its inhaled formulation, the water-soluble, positively charged, aminoglycoside amikacin is encased in a liposomal shell that protects it from negatively charged CF sputum and enables sustained release of the antibiotic.[69] This inhaled formulation has shown promise in recent clinical trials. A randomized, placebo-controlled, phase II trial demonstrated improvements in FEV_1 in the treatment group after 28 days of once-daily administration. A treatment effect of 0.125 L FEV_1 persisted for the following 28 days off of medication in the high-dose group, and improvements in lung function persisted during open-label follow-up consisting of six cycles of 28 days on/56 days off high-dose treatment.[70] The results of a phase III trial comparing inhaled amikacin with TIS are unpublished but were summarized in a recent review.[69] Over three 28-day on/off cycles, once-daily liposomal amikacin was noninferior to twice-daily TIS in terms of relative change in FEV_1. The therapy was well tolerated and associated with higher quality of life scores among participants. Additional phase III trials are underway,[27] findings of which will be important to establish the safety of long-term liposomal amikacin. Given that the drug is cleared by alveolar macrophages, there is a theoretic concern of an immunosuppressive effect, although increased rates of infection have not been seen in trials conducted to date.[69]

Continuous and Continuous Alternating Therapy

Given the existing evidence, a 2011 Cochrane review concluded that inhaled antibiotics improve pulmonary function and reduce exacerbation rates.[48] Alternating month therapy has been the most extensively studied, and is the standard recommended treatment strategy, with a goal of reducing treatment burden, cost,[71] and the development of antibiotic resistance.[26] Indeed, emerging resistance to antibiotics has been demonstrated with even short-term use of inhaled antibiotics,[48] although this does not seem to diminish their efficacy.[24] Trials of continuous antibiotic administration performed in the 1980s showed benefit to this approach, but adequate head-to-head studies with modern nebulized antibiotic formulations have not been done.[71]

With the recent availability of multiple nebulized antibiotic options, CF providers frequently advocate continuous-alternating therapy (the use of different antibiotics in sequence),[72] with the goal of optimizing treatment effect while reducing resistance. A phase III trial of alternating TIS and AZLI compared with alternating TIS and placebo showed nonsignificant trends toward decreased APE and increased FEV₁. The study was underpowered because of difficulty recruiting patients, partially related to widespread use of continuous-alternating therapy before the trial.[73]

Chronic Oral Antibiotics

Data are lacking to support the use of antipseudomonal oral antibiotics for long-term treatment of chronic *P aeruginosa* infection. Although the concern for increased antibiotic resistance with chronic antimicrobial use exists, a Cochrane review concluded that the evidence is insufficient to validate this concern.[21] An additional concern has been raised regarding the impact of long-term systemic antibiotics on the host microbiome.[74] In the absence of evidence, recommendations from expert groups about chronic oral antipseudomonal antibiotics are guarded.[24,25]

The exception to this is the chronic use of oral azithromycin for patients 6 years and older with chronic *P aeruginosa* infection, a treatment strategy that has been previously reviewed in detail and has been shown in multiple trials to improve lung function and decrease exacerbation frequency. Because *P aeruginosa* is not susceptible to macrolides on standard sensitivity testing, a variety of mechanisms are thought to be involved, including effects on inflammation, bacterial virulence, sputum rheology, and ion transport.[75]

TREATMENT OF ACUTE PULMONARY EXACERBATIONS

APEs are a hallmark of CF, and although the pathophysiology is not entirely clear, a change in growth and virulence factors among bacterial subpopulations may play a role.[1] APEs are typically marked by increases in some combination of pulmonary and systemic symptoms, with evidence of decline in lung function.[29] Antibiotics are administered as standard of care during APEs[20,23,29] based on an accumulation of clinical experience[24] despite limited placebo-controlled data to support their use.[76] A multitude of antibiotic options are available to the CF provider in the approach to APEs (see **Table 1**), and a comprehensive review of the available antipseudomonal antibiotics has been recently published.[20] The ensuing discussion highlights some of the considerations in making treatment decisions.

The Use of Antimicrobial Susceptibility Testing to Guide Therapy

Traditionally, antibiotic therapy for the patient is determined by antimicrobial susceptibility testing of a few pure colonies of an isolated pathogen against multiple antibiotics within the clinical microbiology laboratory. Interpretive criteria for susceptibility breakpoints use the minimum inhibitory concentration (MIC) of antibiotic that prevents bacterial growth, pharmacokinetic/pharmacodynamic (PK/PD) drug information, and clinical outcome studies to determine whether a particular organism is susceptible or resistant to different antibiotics (**Fig. 1**).[77]

This susceptibility testing method is problematic in patients with CF for several reasons. First, antibiotics are increasingly delivered via inhalation at high concentrations so the traditional PK/PD data derived from intravenous or oral administration are less relevant to susceptibility determination.[77] Second, chronically infected patients develop phenotypically diverse *P aeruginosa* in the lung over time, including strains with variable susceptibility patterns and metabolic phenotypes.[9,78,79] Choosing a single or few bacterial colonies on which to do susceptibility testing is unlikely to represent the entire bacterial population in the lung, resulting in incomplete data. This is increasingly true the longer the patient is infected and exposed to multiple courses of different antibiotics. Susceptibility testing may play a more valuable role during attempts at eradication after the first positive *P aeruginosa* culture as suggested by effective eradication programs, and this deserves further study.[80] Third, the standard susceptibility testing methods with growth on either an agar plate or in liquid broth do not adequately capture the complex growth conditions of the CF lung. Finally, evidence shows no correlation with bacterial susceptibility testing and clinical outcomes.[81] A retrospective study of 77 patients receiving intravenous tobramycin and ceftazidime for APE found no correlation between the susceptibility of *P aeruginosa* isolate to the administered drugs and treatment outcomes.[81] A second study of 52 children came to a similar conclusion.[82]

Novel approaches to antimicrobial susceptibility testing attempt to better correlate laboratory data with in vivo growth conditions. Biofilm inhibitory concentrations are measured with bacteria growing on a plastic surface that is immersed in liquid containing the antibiotic.[83] A retrospective study of 110 patients treated with antibiotics during APE found a trend toward better clinical outcomes in patients treated with antibiotics that exhibited higher antibiofilm activity.[83] However,

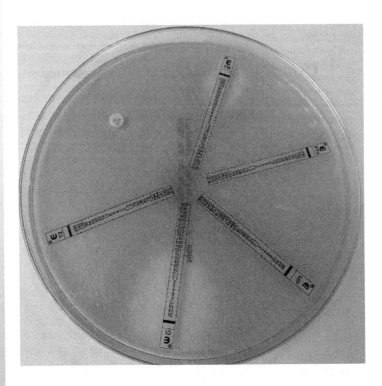

Fig. 1. Antibiotic susceptibility testing for *Pseudomonas aeruginosa*. E-test method revealing multiple MICs to different antibiotics on a single Meuller-Hinton agar plate. In this case the isolate is resistant to tobramycin (TM), meropenem (MP), ceftazidime (TZ), and pipercillin tazobactam (PTc), and susceptible to colistin (Cl).

a Cochrane review examining the evidence comparing standard susceptibility testing with biofilm susceptibility testing found no evidence that biofilm testing was superior based on the primary outcomes of *P aeruginosa* density in the sputum and patient lung function.[84] This recommendation drew from two randomized controlled trials, one with 39 stable patients, and the other with 39 patients who experienced 79 APEs.[85,86] In both studies, patients were given 14 days of antibiotics based either on conventional susceptibility testing, or biofilm susceptibility testing, and no differences in bacterial sputum density or clinical outcomes were observed comparing the two groups.[85,86]

The current method of biofilm susceptibility testing has not completely solved the problem of recreating the in vivo environment, because growth on plastic likely does not replicate the metabolic conditions of growth encased in sputum. Recent data suggest this growth pattern differs from that of biofilms and has unique metabolic properties.[87] These properties can be recreated with growth in an artificial gel and in vitro susceptibility techniques show these aggregates to be highly resistant to antibiotics.[87] Whether antibiotic susceptibility testing under these conditions can be used to guide therapy, and is a better predictor of clinical outcomes, is an important area of further study.

Another challenge for patients chronically infected with *P aeruginosa* is the development of

strains resistant to multiple antibiotics. In such situations, the testing of combinations of different antibiotics for synergy may theoretically provide guidance as to the appropriate antibiotic regimen.[88] Multiple studies have documented that certain combinations of antibiotics provide synergistic activity compared with each antibiotic alone, especially β-lactam drugs combined with agents from other classes (reviewed in Ref.[88]). However, the one randomized clinical trial that compared outcomes in patients whose isolates had synergy testing to guide therapy compared with patients who did not (total numbers for both groups = 251) found no benefit to the use of synergy testing with regard to either clinical outcomes or reductions in bacterial density in sputum. Therefore, synergy testing is not currently recommended for routine clinical care.[29]

Route of Antibiotic Administration

Oral and inhaled antipseudomonal antibiotics are frequently used in the management of CF APEs, especially for episodes of lesser severity.[20] Two recent Cochrane reviews found insufficient evidence to support antibiotic delivery via these two routes.[21,89] When used as additive therapy during APEs requiring intravenous antibiotics, CFF and ECFS guidelines call for caution when considering the use of two routes of antibiotics simultaneously, particularly when agents come from the same class, because of concerns regarding cumulative drug toxicity.[23,29] Additionally, inhaled antibiotics may be ineffective during APEs because of increased mucus production preventing the delivery of medication,[23] and cationic moieties of aminoglycosides may not penetrate negatively charged sputum.[90] Concerns related to electric charges may be abated with the use of liposomal preparations of newer nebulized antibiotics, as previously discussed.[69]

Single Versus Double Coverage of *Pseudomonas aeruginosa*

By convention, when intravenous antibiotics are used in the treatment of APEs, two antibiotics with different mechanisms of action against *P aeruginosa* are administered to ensure adequate coverage and avoid selection of resistant organisms.[29] An antibiotic utilization survey of accredited CFF centers revealed that combination therapy with a β-lactam and an aminoglycoside was the most common strategy, used by 95.5% of centers.[91] Studies comparing monotherapy with combination therapy have been the subject of Cochrane[92] and CFF[29] reviews, with both groups concluding that the data are insufficient to issue an evidence-based recommendation. Available studies are decades old and suffer from methodologic flaws.[92] Pending better data, the CFF[29] and CFT[24] recommend double-coverage of *P aeruginosa* as the standard of care for APE.

Antibiotic Dosing Considerations

Dosing of antipseudomonal antibiotics in patients with CF differs from that in the non-CF population. Patients with CF have higher volumes of distribution, increased clearance leading to lower elimination half-lives, higher MIC isolates of *P aeruginosa*, and difficulty achieving target concentrations in the lung because of mucus characteristics.[20]

Aminoglycosides exert their effects through concentration-dependent killing, and the higher serum concentrations achieved through once-daily dosing have been shown to be clinically effective while potentially reducing nephrotoxicity.[28] Tobramycin is the preferred aminoglycoside in CF because of an extensive literature supporting clinical effect, dosing, and monitoring strategies.[30] Recommended dosing of tobramycin is 10 mg/kg once daily to achieve peak and trough concentrations of 20 to 40 mg/L and less than 1 mg/L, respectively.[30] Amikacin is used less frequently, and gentamicin is typically avoided given an increased risk of nephrotoxicity in relation to other aminoglycosides.[24,30]

β-Lactams demonstrate time-dependent killing; a longer time during which the concentration is above a MIC threshold leads to improved effectiveness. This has led to interest in extended-interval (eg, dose given over 4 hours) and continuous infusions, although a paucity of data currently exist to guide best-practice, and the CFF has called for further study in this area.[29]

The CFF, ECFS, and CFT have issued specific dosing, monitoring, and PK/PD considerations for these and other classes of antibiotics.[20,23,24,29]

Duration of Treatment

There is no clear treatment standard for duration of antibiotic therapy for APEs, and treatment approaches vary between 10 and 21 days,[24,93] with a median and mode of 14 days in accredited CFF centers.[94] A variety of indicators are used to gauge response to therapy including patient symptoms, FEV$_1$, oxygenation, and inflammatory markers, all of which are used to guide therapy.[93] Longer courses are typically administered to patients with more severe exacerbations and sluggish recovery.[93] To date, C-reactive protein is the biomarker that has consistently shown the most promise as a surrogate end point to guide decision making because it typically increases in APE and decreases with treatment.[95] A 2013 Cochrane review found no trials eligible for inclusion and accordingly, no evidence-based recommendations about treatment duration are available.[93] In the absence of data, a minimum of 10 to 14 days of treatment is consistent with practice norms,[24] with modifications based on patient-specific factors including response to treatment, severity of illness, and drug toxicity.

Location of Treatment

Mild APEs are commonly managed at home with nonparenteral antibiotics.[24] With the availability of indwelling catheters, home treatment has become an option for more severe APE's. Home treatment may improve quality of life, reduce cost of care, and minimize exposure to nosocomial pathogens.[96] However, if acute treatment occurs at home, patients and providers may be unable to address the complexity of issues that arise during periods of worsening health. For example, optimization of airway clearance and nutrition are important components of treatment plans for APEs. Additionally, monitoring for drug toxicity, respiratory decline, and impact of an APE on the control of comorbid conditions (eg, CF-related diabetes) is more challenging at home. Data are lacking to guide decision making related to location of care,[96] and the CFF recommends against outpatient treatment when intravenous therapy is necessary unless adequate resources in the home setting can be ensured.[29]

SUMMARY

The prevalence of *P aeruginosa* in patients with CF is 90% by adulthood, and clear epidemiologic links between chronic infection and morbidity and mortality have been described.[34,35] Addressing the burden of disease attributable to *P aeruginosa* requires attention to prevention, eradication on first growth, long-term treatment of chronic infection, and aggressive and appropriate intervention for APE. Specific treatment approaches vary across centers and continents, and many research questions remain to determine best practice as more treatment options become available.

Despite the uncertainty, there is much consensus in the CF community. Prevention and early identification of *P aeruginosa* are critical, and stand to improve with the advent of new vaccines and laboratory methods. It is important that laboratories continue to work to develop novel approaches to better correlate in vitro bacterial testing with clinical outcomes. Genomic study of whole bacterial populations in the lung is an interesting approach that may reveal novel susceptibility information about the entire pulmonary microbiome to help guide therapy (see Huang YJ, LiPuma JJ: The Microbiome in Cystic Fibrosis, in this issue).

Finally, once the organism is identified, a variety of treatment options are available and appropriate for acute and chronic *P aeruginosa* infection with and without APE. Aggressive use of antipseudomonal antibiotics is the standard of care for APE in CF, and like all clinical decisions, providers must take into account specific patient characteristics when making treatment decisions related to antibiotic selection, route and duration of administration, and location of care.

REFERENCES

1. Murray TS, Kazmierczak BI. Chronic vs acute *Pseudomonas aeruginosa* infection states. In: Vasil M, Darwin A, editors. Regulation of bacterial virulence. Washington, DC: ASM Press; 2013. p. 21–39.
2. Jarvis S, Ind P, Thomas C, et al. Microbial contamination of domiciliary nebulisers and clinical implications in chronic obstructive pulmonary disease. BMJ Open Respir Res 2014;1(1):e000018.
3. Saiman L, Siegel JD, LiPuma JJ, et al. Infection prevention and control guideline for cystic fibrosis: 2013 update. Infect Control Hosp Epidemiol 2014; 35:S1–67.
4. Döring G. Vaccine development for patients with cystic fibrosis. Expert Rev Vaccines 2012;11:259–61.
5. Sharma A, Krause A, Worgall S. Recent developments for *Pseudomonas* vaccines. Hum Vaccin 2011;7:999–1011.
6. Moore R, Kyd JM, Carzino R, et al. Mucosal and systemic antibody responses to potential *Pseudomonas aeruginosa* vaccine protein antigens in young children with cystic fibrosis following colonization and infection. Hum Vaccin Immunother 2013;9:506–14.
7. Döring G, Meisner C, Stern M. A double-blind randomized placebo-controlled phase III study of a *Pseudomonas aeruginosa* flagella vaccine in cystic fibrosis patients. Proc Natl Acad Sci U S A 2007; 104:11020–5.
8. Johansen HK, Gøtzsche PC. Vaccines for preventing infection with *Pseudomonas aeruginosa* in cystic fibrosis. Cochrane Database Syst Rev 2013;(6): CD001399.
9. Clark ST, Caballero JD, Cheang M, et al. Phenotypic diversity within a *Pseudomonas aeruginosa* population infecting an adult with cystic fibrosis. Sci Rep 2015;5:10932.
10. Westritschnig K, Hochreiter R, Wallner G, et al. A randomized, placebo-controlled phase I study assessing the safety and immunogenicity of a *Pseudomonas aeruginosa* hybrid outer membrane protein OprF/I vaccine (IC43) in healthy volunteers. Hum Vaccin Immunother 2013;10:170–83.
11. Farjah A, Owlia P, Siadat SD, et al. Immunological evaluation of an alginate-based conjugate as a vaccine candidate against *Pseudomonas aeruginosa*. APMIS 2015;123:175–83.
12. ClinicalTrials.gov. Anti-pseudomonas IgY to prevent infections in cystic fibrosis (PseudIgY). Available at: https://clinicaltrials.gov/ct2/show/NCT00633191. Accessed July 5, 2015.
13. ClinicalTrials.gov. Efficacy Study of IgY (antibody against pseudomonas) in cystic fibrosis patients (PsAer-IgY). Available at: https://clinicaltrials.gov/ct2/show/NCT01455675. Accessed July 5, 2015.
14. Nilsson E, Larsson A, Olesen HV, et al. Good effect of IgY against *Pseudomonas aeruginosa* infections in cystic fibrosis patients. Pediatr Pulmonol 2008; 43:892–9.
15. Smyth AR, Walters S. Prophylactic anti-staphylococcal antibiotics for cystic fibrosis. Cochrane Database Syst Rev 2014;(11):CD001912.
16. Tramper-Stranders GA, Wolfs TF, van Haren Noman S, et al. Controlled trial of cycled antibiotic prophylaxis to prevent initial *Pseudomonas aeruginosa* infection in children with cystic fibrosis. Thorax 2010;65:915–20.
17. Geller DE. Aerosol antibiotics in cystic fibrosis. Respir Care 2009;54:658–70.
18. Aptalis Press Releases. Aptalis pharma, Inc. Announces results of phase 3 studies of Aeroquin (levofloxacin solution for inhalation) among patients with cystic fibrosis and chronic lung infection. 2013.

Available at: http://aptalispharma.mwnewsroom. com/press-releases/aptalis-pharma-inc-announces-results-of-phase-3–971086. Accessed July 5, 2015.

19. ClinicalTrials.gov. Ciprofloxacin dry powder for inhalation in non-cystic fibrosis bronchiectasis (Non-CF BE) (RESPIRE 1). Available at: https://clinicaltrials. gov/ct2/show/NCT01764841. Accessed July 5, 2015.

20. Zobell JT, Young DC, Waters CD, et al. Optimization of anti-pseudomonal antibiotics for cystic fibrosis pulmonary exacerbations: VI. Executive summary. Pediatr Pulmonol 2013;48:525–37.

21. Remmington T, Jahnke N, Harkensee C. Oral anti-pseudomonal antibiotics for cystic fibrosis. Cochrane Database Syst Rev 2013;(10):CD005405.

22. Mogayzel PJ, Naureckas ET, Robinson KA, et al. Cystic fibrosis foundation pulmonary guidelines: pharmacologic approaches to prevention and eradication of initial *Pseudomonas aeruginosa* infection. Ann Am Thorac Soc 2014;11:1640–50.

23. Döring G, Flume P, Heijerman H, et al. Treatment of lung infection in patients with cystic fibrosis: current and future strategies. J Cyst Fibros 2012;11:461–79.

24. UK Cystic Fibrosis Trust Antibiotic Working Group. Antibiotic treatment for cystic fibrosis. 3rd edition. Bomley (United Kingdom): Cystic Fibrosis Trust; 2009.

25. Mogayzel PJ, Naureckas ET, Robinson KA, et al. Cystic fibrosis foundation pulmonary guidelines: chronic medications for maintenance of lung health. Am J Respir Crit Care Med 2013;187:680–9.

26. Heijerman H, Westerman E, Conway S, et al. Inhaled medication and inhalation devices for lung disease in patients with cystic fibrosis: a European consensus. J Cyst Fibros 2009;8(5):295–315.

27. Cystic Fibrosis Foundation. Drug development pipeline: arikace. Available at: http://www.cff.org/research /DrugDevelopmentPipeline/. Accessed July 5, 2015.

28. Smyth AR, Bhatt J. Once-daily versus multiple-daily dosing with intravenous aminoglycosides for cystic fibrosis. Cochrane Database Syst Rev 2012;(2): CD002009.

29. Flume PA, Mogayzel PJ, Robinson KA, et al. Cystic fibrosis pulmonary guidelines: treatment of pulmonary exacerbations. Am J Respir Crit Care Med 2009;180:802–8.

30. Young DC, Zobell JT, Stockmann C, et al. Optimization of anti-pseudomonal antibiotics for cystic fibrosis pulmonary exacerbations: V. Aminoglycosides. Pediatr Pulmonol 2013;48:1047–61.

31. Zobell JT, Waters CD, Young DC, et al. Optimization of anti-pseudomonal antibiotics for cystic fibrosis pulmonary exacerbations: II. Cephalosporins and penicillins. Pediatr Pulmonol 2013;48:107–22.

32. Zobell JT, Young DC, Waters CD, et al. Optimization of anti-pseudomonal antibiotics for cystic fibrosis pulmonary exacerbations: I. Aztreonam and carbapenems. Pediatr Pulmonol 2012;47:1147–58.

33. Antoniu SA, Cojocaru I. Inhaled colistin for lower respiratory tract infections. Expert Opin Drug Deliv 2012;9:333–42.

34. Li Z, Kosorok MR, Farrell PM, et al. Longitudinal development of mucoid *Pseudomonas aeruginosa* infection and lung disease progression in children with cystic fibrosis. JAMA 2005;293:581–8.

35. Langton Hewer SC, Smyth AR. Antibiotic strategies for eradicating *Pseudomonas aeruginosa* in people with cystic fibrosis. Cochrane Database Syst Rev 2014;(11):CD004197.

36. Stuart B, Lin JH, Mogayzel PJ. Early eradication of *Pseudomonas aeruginosa* in patients with cystic fibrosis. Paediatr Respir Rev 2010;11:177–84.

37. Valerius NH, Koch C, Hoiby N. Prevention of chronic *Pseudomonas aeruginosa* colonisation in cystic fibrosis by early treatment. Lancet 1991;338:725–6.

38. Gibson RL, Emerson J, McNamara S, et al. Significant microbiological effect of inhaled tobramycin in young children with cystic fibrosis. Am J Respir Crit Care Med 2003;167:841–9.

39. Treggiari MM, Retsch-Bogart G, Mayer-Hamblett N, et al. Comparative efficacy and safety of 4 randomized regimens to treat early *Pseudomonas aeruginosa* infection in children with cystic fibrosis. Arch Pediatr Adolesc Med 2011;165(9):847–56.

40. Tiddens HA, De Boeck K, Clancy JP, et al. Open label study of inhaled aztreonam for *Pseudomonas* eradication in children with cystic fibrosis: the ALPINE study. J Cyst Fibros 2015;14:111–9.

41. Ali H, Orchard C, Mariveles M, et al. Effective strategies for managing new *Pseudomonas* cultures in adults with cystic fibrosis. Eur Respir J 2015;46: 862–5.

42. Murray TS, Egan M, Kazmierczak BI. *Pseudomonas aeruginosa* chronic colonization in cystic fibrosis patients. Curr Opin Pediatr 2007;19:83–8.

43. ECFS-Clinical Trials Network. Trial of optimal therapy for *Pseudomonas* eradication in cystic fibrosis (TORPEDO-CF). Available at: https://www.ecfs.eu/ctn/ torpedo-cf. Accessed July 5, 2015.

44. ClinicalTrials.gov. Optimizing treatment for early *Pseudomonas aeruginosa* infection in cystic fibrosis (OPTIMIZE). Available at: https://clinicaltrials.gov/ ct2/show/NCT02054156. Accessed July 5, 2015.

45. Pressler T, Bohmova C, Conway S, et al. Chronic *Pseudomonas aeruginosa* infection definition: EuroCareCF working group report. J Cyst Fibros 2011;10:S75–8.

46. Bendiak GN, Ratjen F. The approach to *Pseudomonas aeruginosa* in cystic fibrosis. Semin Respir Crit Care Med 2009;30:587–95.

47. di Sant'Agnese PE, Andersen DH. Celiac Syndrome. IV. Chemotherapy in infections of the respiratory tract associated with cystic fibrosis of the pancreas; observations with penicillin and drugs of the sulfonamide group, with special reference to penicillin aerosol. Am J Dis Child 1946;72:17–61.

48. Ryan G, Singh M, Dwan K. Inhaled antibiotics for long-term therapy in cystic fibrosis. Cochrane Database Syst Rev 2011;(3):CD001021.

49. Ramsey BW, Pepe MS, Quan JM, et al. Intermittent administration of inhaled tobramycin in patients with cystic fibrosis. N Engl J Med 1999;340:23–30.

50. Bowman CM. The long-term use of inhaled tobramycin in patients with cystic fibrosis. J Cyst Fibros 2002;1:194–8.

51. Sawicki GS, Signorovitch JE, Zhang J, et al. Reduced mortality in cystic fibrosis patients treated with tobramycin inhalation solution. Pediatr Pulmonol 2012;47:44–52.

52. Harrison MJ, McCarthy M, Fleming C, et al. Inhaled versus nebulised tobramycin: a real world comparison in adult cystic fibrosis. J Cyst Fibros 2014;13: 692–8.

53. Fiel SB. Aerosolized antibiotics in cystic fibrosis: an update. Expert Rev Respir Med 2014;8:305–14.

54. Konstan MW, Geller DE, Minic P, et al. Tobramycin inhalation powder for Pseudomonas aeruginosa infection in cystic fibrosis: the EVOLVE trial. Pediatr Pulmonol 2011;46:230–8.

55. Galeva I, Konstan MW, Higgins M, et al. Tobramycin inhalation powder manufactured by improved process in cystic fibrosis: the randomized EDIT trial. Curr Med Res Opin 2013;29:947–56.

56. Konstan MW, Flume PA, Kappler M, et al. Safety, efficacy, and convenience of tobramycin inhalation powder in cystic fibrosis patients: the EAGER trial. J Cyst Fibros 2011;10:54–61.

57. Retsch-Bogart GZ, Quittner AL, Gibson RL, et al. Efficacy and safety of inhaled aztreonam lysine for airway pseudomonas in cystic fibrosis. Chest 2009;135:1223–32.

58. McCoy KS, Quittner AL, Oermann CM, et al. Inhaled aztreonam lysine for chronic airway Pseudomonas aeruginosa in cystic fibrosis. Am J Respir Crit Care Med 2008;178:921–8.

59. Oermann CM, Retsch-Bogart GZ, Quittner AL, et al. An 18-month study of the safety and efficacy of repeated courses of inhaled aztreonam lysine in cystic fibrosis. Pediatr Pulmonol 2010;45:1121–34.

60. Assael BM, Pressler T, Bilton D, et al. Inhaled aztreonam lysine vs. inhaled tobramycin in cystic fibrosis: a comparative efficacy trial. J Cyst Fibros 2013;12: 130–40.

61. Hodson ME, Gallagher CG, Govan JR. A randomised clinical trial of nebulised tobramycin or colistin in cystic fibrosis. Eur Respir J 2002;20:658–64.

62. FDA. Alert: colistimethate. Available at: http://www.fda. gov/downloads/Drugs/DrugSafety/PostmarketDrug SafetyInformationforPatientsandProviders/UCM124 894.pdf. Accessed July 5, 2015.

63. Schuster A, Haliburn C, Döring G, et al. Safety, efficacy and convenience of colistimethate sodium dry powder for inhalation (Colobreathe DPI) in patients with cystic fibrosis: a randomized study. Thorax 2013;68:344–50.

64. Geller DE, Flume PA, Staab D, et al. Levofloxacin inhalation solution (MP-376) in patients with cystic fibrosis with Pseudomonas aeruginosa. Am J Respir Crit Care Med 2011;183:1510–6.

65. Elborn JS, Geller D, Conrad D. Phase 3 trial of inhaled levofloxacin (Aeroquin, MP-376, APT-1026) vs tobramycin inhalation solution (TIS) in intensively treated CF patients over 6 months. J Cyst Fibros 2013;12:S35.

66. Stass H, Weimann B, Nagelshmitz J, et al. Tolerability and pharmokinetic properties of ciprofloxacin dry powder inhalation in patients with cystic fibrosis: a phase I, randomized, dose-escalation study. Clin Ther 2013;35:1571–81.

67. Stass H, Delesen H, Nagelschmitz J, et al. Safety and pharmokinetics of ciprofloxacin dry powder for inhalation in cystic fibrosis: a phase I, randomized, single-dose, dose-escalation study. J Aerosol Med Pulm Drug Deliv 2015;28:106–15.

68. Dorkin H, Criollo M, Reimnitz R, et al. Randomized, double-blind, placebo-controlled, multicenter study to evaluate the safety and efficacy of inhaled ciprofloxacin compared with placebo in patients with cystic fibrosis: a phase IIb study of ciprofloxacin dry powder for inhalation (DPI). Pediatr Pulmonol 2011;46:296.

69. Waters V, Ratjen F. Inhaled liposomal amikacin. Expert Rev Respir Med 2014;8:401–9.

70. Clancy JP, Dupont L, Konstan MW, et al. Phase II studies of nebulised arikace in CF patients with Pseudomonas aeruginosa infection. Thorax 2013; 68:818–25.

71. Lo D, VanDevanter DR, Flume P, et al. Aerosolized antibiotic therapy for chronic cystic fibrosis airway infections: continuous or intermittent? Respir Med 2011;105:S9–17.

72. Greenberg J, Palmer J, Chan W, et al. A real world assessment of patient experience with tobramycin inhalation powder (TIP) among patients with cystic fibrosis. Pediatr Pulmonol 2014;49(S38):377.

73. Flume PA, Clancy JP, Retsch-Bogart GZ, et al. Aztreonam for inhalation solution and tobramycin inhalation solution continuous alternating therapy for cystic fibrosis patients with chronic Pseudomonas aeruginosa infection: a randomized, double-blind, placebo-controlled trial. Pediatr Pulmonol 2015; 50(S41):352.

74. Waters V, Smyth A. Cystic fibrosis microbiology: advances in antimicrobial therapy. J Cyst Fibros 2015; 14(5):551–60.

75. McArdle JR, Talwalkar JS. Macrolides in cystic fibrosis. Clin Chest Med 2007;28:347–60.

76. Regelmann WE, Elliott GR, Warwick WJ, et al. Reduction of sputum Pseudomonas aeruginosa density by antibiotics improves lung function in

cystic fibrosis more than do bronchodilators and chest physiotherapy alone. Am Rev Respir Dis 1990;141:914–21.

77. Turnidge J, Paterson DL. Setting and revising anti-bacterial susceptibility breakpoints. Clin Microbiol Rev 2007;20:391–408.

78. Foweraker JE, Laughton CR, Brown DFJ, et al. Phenotypic variability of *Pseudomonas aeruginosa* in sputa from patients with acute infective exacerbation of cystic fibrosis and its impact on the validity of antimicrobial susceptibility testing. J Antimicrob Chemother 2005;55:921–7.

79. Hogardt M, Heesemann J. Adaptation of *Pseudomonas aeruginosa* during persistence in the cystic fibrosis lung. Int J Med Microbiol 2010;300:557–62.

80. Foweraker JE, Govan JR. Antibiotic susceptibility testing in early and chronic respiratory infections with *Pseudomonas aeruginosa*. J Cyst Fibros 2012; 12:302.

81. Smith AL, Fiel SB, Mayer-Hamblett N, et al. Susceptibility testing of *Pseudomonas aeruginosa* isolates and clinical response to parenteral antibiotic administration: lack of association in cystic fibrosis. Chest 2003;123:1495–502.

82. Hurley MN, Ariff AH, Bertenshaw C, et al. Results of antibiotic susceptibility testing do not influence clinical outcome in children with cystic fibrosis. J Cyst Fibros 2012;11:288–92.

83. Keays T, Ferris W, Vandemheen KL, et al. A retrospective analysis of biofilm antibiotic susceptibility testing: a better predictor of clinical response in cystic fibrosis exacerbations. J Cyst Fibros 2009; 8:122–7.

84. Waters V, Ratjen F. Standard versus biofilm antimicrobial susceptibility testing to guide antibiotic therapy in cystic fibrosis. Cochrane Database Syst Rev 2015;(11):CD009528.

85. Yau YC, Ratjen F, Tullis E, et al. Randomized controlled trial of biofilm antimicrobial susceptibility testing in cystic fibrosis patients. J Cyst Fibros 2015;14:262–6.

86. Moskowitz S, Emerson J, McNamara S, et al. Randomized trial of biofilm testing to select antibiotics for cystic fibrosis airway infection. Pediatr Pulmonol 2011;46:184–92.

87. Staudinger BJ, Muller JF, Halldórsson S, et al. Conditions associated with the cystic fibrosis defect promote chronic *Pseudomonas aeruginosa* infection. Am J Respir Crit Care Med 2014;189:812–24.

88. Doern CD. When does 2 plus 2 equal 5? a review of antimicrobial synergy testing. J Clin Microbiol 2014; 52:4124–8.

89. Ryan G, Jahnke N, Remmington T. Inhaled antibiotics for pulmonary exacerbations in cystic fibrosis. Cochrane Database Syst Rev 2012;(12):CD008319.

90. Gaspar MC, Couet W, Olivier JC, et al. *Pseudomonas aeruginosa* infection in cystic fibrosis lung disease and new perspectives of treatment: a review. Eur J Clin Microbiol Infect Dis 2013;32: 1231–52.

91. Prescott WA. National survey of extended-interval aminoglycoside dosing in pediatric cystic fibrosis pulmonary exacerbations. J Pediatr Pharmacol Ther 2011;16:262–9.

92. Elphick HE, Tan AA. Single versus combination intravenous antibiotic therapy for people with cystic fibrosis. Cochrane Database Syst Rev 2005;(2): CD002007.

93. Plummer A, Wildman M. Duration of intravenous antibiotic therapy in people with cystic fibrosis. Cochrane Database Syst Rev 2013;(5):CD006682.

94. Cystic Fibrosis Foundation, Cystic Fibrosis Foundation Patient Registry. 2013 annual data report to the center directors. Bethesda (MD): The Foundation; 2014.

95. Shoki AH, Mayer-Hamblett N, Wilcox PG, et al. Systematic review of blood biomarkers in cystic fibrosis pulmonary exacerbations. Chest 2013;144:1659–70.

96. Balaguer A, González de Dios J. Home versus hospital intravenous antibiotic therapy for cystic fibrosis. Cochrane Database Syst Rev 2012;(3):CD001917.

Nontuberculous Mycobacterial Infections in Cystic Fibrosis

Stacey L. Martiniano, MD[a], Jerry A. Nick, MD[b,c],
Charles L. Daley, MD[b,c],*

KEYWORDS

- Cystic fibrosis • Nontuberculous mycobacteria • *Mycobacterium avium* complex
- *Mycobacterium abscessus* complex

KEY POINTS

- Nontuberculous mycobacterial (NTM) lung infections appear to be increasing in patients with cystic fibrosis (CF).
- *Mycobacterium avium* complex and *Mycobacterium abscessus* complex are the most frequently encountered NTM respiratory pathogens in patients with CF in most areas.
- Diagnosis of NTM lung disease in patients with CF generally follows American Thoracic Society and Cystic Fibrosis Foundation guidelines, with an emphasis on evaluating and treating all known comorbidities.
- Therapy for NTM in patients with CF depends on the species, resistance pattern, and extent of disease.
- Optimal management of patients with CF and NTM lung disease requires carefully considered treatment of both conditions.

INTRODUCTION

Nontuberculous mycobacteria (NTM) have emerged as important pathogens in the setting of cystic fibrosis (CF) lung disease. Although historically CF has been considered a fatal disease of childhood, improvements in therapy have resulted in the oldest and healthiest CF population in history. However, as the disease phenotype has changed in response to improved treatment, it appears that susceptibility to NTM has increased.[1–3] This article reviews the epidemiology, diagnosis, treatment, and prevention of NTM lung disease in people living with CF.

EPIDEMIOLOGY

The CF population has an especially high risk for NTM infection and poses unique challenges with regard to diagnosis, treatment, and prevention.[4] Although the NTM isolation rate in the general population in North America ranges from approximately 6 to 22 per 100,000 and the NTM disease rate from 5 to 10 per 100,000,[5] there is a 1000-fold greater prevalence of NTM in respiratory cultures from patients with CF. The reported prevalence of positive NTM cultures and/or NTM disease within various CF patient cohorts or at single centers varies dramatically,[6,7] but in the

Disclosures: The authors are supported by the Cystic Fibrosis Foundation Research Development Grant (NICK15R0).
[a] Department of Pediatrics, Children's Hospital Colorado, University of Colorado Denver School of Medicine, 13123 East 16th Avenue, Box B-395, Aurora, CO 80045, USA; [b] Department of Medicine, National Jewish Health, 1400 Jackson Street, Denver, CO 80206, USA; [c] Department of Medicine, University of Colorado Anschutz Medical Campus, 13001 E. 17th Place, Aurora, CO 80045, USA
* Corresponding author. Department of Medicine, National Jewish Health, 1400 Jackson Street, Denver, CO 80206.
E-mail address: daleyc@njhealth.org

Clin Chest Med 37 (2016) 83–96
http://dx.doi.org/10.1016/j.ccm.2015.11.001

largest studies the overall prevalence is 6% to 13%.[1,3,8–12] In a recent review of data from the US CF Patient Registry, the median state prevalence of NTM in patients with CF was 12%, although this ranged from 0% to 28% (**Fig. 1**). Significant spacial clustering of NTM was detected in Wisconsin, Arizona, Florida, and Maryland.[13]

The prevalence of NTM infection appears to be increasing within the CF population,[1–3,14–17] as it is in the general population.[18,19] For example, among patients with CF in Israel, NTM infection prevalence increased threefold from 5% in 2003% to 14.5% in 2011.[16] The reasons for the increase in prevalence are uncertain but culture techniques, increased physician awareness, and more frequent diagnosis of "nonclassic" forms of CF in adulthood may contribute to the apparent increase in NTM prevalence observed in this population.[14]

Most NTM species recovered in CF samples in the United States are from either the *Mycobacterium avium* complex (MAC) or the *Mycobacterium abscessus* complex (MABSC).[12] MAC has historically been the most common NTM isolated from respiratory specimens,[20–23] and in the largest US survey it was present in up to 72% of patients with NTM-positive sputum cultures.[9] Among patients with CF in the US Patient Registry during 2010 to 2011, 60% of positive cultures were for MAC, although this ranged by state, from 29% in Louisiana to 100% in Nebraska and Delaware.[12]

The percentage of MABSC reported in patients with CF with NTM-positive sputum cultures has ranged between 16% and 68%,[3,8,9,24] and it appears that the proportion of MABSC is increasing,[1,2,25] with some centers reporting a greater frequency than MAC. In part, this variation may be due to geographic factors, as MABSC appears especially prevalent in Europe,[3,8,24,25] and *Mycobacterium simiae* and MABSC are the most common species isolated in Israel.[16,26] Differences in relative prevalence of MAC and MABSC may also relate to the age of the cohorts studied, as MAC is more often associated with older patients with CF, often diagnosed in adulthood, whereas MABSC is frequently seen in younger patients and those with more severe lung disease.[3,27]

Less frequently isolated species include *Mycobacterium kansasii*[7,8,21,23] and *Mycobacterium fortuitum*.[8,22,28,29]

Individual Risk Factors for Nontuberculous Mycobacteria in Cystic Fibrosis

Our understanding of individual risk factors for NTM in patients with CF is incomplete, as most reports have studied relatively small cohorts from

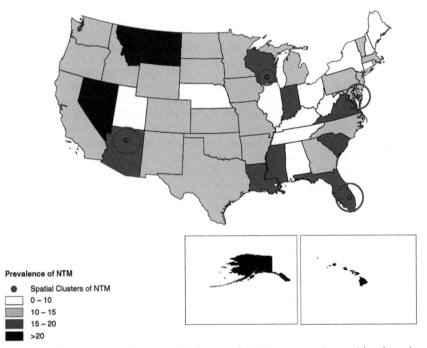

Prevalence of NTM

- ● Spatial Clusters of NTM
- ☐ 0 – 10
- ▨ 10 – 15
- ▤ 15 – 20
- ■ >20

Fig. 1. State-level prevalence and significant (*P*<.05) clusters of NTM among patients with cultured cystic fibrosis, 2010 to 2011. (*Reprinted with* permission of the American Thoracic Society. Copyright © 2015 American Thoracic Society. *From* Adjemian J, Olivier KN, Prevots DR. Nontuberculous mycobacteria among patients with cystic fibrosis in the United States: screening practices and environmental risk. Am J Respir Crit Care Med 2014;190:581–6. The American Journal of Respiratory and Critical Care Medicine is an official journal of the American Thoracic Society.)

single centers or specific geographic areas, often leading to contradictory conclusions. The largest population studies have reported that the increased prevalence of NTM isolation[2,9,10,22,25,26] and NTM disease[26,28] is strongly linked to older age and relatively milder lung disease.[9] A very high prevalence has been reported in adult patients with a "nonclassic" form of CF resulting from residual function mutations.[20,30,31] It is worth noting, however, that other studies have reported the opposite conclusions, in particular that NTM is common in severe lung disease.[10,26,28,32] For example, in Israel, NTM infection was associated with a known "severe" Cystic Fibrosis Transmembrane Conductance Regulator (CFTR) genotype and pancreatic insufficiency.[16]

The presence of *Aspergillus fumigatus*[2,16,26,33–35] and allergic bronchopulmonary aspergillosis (ABPA)[16,36,37] have been associated with increased risk for NTM. Coinfection with *Pseudomonas aeruginosa* has been associated with decreased prevalence of NTM in some studies,[9,23] and higher rates of *P. aeruginosa* coinfection in others.[26] These divergent findings may relate in part to differences in study methodology, as many reports have not distinguished between a positive NTM culture and the presence of NTM disease, and often MAC and MABSC are combined within both adult and pediatric populations.

Although increased survival may indirectly result in greater NTM prevalence through longer cumulative exposure,[38] a greater concern is the possibility that various medications and CF treatment strategies have contributed to the apparent increase in NTM prevalence within this population. Although these reports are not entirely consistent in their conclusions, they have served to heighten awareness of the potential for unforeseen consequences of many therapies in common use. In particular, administration of systemic steroids, often in the context of ABPA treatment, has been associated with increased prevalence of NTM,[26,34,36,37] as well as high-dose ibuprofen.[26] However, other studies have failed to see an increase in NTM-positive cultures with steroid use,[10,26,39] or even an association with decreased NTM.[40]

Use of azithromycin, an antibiotic with anti-inflammatory properties, also has been associated with an increased,[26,41] decreased,[42] or unchanged prevalence of NTM.[39,43,44] Likewise, higher use of antipseudomonal antibiotics has been linked to increased NTM in some,[7,26] but not all reports.[27]

Environmental Risk Factors

Atmospheric conditions appear to explain more of the variation in NTM disease prevalence than individual behaviors in patients with CF in the United States.[45] Among patients with CF at 21 geographically diverse CF centers in the United States, average annual atmospheric water vapor content was significantly predictive of center prevalence ($P = .0019$). The only individual risk factor associated with incident infection was indoor swimming (odds ratio [OR] 5.9, 95% confidence interval [CI] 1.3–26.1). In a review of the prevalence of NTM in the US Patient Registry, high saturated vapor pressure was associated with an increased risk for NTM (OR 1.06, 95% CI 1.02–1.1).[12]

DIAGNOSIS OF NONTUBERCULOUS MYCOBACTERIA LUNG DISEASE IN CYSTIC FIBROSIS

Given the ubiquitous nature of NTM, isolation of an NTM from a respiratory specimen is not synonymous with disease, nor is it necessarily an indication to initiate treatment. Current American Thoracic Society and Infectious Diseases Society of America (ATS/IDSA) criteria for the diagnosis of NTM lung disease calls for the presence of 2 or more positive cultures, in the setting of characteristic clinical symptoms and radiographic findings, and the exclusion of other diseases.[4] These guidelines have not been validated in any patient population, and are particularly challenging in the setting of CF, where radiographic signs suggestive of NTM are common, and identical clinical symptoms can occur due to the near universal presence of coinfections with virulent pathogens, such as *P aeruginosa* and *Staphylococcus aureus*.[14]

The primary clinical question for a patient who has cultured positive for a species of NTM on more than one occasion is whether this represents an indolent infection, or actual NTM disease, which may benefit from treatment. Patients who are smear-positive for NTM are more likely to have NTM disease,[23,26] as well as those who demonstrate progression by computed tomography (CT) of the chest of typical findings associated with NTM.[40] Unfortunately, many of the radiographic findings consistent with NTM infection are nonspecific, such as nodules and centrilobular nodules with a tree-in-bud appearance (**Fig. 2**). The presence of cavitation is the most important radiographic finding, as it is a reflection of tissue destruction (**Fig. 3**).

Unexpectedly rapid decline in lung function, specifically, forced expiratory volume in 1 second (FEV_1), is frequently associated with NTM disease in patients with positive cultures for NTM.[28,46,47] In a recent retrospective study, the cohort of patients with NTM disease demonstrated a mean decline in FEV_1 for a year before initial recovery of NTM in

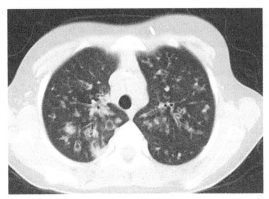

Fig. 2. Radiographic findings of NTM disease in CF. The patient is an 11-year-old with CF and history of chronic *Pseudomonas* infection. In addition, he has had multiple cultures that were positive for *M abscessus* subspecies *abscessus*. Despite several courses of prolonged intravenous, oral, and inhaled drugs he remained culture positive. The CT shows diffuse bronchiectasis, airway wall thickening, extensive mucus plugging, and scattered nodules including centrilobular nodules with a tree-and-bud appearance. The patient had a positive acid-fast smear at the time of this CT.

their sputum.[48] Whereas patients with indolent infection, or patients who apparently cleared the infection after a single positive culture demonstrated a stable FEV$_1$ for a year before, and 3 years

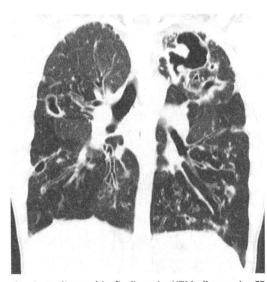

Fig. 3. Radiographic findings in NTM disease in CF. The patient is a 33-year-old diagnosed with CF as an adult. After several years of multidrug therapy for *M avium* complex, the isolate developed macrolide resistance. The CT shows a large left upper lobe cavity with additional smaller cavitary lesions on the right. Note the airways running into the smaller cavities.

after, the initial positive culture.[48] Suggested criteria for the diagnosis of NTM disease in CF is outlined in **Box 1**.[49]

Laboratory Identification of Nontuberculous Mycobacteria in the Cystic Fibrosis Sputum

Historically, descriptions of NTM infection in patients with CF were relatively uncommon,[10,21,22] in part due to the lack of laboratory methodology specific to CF. Recovery of NTM from CF sputum samples was difficult because of culture overgrowth by *P aeruginosa* and other CF microbes before the slower-growing mycobacteria could be detected.[50–52] Development of effective sample decontamination protocols to remove conventional bacteria and fungi has allowed for improved culture-based detection of mycobacteria in CF samples.[53,54]

Currently, the standard approach to decontamination involves 2 steps[51] to avoid excessive decontamination, which can reduce NTM viability in samples.[55] Decontamination is first performed with N-Acetyl L-cysteine-NaOH, before mycobacterial culture.[51,53,54,56] Samples that remain contaminated can then be treated with 5% oxalic acid or alternatively 1% chlorhexidine, which may permit recovery of NTM, although with reduced sensitivity.[50,56–58] A recent study reported the use of a novel culture medium for rapidly growing mycobacteria (RGM) in patients with CF that does not require decontamination.[59] Of 118 isolates of RGM, all but one grew on the agar. RGM were recovered from 54 sputum samples using the RGM media compared with only 17 samples using the control agar.

Both liquid and solid media are recommended for culturing NTM with incubation for at least 6 weeks.[56] Once NTM has been detected in culture, it is critical that the organism is properly speciated, as treatment varies depending on the species. New methods of rapid specification are available, including line probe assays, partial gene sequencing, multilocus sequencing, and matrix-assisted laser desorption ionization-time-of-flight (MALDI-TOF) mass spectrometry. Line probe assays are easy to perform and allow identification of the most frequently encountered NTM; however, these assays are unable to distinguish the different subspecies of MABSC.[60] Partial sequencing allows a higher level of discrimination than line probe assays but requires access to sequencing facilities: 16S rRNA allows discrimination to the species level for most species, whereas *hsp*65, *rpo*B genes, and the 16S-23S internal transcribed spacer allow discrimination to the subspecies level. Sequencing of multiple loci allows

---

Box 1
Suggested criteria for the diagnosis of nontuberculous mycobacteria (NTM) disease in cystic fibrosis (CF)

All 3 criteria should be met before treatment.

1. Positive acid-fast bacilli cultures on at least 2 separate occasions, from either sputum or bronchoalveolar lavage.

2. Clinical, spirometric, and radiographic findings consistent with NTM infection. At least 1 must be present, including

   - Unexplained loss in lung function

   - Increased respiratory symptoms (cough, sputum production, dyspnea, hemoptysis)

   - Constitutional symptoms such as fever, fatigue, night sweats, or weight loss

   - Progression of radiographic features consistent with NTM infection (cavitary disease, single or multiple nodules, tree-in-bud opacities, parenchymal consolidation)

3. Exclusion of other comorbidities common in CF, including adequate treatment of

   - Coinfections, such as *Pseudomonas aeruginosa* and *Staphylococcus aureus*

   - Airway clearance therapy

   - Nutritional deficiencies

   - CF-related diabetes

   - Reactive airway disease and allergic bronchopulmonary aspergillosis

   - CF sinus disease

---

excellent discrimination of the various MABSC subspecies. MALDI-TOF mass spectrometry is a new tool for NTM identification but cannot provide the level of subspecies discrimination given by sequencing.[61]

Drug Susceptibility Testing

The ATS, IDSA, and the Clinical and Laboratory Standards Institute (CLSI) have published recommendations for drug susceptibility testing of the most commonly encountered NTM.[4,62] Except in a few instances, the laboratory-defined cutoffs for resistance have not been validated clinically.

In the setting of MAC infections, resistance to macrolides has been associated with poor clinical outcomes, so current recommendations are to perform susceptibility testing on all initial isolates.[4,62] In addition, repeat testing should be performed if there is failure to convert the culture to negative after 6 months of treatment, when MAC is recultured after completion of treatment (recurrence), or when MAC is recultured after conversion while on treatment (failure).[56]

For RGM, microdilution methods are recommended, although there are no studies that have associated minimum inhibitory concentration (MIC) breakpoints with clinical outcomes in the setting of pulmonary infections.[62] Antimicrobials that should be tested against RGM are amikacin,

tobramycin (for *Mycobacterium chelonae*), cefoxitin, ciprofloxacin, clarithromycin, doxycycline (or minocycline), imipenem, linezolid, moxifloxacin, and trimethoprim-sulfamethoxazole.[62]

Some RGM (*Mycobacterium fortuitum*, *Mycobacterium abscessus* subspecies *abscessus*, and *Mycobacterium abscessus* subspecies *bolettii*) contain an erythromycin resistance methylase (*erm*) gene that causes inducible resistance to macrolides.[63] It is currently recommended that the final reading for macrolide resistance be at least 14 days after inoculation unless resistance (MIC ≥ 8 μg/mL) is noted earlier.[62] Alternatively, molecular identification of a complete, functional gene versus a truncated, nonfunctional gene can be performed.

SCREENING FOR NONTUBERCULOUS MYCOBACTERIA IN THE CYSTIC FIBROSIS POPULATION

NTM are often first detected in a CF sputum sample in the absence of clinical suspicion, as part of routine screening; the optimal frequency for such screening is not known. Among patients with CF 12 years of age or older in the US CF Patient Registry, 58% had mycobacterial cultures of which 14% were positive.[12] Not all of these individuals had NTM lung disease, as small quantities of NTM from the environment may intermittently be present in the CF airway, but not result in NTM pulmonary disease.[9,40,48] Cultures for NTM should be performed annually in spontaneously expectorating patients with a stable clinic course. In the absence of clinical features suggestive of NTM pulmonary disease in individuals unable to spontaneously produce sputum, screening is not required.[56]

Screening also may be considered in several other situations, such as before the initiation of chronic macrolide therapy,[14,40] which has been associated with increased development of resistance to the antibiotic.[64,65] Screening more than once a year also may be considered in various patients deemed to be at higher risk for acquiring the infection, or in which the infection could have more severe consequences. In particular, older patients, those with advanced lung disease awaiting transplantation, and those with previous NTM-positive cultures. Conversely, in small children and individuals not capable of producing a sputum sample, and with no recognized risk factors or clinical symptoms, NTM screening can be deferred.

Nearly all studies reporting prevalence of NTM in the CF population have used acid-fast bacilli (AFB) smear and culture from sputum, either induced or spontaneously produced. Although NTM can, on occasion, be detected through laryngeal suction, oropharyngeal swabs, or gastric aspirate,[21,28,34,66] these methods have not been validated for NTM detection. The use of oropharyngeal swabs is not recommended.[56] Skin testing for delayed-type hypersensitivity against NTM antigens does not appear sufficiently sensitive or specific to use for screening.[21,29,67]

In the future, it is likely that culture-independent methods of NTM detection will be used. In particular, molecular techniques can be performed rapidly, and are extremely sensitive and specific for the detection of NTM in sputum,[68–70] although not yet validated in the setting of CF. Use of serologic assays, such as immunoglobulin (Ig)G against Mycobacterium antigen A60 for NTM surveillance appear promising,[71,72] but currently lack validation in the CF population. A recent study from Sweden reported that anti-MABSC IgG ELISA was sixfold higher in patients with CF with MABSC pulmonary disease compared with those without disease: the sensitivity of the assay was 95% and the specificity was 73%.[73]

TREATMENT OF NONTUBERCULOUS MYCOBACTERIA LUNG DISEASE

Treatment of NTM pulmonary disease in CF should be based on ATS/IDSA guidelines that were developed for the general population,[4] as well as guidelines developed under the sponsorship of the US CF Foundation (CFF) and the European CF Society specific to individuals with CF.[56]

Treatment of Mycobacterium avium Complex Lung Disease

Initial treatment for noncavitary NTM disease due to MAC uses a macrolide, rifamycin, and ethambutol.[4] Frequently, azithromycin is the macrolide chosen due to better tolerance, a long history of use in CF lung disease, and fewer interactions with rifampicin and other drugs metabolized through the CYP3A enzyme system compared with clarithromycin.[74] Although azithromycin has recently been shown to reduce macrophage autophagy of M abscessus,[41] this potential detriment has not been evaluated in patients with NTM disease. Additionally, chronic azithromycin therapy has been shown to have benefits in people with CF felt to be due to immunomodulatory properties of the drug, in particular those patients with P aeruginosa.[75–78]

Intermittent oral antibiotic therapy (ie, 3 times weekly) is recommended for non–CF-related MAC lung disease with less extensive disease and recent studies have demonstrated success rates similar to daily therapy but with less drug intolerance.[79,80] However, intermittent therapy is not recommended in CF due to the presence of underlying lung disease and concerns of reduced absorption of antimycobacterials and altered pharmacokinetics in CF.[56,81]

To date, only the presence of resistance to macrolides has been shown to correlate with worse clinical outcomes.[4] In non CF patients with macrolide-resistant MAC lung disease was associated with a very low culture conversion rate.[65] Surgical resection and use of injectable aminoglycosides for more than 6 months increased the culture conversion rate to 79% from 5%. In patients with CF with MAC that is macrolide-resistant, or who are systemically ill, are AFB smear positive, or have evidence of a cavitary lesion on chest imaging, a 1-month to 3-month course of intravenous daily amikacin may be added at the beginning of the treatment course along with the standard 3 oral antibiotics. Patients within this category should generally be managed in collaboration with an expert in the treatment of NTM disease and CF.

Treatment of Mycobacterium abscessus Complex Lung Disease

Typically, treatment regimens for MABSC are divided into an initial intensive phase followed by a continuation phase. The intensive phase consists of 3 to 12 weeks of 3 antibiotics, including intravenous amikacin, cefoxitin, imipenem, or tigecycline, in addition to oral antibiotics.[56] After intravenous therapy, patients usually continue on prolonged chronic suppressive therapy with oral and inhaled treatments with adjustments of therapy based on microbiologic, clinical, and radiographic responses.[82] In some patients, intermittent courses of intravenous antibiotics are required to control the infection. Changes to the drug regimen are common, due to patient tolerance, side effects, and lack of efficacy (**Fig. 4**). These patients also should be generally managed in collaboration with an expert in the treatment of NTM disease and CF.

MABSC can be divided into 3 subspecies, including *M abscessus*, *Mycobacterium bolettii*, and *Mycobacterium massiliense*.[83] *M abscessus* subspecies *abscessus* and subspecies *bolettii* contain an *erm*[41] gene, which can result in inducible macrolide resistance. *M massiliense* has a truncated nonfunctional gene so the organism does not develop inducible macrolide resistance. There are significant differences in treatment outcomes for *M abscessus* subspecies *abscessus* and subspecies *massiliense* in both patients with CF and without CF. In a study from France, clarithromycin-based regimens led to mycobacterial eradication in 100% of patients with *M massiliense* but only 27% of patients with *M abscessus* (*P* = .009).[84] These differences are presumably related to the development of inducible macrolide resistance in subspecies *abscessus* but not in *massiliense*. Whether a macrolide should be continued in the face of potential inducible resistance is not known, but given the potential immunomodulatory benefits in CF lung disease, most providers maintain the macrolide in the treatment regimen.

Monitoring of Drug Toxicity and Clinical Response

Routine monitoring of drug toxicity is essential, and a plan for monitoring should be set in place at the initiation of treatment. Patients with CF are commonly treated with aminoglycosides for other lung pathogens, and therefore prone to auditory-vestibular toxicity and renal injury, making baseline and regular audiology evaluations and monitoring of renal function essential. Even among oral agents, the potential for drug-related side effects and toxicity is considerable, including bone marrow suppression, hepatitis, and QT prolongation. Of particular concern is change in visual acuity due to ethambutol. Patients are recommended to monitor their vision daily and the drug should be discontinued immediately at the first sign of vision disturbance.[49]

Therapeutic Drug Monitoring

Recommended dosages of antimycobacterials are based on pharmacokinetic (PK) and pharmacodynamic (PD) data from healthy volunteers and patients with tuberculosis. In patients with non-CF NTM disease, 48% of patients had low serum concentrations of ethambutol, 56% for clarithromycin, and 35% for azithromycin, despite using ATS/IDSA recommended doses.[74] In one small case-series, researchers demonstrated that serum levels of oral agents for the treatment of NTM are usually far below the target range in patients with CF and in one case in which treatment was failing, increasing the dose to achieve therapeutic levels was associated with eradication of the organism.[81] Based on these studies and others, it appears that the dosing of patients with both CF and non-CF NTM disease may in some cases be

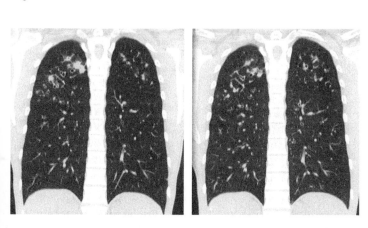

Fig. 4. Treatment response to *M abscessus* subspecies *abscessus*. A 21-year-old with history of previous diagnosis and treatment of *M avium* complex and *Pseudomonas* infections. Despite several rounds of intravenous antimycobacterial therapy, he remained culture positive. He was placed on a "suppressive" regimen of inhaled amikacin, clofazimine, and clarithromycin and his CT scan was repeated after 1 year. The CT scan on the left shows upper lobe predominate bronchiectasis with mucus plugging and nodules. Follow-up CT 1 year later shows that the nodules had diminished in size but he remained culture positive. His spirometric values remained stable.

subtherapeutic, possibly contributing to poor response to treatment.[81]

Challenges to optimal dosing of patients with CF include malabsorption of drug, impaired gastric motility, larger volume of distribution, increased metabolic rate, and potentially increased elimination.[85–87] In addition, drug-drug interactions may occur among various medications used to treat NTM; in particular, rifampin may increase the metabolism of macrolides and moxifloxacin.[74,88] Currently, it is standard practice to monitor amikacin serum levels when administered intravenously. Although sufficient evidence is not available to recommend routine drug monitoring in all patients with CF, it should be considered in the setting of treatment failure, or when multiple drug interactions are possible.[89] In all patients with CF, it must be emphasized that currently available antibiotics have significant limitation in achieving bacteriostatic concentrations within mucus plugs lodged in the airway,[90] thus intensive airway clearance is an essential component of treatment.

NONPHARMACOLOGIC TREATMENT OPTIONS

In addition to pharmacologic treatment of NTM infection, nonpharmacologic therapies for underlying CF lung disease that primarily target clearance of airway mucus obstruction are essential. All NTM treatment regimens need to be part of a comprehensive CF care plan that includes effective airway clearance, nutrition management, and treatment of CF comorbidities, such as sinus disease and CF-related diabetes. This care is most effectively delivered at a CF Care Center, which uses a multidisciplinary approach, providing access to a respiratory therapist, dietitian, and social worker, in addition to nurses and physicians experienced in CF care. The CF Care Centers can be located at http://www.cff.org/LivingWithCF/CareCenterNetwork/CFFoundation-accreditedCareCenters/.

SURGICAL TREATMENT OPTIONS

Surgical resection (pneumonectomy, lobectomy, or segmentectomy) may be a consideration as adjuvant therapy to medical treatment of NTM pulmonary disease. Patients with MABSC lung disease but without CF have been reported to have a higher rate of sustained culture conversion after surgery than with antimicrobial therapy alone.[91,92] In patients with CF, often there is a lobe with a greater burden of disease; however, disease is generally diffuse and bronchiectasis eventually will involve all lobes. It is difficult to identify, with certainty, a focus of NTM infection in the setting of coinfection with typical CF pathogens, such as P aeruginosa and S aureus, and patients with CF with a history of NTM are at very high risk to acquire a second NTM in their lifetime (**Fig. 5**).[48] In rare circumstances, a patients with CF with NTM disease may be identified who is a good candidate to benefit from lung resection, but only in combination with intensive preoperative and postoperative medical treatment, and in the hands of an experienced thoracic surgeon.[4,93,94]

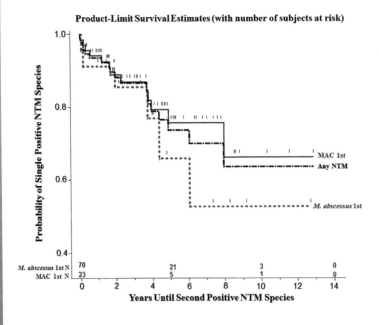

Fig. 5. Probability of detecting a second NTM species after culturing a first NTM. Following an initial positive culture, 24% of subjects with MAC initially grew a second NTM species during 5 years of follow-up, whereas 34% with M abscessus first grew a second NTM species at 5 years. Overall, 26% of subjects grew a second NTM species at 5 years and 36% at 10 years. Kaplan-Meier analysis, separated by initial positive NTM culture species. (Reprinted with permission of the American Thoracic Society. Copyright © 2014 American Thoracic Society. From Martiniano SL, Sontag MK, Daley CL, et al. Clinical significance of a first positive nontuberculous mycobacteria culture in cystic fibrosis. Ann Am Thorac Soc 2014;11:36–44.)

TREATMENT OUTCOMES AND IMPACT OF NONTUBERCULOUS MYCOBACTERIA LUNG DISEASE

Treatment success is generally defined by sustained culture conversion for at least 12 months.[4,92] Rates of successful therapy appear to vary dramatically, based on NTM species, patterns of antibiotic resistance, and severity of disease, as seen in prospective trials in patients with NTM lung disease. In a recent retrospective review of patients with CF from Colorado, the rate of sustained culture conversion in response to initial treatment of MABSC (subspecies not designated) was 45%, and response to treatment of MAC was 60%.[48] The issue of treatment failure is particularly problematic in the context of CF. General considerations in the evaluation of treatment failure include antibiotic resistance, inadequate dosing, and/or poor absorption of antibiotics, suboptimal airway clearance, lack of adherence to the prescribed medications, and the contribution of other comorbidities, including exacerbations of other chronic infections, chronic aspiration, and CF-related diabetes.

RECOMMENDATIONS FOR FOLLOW-UP

After a person with CF has been identified as having a positive NTM culture, close surveillance is warranted, with repeat sputum cultures obtained regularly.[4] Additionally, people with CF with clinical decline or radiographic progression of lung disease that is unresponsive to treatment of typical CF pathogens should be evaluated for NTM. This is particularly important in patients previously infected with an NTM or treated for NTM pulmonary disease, as the presence of a second NTM is a relatively common occurrence. Many previous trials have noted the presence of individuals with more than one species of NTM recovered from their sputum.[1,2,9,22,25–27,95] In patients from the Colorado CF center, we found that MAC was typically the first identified NTM, but a subsequent positive culture for M abscessus was common, whereas subjects who first cultured M abscessus also had a high rate of secondary positive cultures for MAC.[48] Remarkably, 26% of subjects were identified with a second NTM species at 5 years and 36% at 10 years (see **Fig. 5**). These findings support the need for lifelong strategies for NTM surveillance and management in patients with CF who present with a positive NTM culture.

LUNG TRANSPLANTATION IN CYSTIC FIBROSIS AND NONTUBERCULOUS MYCOBACTERIA

Bilateral lung transplantation is an option considered by patients with CF who develop severe bronchiectasis and end-stage lung disease, generally described as an FEV_1 consistently below 30% predicted, a rapid decline in FEV_1, or presence of increased frequency or severity of pulmonary exacerbations.[96] In 2006, the International Society for Heart and Lung Transplantation included colonization with highly resistant or highly virulent bacteria, fungi, or mycobacteria in the list of relative contraindications for lung transplantation.[97]

NTM-positive cultures and NTM pulmonary disease have been reported at a higher prevalence in patients with CF referred for lung transplantation compared with patients without CF.[32] Case reports of death due to disseminated M abscessus after lung transplantation in adult and pediatric patients with CF have been described in people with pretransplant infection,[98–100] although several patients have been described in whom preexisting NTM was not detected but then was a source of posttransplant morbidity and mortality.[99,101,102]

Investigators from the University of North Carolina described a 19.7% prevalence rate of NTM isolated from respiratory cultures from patients with CF referred for transplantation.[32] After transplantation, NTM disease prevalence was low, but a cause of significant morbidity, although no increase in mortality. In a follow-up study, the center reported 13 patients between 1992 and 2012 with at least one pretransplant culture positive for M abscessus (6 were smear positive).[103] Three patients developed M abscessus–related complications with clearance of the organism following treatment. Survival after transplantation was 77% at 1 year, 64% at 3 years, and 50% at 5 years. None of the patients died from M abscessus.

A group from Denmark reviewed 52 patients with CF who underwent lung transplantation, describing a 21% prevalence of NTM-positive cultures pretransplantation and a 17% prevalence of pretransplant NTM pulmonary disease.[104] With perioperative medical treatment, 67% of their patients were alive at follow-up and no deaths had been attributed to NTM infection; however, morbidity, including wound infections, was described. Wound infections from M abscessus posttransplantation also have been reported from Sweden in patients with CF with pretransplant M abscessus.[102]

Based on these studies, it is currently recommended that infection with NTM, even M abscessus, should not be an absolute contraindication to lung transplantation, although morbidity is to be expected.[56] Consensus opinion is that aggressive and prolonged courses of multiple antimycobacterial agents before transplantation, perioperatively, and after transplantation are critical to improving outcomes in these patients.[99,105]

The decision to proceed with lung transplantation in patients with active MABSC disease should be made individually by each transplant program; currently most programs decline to perform the transplant under this circumstance.

INFECTION PREVENTION

Infections with NTM have historically been thought to be from environmental exposure[8,106]; however, recently, the potential for patient-to-patient spread within CF centers has been described[95,107–109] with devastating consequences.[109] Five patients who had overlapping clinical encounters at the University of Washington CF Center were found to have identical isolates of *M abscessus* subspecies *massiliense* by PFGE (pulsed-field gel electrophoresis) and repetitive unit-sequence–based polymerase chain reaction pattern.[109] In the United Kingdom, another group used whole-genome sequencing as well as analysis of antibiotic resistance patterns to identify 2 clustered outbreaks of *M abscessus* subspecies *massiliense*.[108] Both groups suspected indirect person-to-person spread within the clinic and hospital setting. On the other hand, a recent report from the United Kingdom could not demonstrate cross-transmission of *M abscessus* within a cohort of pediatric patients with CF except between one sibling pair.[110]

Based on these recent reports, the CF Foundation recommends that all health care personnel implement contact precautions (ie, wear a gown and gloves) when caring for all people with CF, regardless of respiratory culture results, in both ambulatory and inpatient settings.[111] Additionally, they recommend that molecular typing of all NTM isolates be performed if there is a suspected patient-to-patient transmission event.

SUMMARY/DISCUSSION

The prevalence of pulmonary NTM infections appears to be increasing in patients living with CF and, based on current trends, it seems likely that NTM infections will continue to increase. The steady improvement in survival achieved over the past 2 decades will likely lead to a greater proportion of the CF population resembling the phenotype best suited to MAC infection; those with less severe CFTR mutations and greater age. Likewise, it appears that the prevalence of MABSC is increasing possibly due to patient-to-patient transmission and that children and patients with more severe pulmonary disease are at risk.

Diagnosis of NTM disease in the setting of CF can be difficult given the overlapping clinical and radiographic findings caused by common CF pathogens and because isolation of NTM may or may not be associated with progressive disease. As treatment may not be necessary in all cases, CF-specific diagnostic criteria are greatly needed.

Treatment presents a significant burden on the patient and health care system,[112] requiring a prolonged multidrug regimen, often including several months of multiple intravenous antibiotics and associated with frequent drug-related toxicities. For patients with CF, this treatment burden comes in addition to existing time-intensive and cost-intensive regimens of medications and airway clearance. Given the increasing common morbidity caused by NTM disease, a significant investment in NTM-related research will be required over the next decades.

REFERENCES

1. Roux A-L, Catherinot E, Ripoll F, et al, Jean-Louis Herrmann for the OMAG. Multicenter study of prevalence of nontuberculous mycobacteria in patients with cystic fibrosis in France. J Clin Microbiol 2009; 47:4124–8.
2. Esther CR Jr, Esserman DA, Gilligan P, et al. Chronic *Mycobacterium abscessus* infection and lung function decline in cystic fibrosis. J Cyst Fibros 2010;9:117–23.
3. Qvist T, Pressler T, Hoiby N, et al. Shifting paradigms of nontuberculous mycobacteria in cystic fibrosis. Respir Res 2014;15:41.
4. Griffith DE, Aksamit T, Brown-Elliott BA, et al. An official ATS/IDSA statement: diagnosis, treatment, and prevention of nontuberculous mycobacterial diseases. Am J Respir Crit Care Med 2007;175: 367–416.
5. Prevots DR, Marras TK. Epidemiology of human pulmonary infection with nontuberculous mycobacteria: a review. Clin Chest Med 2015;36:13–34.
6. Andre E, Degraux J, Simon A, et al. Absence of non-tuberculous mycobacteria recovery in sputum of cystic fibrosis patients despite adequate decontamination: a possible role of specific antimicrobial therapy used in our centre. Clin Microbiol Infect 2010;16:S33–4.
7. Torrens JK, Dawkins P, Conway SP, et al. Nontuberculous mycobacteria in cystic fibrosis. Thorax 1998;53:182–5.
8. Sermet-Gaudelus I, Le Bourgeois M, Pierre-Audigier C, et al. Mycobacterium abscessus and children with cystic fibrosis. Emerg Infect Dis 2003;9:1587–91.
9. Olivier KN, Weber DJ, Wallace RJ Jr, et al, Nontuberculous Mycobacteria in Cystic Fibrosis Study Group. Nontuberculous mycobacteria. I: multicenter prevalence study in cystic fibrosis. Am J Respir Crit Care Med 2003;167:828–34.

10. Aitken ML, Burke W, McDonald G, et al. Nontuberculous mycobacterial disease in adult cystic fibrosis patients. Chest 1993;103:1096–9.

11. Valenza G, Tappe D, Turnwald D, et al. Prevalence and antimicrobial susceptibility of microorganisms isolated from sputa of patients with cystic fibrosis. J Cyst Fibros 2008;7:123–7.

12. Adjemian J, Olivier KN, Prevots DR. Nontuberculous mycobacteria among patients with cystic fibrosis in the United States: screening practices and environmental risk. Am J Respir Crit Care Med 2014;190:581–6.

13. Adjemian J, Olivier KN, Seitz AE, et al. Spatial clusters of nontuberculous mycobacterial lung disease in the United States. Am J Respir Crit Care Med 2012;186(6):553–8.

14. Leung JM, Olivier KN. Nontuberculous mycobacteria in patients with cystic fibrosis. Semin Respir Crit Care Med 2013;34:124–34.

15. Qvist T, Gilljam M, Jonsson B, et al, Scandinavian Cystic Fibrosis Study Consortium (SCFSC). Epidemiology of nontuberculous mycobacteria among patients with cystic fibrosis in Scandinavia. J Cyst Fibros 2015;14:46–52.

16. Bar-On O, Mussaffi H, Mei-Zahav M, et al. Increasing nontuberculous mycobacteria infection in cystic fibrosis. J Cyst Fibros 2015;14:53–62.

17. Raidt L, Idelevich EA, Dubbers A, et al. Increased prevalence and resistance of important pathogens recovered from respiratory specimens of cystic fibrosis patients during a decade. Pediatr Infect Dis J 2015;34:700–5.

18. Adjemian J, Olivier KN, Seitz AE, et al. Prevalence of nontuberculous mycobacterial lung disease in U.S. Medicare beneficiaries. Am J Respir Crit Care Med 2012;185:881–6.

19. Prevots DR, Shaw PA, Strickland D, et al. Nontuberculous mycobacterial lung disease prevalence at four integrated health care delivery systems. Am J Respir Crit Care Med 2010;182:970–6.

20. Rodman DM, Polis JM, Heltshe SL, et al. Late diagnosis defines a unique population of long-term survivors of cystic fibrosis. Am J Respir Crit Care Med 2005;171:621–6.

21. Hjelte L, Petrini B, Kallenius G, et al. Prospective study of mycobacterial infections in patients with cystic fibrosis. Thorax 1990;45:397–400.

22. Kilby JM, Gilligan PH, Yankaskas JR, et al. Nontuberculous mycobacteria in adult patients with cystic fibrosis. Chest 1992;102:70–5.

23. Esther CR Jr, Henry MM, Molina PL, et al. Nontuberculous mycobacterial infection in young children with cystic fibrosis. Pediatr Pulmonol 2005;40:39–44.

24. Seddon P, Fidler K, Raman S, et al. Prevalence of nontuberculous mycobacteria in cystic fibrosis clinics, United Kingdom, 2009. Emerg Infect Dis 2013;19:1128–30.

25. Pierre-Audigier C, Ferroni A, Sermet-Gaudelus I, et al. Age-related prevalence and distribution of nontuberculous mycobacterial species among patients with cystic fibrosis. J Clin Microbiol 2005;43:3467–70.

26. Levy I, Grisaru-Soen G, Lerner-Geva L, et al. Multicenter cross-sectional study of nontuberculous mycobacterial infections among cystic fibrosis patients, Israel. Emerg Infect Dis 2008;14:378–84.

27. Catherinot E, Roux AL, Vibet MA, et al, OMA Group. Mycobacterium avium and Mycobacterium abscessus complex target distinct cystic fibrosis patient subpopulations. J Cyst Fibros 2013;12:74–80.

28. Fauroux B, Delaisi B, Clement A, et al. Mycobacterial lung disease in cystic fibrosis: a prospective study. Pediatr Infect Dis J 1997;16:354–8.

29. Hjelt K, Hojlyng N, Howitz P, et al. The role of mycobacteria other than tuberculosis (MOTT) in patients with cystic fibrosis. Scand J Infect Dis 1994;26:569–76.

30. Keating CL, Liu X, Dimango EA. Classic respiratory disease but atypical diagnostic testing distinguishes adult presentation of cystic fibrosis. Chest 2010;137:1157–63.

31. Nick JA, Chacon CS, Brayshaw SJ, et al. Effects of gender and age at diagnosis on disease progression in long-term survivors of cystic fibrosis. Am J Respir Crit Care Med 2010;182:614–26.

32. Chalermskulrat W, Sood N, Neuringer IP, et al. Nontuberculous mycobacteria in end stage cystic fibrosis: implications for lung transplantation. Thorax 2006;61:507–13.

33. Burgel P, Morand P, Audureau E, et al. Azithromycin and the risk of nontuberculous mycobacteria in adults with cystic fibrosis. Pediatr Pulmonology 2011;46:328.

34. Ager S, O'Brien C, Spencer DA, et al. A retrospective review of non-tuberculous mycobacteria in paediatric cystic fibrosis patients at a regional centre. J Cyst Fibros 2011;10:S36.

35. Paugam A, Baixench M-T, Demazes-Dufeu N, et al. Characteristics and consequences of airway colonization by filamentous fungi in 201 adult patients with cystic fibrosis in France. Med Mycol 2010;48(Suppl 1):S32–6.

36. Mussaffi H, Rivlin J, Shalit I, et al. Nontuberculous mycobacteria in cystic fibrosis associated with allergic bronchopulmonary aspergillosis and steroid therapy. Eur Respir J 2005;25:324–8.

37. Evans JT, Ratnaraja N, Gardiner S, et al. Mycobacterium abscessus in cystic fibrosis: what does it all mean? Clin Microbiol Infect 2011;17:S602.

38. Falkinham JO 3rd. Surrounded by mycobacteria: nontuberculous mycobacteria in the human environment. J Appl Microbiol 2009;107:356–67.

39. Giron RM, Maiz L, Barrio I, et al. Nontuberculous mycobacterial infection in patients with cystic fibrosis: a multicenter prevalence study. Arch Bronconeumol 2008;44:679–84 [in Spanish].

40. Olivier KN, Weber DJ, Lee J-H, et al, Nontuberculous Mycobacteria in Cystic Fibrosis Study Group. Nontuberculous mycobacteria. II: nested-cohort study of impact on cystic fibrosis lung disease. Am J Respir Crit Care Med 2003;167:835–40.

41. Renna M, Schaffner C, Brown K, et al. Azithromycin blocks autophagy and may predispose cystic fibrosis patients to mycobacterial infection. J Clin Invest 2011;121:3554–63.

42. Binder AM, Adjemian J, Olivier KN, et al. Epidemiology of nontuberculous mycobacterial infections and associated chronic macrolide use among persons with cystic fibrosis. Am J Respir Crit Care Med 2013;188:807–12.

43. Catherinot E, Roux AL, Vibet MA, et al, OMA Group. Inhaled therapies, azithromycin and *Mycobacterium abscessus* in cystic fibrosis patients. Eur Respir J 2013;41:1101–6.

44. Radhakrishnan DK, Yau Y, Corey M, et al. Nontuberculous mycobacteria in children with cystic fibrosis: isolation, prevalence, and predictors. Pediatr Pulmonology 2009;44:1100–6.

45. Prevots DR, Adjemian J, Fernandez AG, et al. Environmental risks for nontuberculous mycobacteria. Individual exposures and climatic factors in the cystic fibrosis population. Ann Am Thorac Soc 2014;11:1032–8.

46. Forslow U, Geborek A, Hjelte L, et al. Early chemotherapy for non-tuberculous mycobacterial infections in patients with cystic fibrosis. Acta Paediatr 2003;92:910–5.

47. Leitritz L, Griese M, Roggenkamp A, et al. Prospective study on nontuberculous mycobacteria in patients with and without cystic fibrosis. Med Microbiol Immunol 2004;193:209–17.

48. Martiniano SL, Sontag MK, Daley CL, et al. Clinical significance of a first positive nontuberculous mycobacteria culture in cystic fibrosis. Ann Am Thorac Soc 2014;11:36–44.

49. Martiniano SL, Nick JA. Nontuberculous mycobacterial infections in cystic fibrosis. Clin Chest Med 2015;36:101–15.

50. Whittier S, Olivier K, Gilligan P, et al. Proficiency testing of clinical microbiology laboratories using modified decontamination procedures for detection of nontuberculous mycobacteria in sputum samples from cystic fibrosis patients. The Nontuberculous Mycobacteria in Cystic Fibrosis Study Group. J Clin Microbiol 1997;35:2706–8.

51. Bange FC, Bottger EC. Improved decontamination method for recovering mycobacteria from patients with cystic fibrosis. Eur J Clin Microbiol Infect Dis 2002;21:546–8.

52. Whittier S, Hopfer RL, Knowles MR, et al. Improved recovery of mycobacteria from respiratory secretions of patients with cystic fibrosis. J Clin Microbiol 1993;31:861–4.

53. Steingart KR, Ng V, Henry M, et al. Sputum processing methods to improve the sensitivity of smear microscopy for tuberculosis: a systematic review. Lancet Infect Dis 2006;6:664–74.

54. Brown-Elliott BA, Griffith DE, Wallace RJ Jr. Diagnosis of nontuberculous mycobacterial infections. Clin Lab Med 2002;22:911–25, vi.

55. Buijtels PC, Petit PL. Comparison of NaOH-N-acetyl cysteine and sulfuric acid decontamination methods for recovery of mycobacteria from clinical specimens. J Microbiol Methods 2005;62:83–8.

56. Floto A, ea. Cystic Fibrosis Foundation and European Cystic Fibrosis Society consensus recommendations for the management of nontuberculous mycobacteria in individuals with cystic fibrosis. Thorax, in press.

57. Bange FC, Kirschner P, Bottger EC. Recovery of mycobacteria from patients with cystic fibrosis. J Clin Microbiol 1999;37:3761–3.

58. Ferroni A, Vu-Thien H, Lanotte P, et al. Value of the chlorhexidine decontamination method for recovery of nontuberculous mycobacteria from sputum samples of patients with cystic fibrosis. J Clin Microbiol 2006;44:2237–9.

59. Preece CL, Perry A, Gray B, et al. A novel culture medium for isolation of rapidly-growing mycobacteria from the sputum of patients with cystic fibrosis. J Cyst Fibros 2015. [Epub ahead of print].

60. van Ingen J. Microbiological diagnosis of nontuberculous mycobacterial pulmonary disease. Clin Chest Med 2015;36:43–54.

61. Buchan BW, Riebe KM, Timke M, et al. Comparison of MALDI-TOF MS with HPLC and nucleic acid sequencing for the identification of *Mycobacterium* species in cultures using solid medium and broth. Am J Clin Pathol 2014;141:25–34.

62. CLSI. Susceptibility testing of mycobacteria, nocardia, and other aerobic actinomycetes: approved standard-second edition. CLSI document M24–A2. Wayne (PA): Clinical and Laboratory Standards Institute; 2011.

63. Nash KA, Brown-Elliott BA, Wallace RJ Jr. A novel gene, erm(41), confers inducible macrolide resistance to clinical isolates of *Mycobacterium abscessus* but is absent from *Mycobacterium chelonae*. Antimicrob Agents Chemother 2009;53:1367–76.

64. Doucet-Populaire F, Buriankova K, Weiser J, et al. Natural and acquired macrolide resistance in mycobacteria. Curr Drug Targets Infect Disord 2002;2:355–70.

65. Griffith DE, Brown-Elliott BA, Langsjoen B, et al. Clinical and molecular analysis of macrolide

resistance in *Mycobacterium avium* complex lung disease. Am J Respir Crit Care Med 2006;174: 928–34.

66. Verma N, Spencer D. Disseminated *Mycobacterium gordonae* infection in a child with cystic fibrosis. Pediatr Pulmonology 2012;47:517–8.

67. Mulherin D, Coffey MJ, Halloran DO, et al. Skin reactivity to atypical mycobacteria in cystic fibrosis. Respir Med 1990;84:273–6.

68. Ngan GJ, Ng LM, Jureen R, et al. Development of multiplex PCR assays based on the 16S-23S rRNA internal transcribed spacer for the detection of clinically relevant nontuberculous mycobacteria. Lett Appl Microbiol 2011;52:546–54.

69. Leung KL, Yip CW, Cheung WF, et al. Development of a simple and low-cost real-time PCR method for the identification of commonly encountered mycobacteria in a high throughput laboratory. J Appl Microbiol 2009;107:1433–9.

70. Devine M, Moore JE, Xu J, et al. Detection of mycobacterial DNA from sputum of patients with cystic fibrosis. Ir J Med Sci 2004;173:96–8.

71. Oliver A, Maiz L, Canton R, et al. Nontuberculous mycobacteria in patients with cystic fibrosis. Clin Infect Dis 2001;32:1298–303.

72. Ferroni A, Sermet-Gaudelus I, Le Bourgeois M, et al. Measurement of immunoglobulin G against mycobacterial antigen A60 in patients with cystic fibrosis and lung infection due to *Mycobacterium abscessus*. Clin Infect Dis 2005;40:58–66.

73. Qvist T, Pressler T, Taylor-Robinson D, et al. Serodiagnosis of *Mycobacterium abscessus* complex infection in cystic fibrosis. Eur Respir J 2015; 46(3):707–16.

74. van Ingen J, Egelund EF, Levin A, et al. The pharmacokinetics and pharmacodynamics of pulmonary *Mycobacterium avium* complex disease treatment. Am J Respir Crit Care Med 2012; 186(6):559–65.

75. Clement A, Tamalet A, Leroux E, et al. Long term effects of azithromycin in patients with cystic fibrosis: a double blind, placebo controlled trial. Thorax 2006;61:895–902.

76. Equi A, Balfour-Lynn IM, Bush A, et al. Long term azithromycin in children with cystic fibrosis: a randomised, placebo-controlled crossover trial. Lancet 2002;360:978–84.

77. Saiman L, Marshall BC, Mayer-Hamblett N, et al. Azithromycin in patients with cystic fibrosis chronically infected with *Pseudomonas aeruginosa*: a randomized controlled trial. JAMA 2003;290:1749–56.

78. Wolter J, Seeney S, Bell S, et al. Effect of long term treatment with azithromycin on disease parameters in cystic fibrosis: a randomised trial. Thorax 2002; 57:212–6.

79. Wallace RJ Jr, Brown-Elliott BA, McNulty S, et al. Macrolide/Azalide therapy for nodular/

bronchiectatic *Mycobacterium avium* complex lung disease. Chest 2014;146:276–82.

80. Jeong BH, Jeon K, Park HY, et al. Intermittent antibiotic therapy for nodular bronchiectatic *Mycobacterium avium* complex lung disease. Am J Respir Crit Care Med 2015;191:96–103.

81. Gilljam M, Berning SE, Peloquin CA, et al. Therapeutic drug monitoring in patients with cystic fibrosis and mycobacterial disease. Eur Respir J 1999;14:347–51.

82. Ebert DL, Olivier KN. Nontuberculous mycobacteria in the setting of cystic fibrosis. Clin Chest Med 2002;23:655–63.

83. Cho YJ, Yi H, Chun J, et al. The genome sequence of '*Mycobacterium massiliense*' strain CIP 108297 suggests the independent taxonomic status of the *Mycobacterium abscessus* complex at the subspecies level. PLoS One 2013;8:e81560.

84. Roux AL, Catherinot E, Soismier N, et al, OMA Group. Comparing *Mycobacterium massiliense* and *Mycobacterium abscessus* lung infections in cystic fibrosis patients. J Cyst Fibros 2015;14:63–9.

85. Kearns GL, Trang JM. Introduction to pharmacokinetics: aminoglycosides in cystic fibrosis as a prototype. J Pediatr 1986;108:847–53.

86. de Groot R, Smith AL. Antibiotic pharmacokinetics in cystic fibrosis. Differences and clinical significance. Clin Pharmacokinet 1987;13:228–53.

87. Rey E, Treluyer JM, Pons G. Drug disposition in cystic fibrosis. Clin Pharmacokinet 1998;35: 313–29.

88. Wallace RJ Jr, Brown BA, Griffith DE, et al. Reduced serum levels of clarithromycin in patients treated with multidrug regimens including rifampin or rifabutin for *Mycobacterium avium-M. intracellulare* infection. J Infect Dis 1995;171:747–50.

89. Peloquin CA. Therapeutic drug monitoring in the treatment of tuberculosis. Drugs 2002;62: 2169–83.

90. Moriarty TF, McElnay JC, Elborn JS, et al. Sputum antibiotic concentrations: implications for treatment of cystic fibrosis lung infection. Pediatr Pulmonol 2007;42:1008–17.

91. Jeon K, Kwon OJ, Lee NY, et al. Antibiotic treatment of *Mycobacterium abscessus* lung disease: a retrospective analysis of 65 patients. Am J Respir Crit Care Med 2009;180:896–902.

92. Jarand J, Levin A, Zhang L, et al. Clinical and microbiologic outcomes in patients receiving treatment for *Mycobacterium abscessus* pulmonary disease. Clin Infect Dis 2011;52:565–71.

93. Mitchell JD. Surgical approach to pulmonary nontuberculous mycobacterial infections. Clin Chest Med 2015;36:117–22.

94. Yu JA, Weyant MJ, Mitchell JD. Surgical treatment of atypical mycobacterial infections. Thorac Surg Clin 2012;22:277–85.

95. Jonsson BE, Gilljam M, Lindblad A, et al. Molecular epidemiology of *Mycobacterium abscessus*, with focus on cystic fibrosis. J Clin Microbiol 2007;45: 1497–504.

96. Braun AT, Merlo CA. Cystic fibrosis lung transplantation. Curr Opin Pulm Med 2011;17:467–72.

97. Orens JB, Estenne M, Arcasoy S, et al, Pulmonary Scientific Council of the International Society for Heart and Lung Transplantation. International guidelines for the selection of lung transplant candidates: 2006 update–a consensus report from the Pulmonary Scientific Council of the International Society for Heart and Lung Transplantation. J Heart Lung Transplant 2006;25:745–55.

98. Taylor JL, Palmer SM. *Mycobacterium abscessus* chest wall and pulmonary infection in a cystic fibrosis lung transplant recipient. J Heart Lung Transplant 2006;25:985–8.

99. Zaidi S, Elidemir O, Heinle JS, et al. *Mycobacterium abscessus* in cystic fibrosis lung transplant recipients: report of 2 cases and risk for recurrence. Transpl Infect Dis 2009;11:243–8.

100. Sanguinetti M, Ardito F, Fiscarelli E, et al. Fatal pulmonary infection due to multidrug-resistant *Mycobacterium abscessus* in a patient with cystic fibrosis. J Clin Microbiol 2001;39:816–9.

101. Flume PA, Egan TM, Paradowski LJ, et al. Infectious complications of lung transplantation. Impact of cystic fibrosis. Am J Respir Crit Care Med 1994; 149:1601–7.

102. Gilljam M, Schersten H, Silverborn M, et al. Lung transplantation in patients with cystic fibrosis and *Mycobacterium abscessus* infection. J Cyst Fibros 2010;9:272–6.

103. Lobo LJ, Chang LC, Esther CR Jr, et al. Lung transplant outcomes in cystic fibrosis patients with preoperative *Mycobacterium abscessus* respiratory infections. Clin Transplant 2013;27:523–9.

104. Qvist T, Pressler T, Thomsen VO, et al. Nontuberculous mycobacterial disease is not a contraindication to lung transplantation in patients with cystic fibrosis: a retrospective analysis in a Danish patient population. Transplant Proc 2013;45:342–5.

105. Watkins RR, Lemonovich TL. Evaluation of infections in the lung transplant patient. Curr Opin Infect Dis 2012;25:193–8.

106. Bange FC, Brown BA, Smaczny C, et al. Lack of transmission of *Mycobacterium abscessus* among patients with cystic fibrosis attending a single clinic. Clin Infect Dis 2001;32:1648–50.

107. Harris KA, Kenna DTD, Blauwendraat C, et al. Molecular fingerprinting of *Mycobacterium abscessus* strains in a cohort of pediatric cystic fibrosis patients. J Clin Microbiol 2012;50:1758–61.

108. Bryant JM, Harris SR, Parkhill J, et al. Whole-genome sequencing to establish relapse or re-infection with *Mycobacterium tuberculosis*: a retrospective observational study. Lancet Respir Med 2013;1:786–92.

109. Aitken ML, Limaye A, Pottinger P, et al. Respiratory outbreak of *Mycobacterium abscessus* subspecies *massiliense* in a lung transplant and cystic fibrosis center. Am J Respir Crit Care Med 2012;185:231–2.

110. Harris KA, Underwood A, Kenna DT, et al. Whole-genome sequencing and epidemiological analysis do not provide evidence for cross-transmission of *Mycobacterium abscessus* in a cohort of pediatric cystic fibrosis patients. Clin Infect Dis 2015;60: 1007–16.

111. Saiman L, Siegel JD, LiPuma JJ, et al. Infection prevention and control guideline for cystic fibrosis: 2013 update. Infect Control Hosp Epidemiol 2014; 35(Suppl 1):S1–67.

112. Ballarino GJ, Olivier KN, Claypool RJ, et al. Pulmonary nontuberculous mycobacterial infections: antibiotic treatment and associated costs. Respir Med 2009;103:1448–55.

Nutritional Issues in Cystic Fibrosis

Missale Solomon, MD[a],*, Molly Bozic, MD[b], Maria R. Mascarenhas, MBBS[c]

KEYWORDS

- Cystic fibrosis • Nutritional status • Nutritional assessment • Malnutrition • Pancreatic insufficiency
- Malabsorption • Cystic fibrosis–related diabetes • Enteral nutrition

KEY POINTS

- Patients with cystic fibrosis (CF) are at risk for malnutrition secondary to increased losses from malabsorption and increased energy demands from infections, chronic disease, and decreased oral intake.
- Complications, including pancreatic insufficiency, CF-related diabetes, and CF-related liver disease, place patients with CF at further risk for poor nutritional status.
- Optimizing growth and nutrition has a clear positive influence on lung health and overall survival.
- Comprehensive nutritional assessments at regular intervals are necessary to identify those at risk of nutritional failure even before malnutrition occurs.
- Aggressive nutritional support should be implemented early, and patients should be monitored closely to ensure optimal growth and nutritional status.

INTRODUCTION

The importance of nutritional status in individuals with cystic fibrosis (CF) and the impact on pulmonary function and survival has been well established.[1–3] Clinically characterized by progressive lung disease, nearly 90% of patients with CF have exocrine pancreatic insufficiency and subsequent malabsorption.[4] This malabsorption, along with increased energy requirements and chronic infections, place patients with CF at significant risk for malnutrition. Pancreatic-sufficient (PS) patients with CF are also at risk for poor nutrition and micronutrient deficiencies. Chronic undernutrition and poor growth are well-known causes of mortality and morbidity among patients with CF. This article focuses on nutritional issues in children, adolescents, and adults with CF.

EFFECT OF NUTRITIONAL STATUS ON CYSTIC FIBROSIS LUNG DISEASE AND SURVIVAL

The earliest study to elegantly highlight the relationship between nutritional status and survival in CF was published in 1988 by Corey and colleagues.[5] This retrospective comparative study identified a marked difference in the median survival between patients at 2 centers in Boston and Toronto. Although there was no significant difference in the pulmonary therapy between the centers, the approach to nutritional care was quite different. Adoption of a high-calorie, high-fat diet with aggressive pancreatic enzyme replacement therapy (PERT) by the Toronto team resulted in improved nutritional status, which in turn was associated with significantly better survival. This study did not identify any significant difference in

Disclosures: None.
[a] Drexel University Philadelphia, Philadelphia, PA, USA; [b] Pediatric Gastroenterology, Hepatology & Nutrition, Riley Hospital for Children, Indianapolis, IN, USA; [c] Nutrition, Nutrition Support Service, Clinical Nutrition, The Children's Hospital of Philadelphia, Perelman School of Medicine, University of Pennsylvania, Philadelphia, PA, USA
* Corresponding author. 219 North Broad street, 5th Floor Philadelphia, PA 19107.
E-mail address: missale.solomon@drexelmed.edu

chestmed.theclinics.com

the pulmonary function between the patients in the 2 centers, which suggested a direct detrimental impact of poor nutritional status on survival.

In a 2003 study of nearly 1000 subjects between 3 and 6 years of age, children with a weight for age less than the fifth percentile at 3 years of age had significantly lower pulmonary function at 6 years of age compared with those with a weight for age greater than the 75th percentile at 3 years.[6] A more recent study of more than 3000 pediatric patients with CF prospectively followed outcomes from birth to 18 years of age and found that the weight-for-age percentile at 4 years was associated with improved height and improved pulmonary function, fewer complications, and increased survival at 18 years.[7]

The relationship between nutritional status and pulmonary function seems to be linear to a certain extent. The CF Foundation Patient Registry data consistently show that children and adults with a higher body mass index (BMI) percentile and BMI, respectively, have better lung function. Based on analysis of registry data from 1994 to 2003, the CF Foundation recommends a goal BMI of greater than 50th percentile in children and a BMI greater than or equal to 22 in women and 23 in men.[8] Children with BMIs between the 10th and 25th percentiles are considered at nutritional risk, and those with BMIs less than the 10th percentile are considered to have nutritional failure.[9] A 2-year longitudinal analysis of more than 3000 patients in the German CF patient registry revealed that a greater than 5% decrease in weight for height had a concomitant mean loss of forced expiratory volume in the first second (FEV_1) of 16.5% predicted, whereas patients with improved nutrition showed consistent or even improved FEV_1.[10] The transition from adolescence into adulthood is a critical stage in CF with a mortality peak seen in young adults. This peak follows acceleration in lung function decline even in adolescents with mild lung disease. One of the most important predictors of this decline is a faster rate of decline in BMI during adolescence.[11] Therefore, a more rigorous monitoring of nutritional status and early and aggressive nutritional intervention is crucial during adolescence, even in those with mild lung disease.

LUNG TRANSPLANTATION AND NUTRITIONAL STATUS

Lung transplantation is an established and very effective means of therapy for end-stage lung disease; however, because of the limited organ supply, 20% to 30% of patients die while on the waiting list.[12] Lung transplant candidates are often malnourished; even those with normal weight tend to have depleted lean body mass, which is associated with a higher mortality, while awaiting a lung transplant, and even after transplant.[13] A recent retrospective study investigated the nutritional status in patients with CF before and after transplant and identified that a BMI of 18.5 kg/m^2 or less and a fat-free mass index (FFMI) of 16.7 kg/m^2 or less (men) or 14.6 kg/m^2 or less (women) was associated with impaired survival in lung transplant candidates with CF whereby FFMI is calculated by substituting the fat-free mass (FFM) (which only includes muscle mass and bone mass) for the body mass.[14] Another study identified female sex as a risk factor for increased waiting-list mortality, such that the combination of BMI less than 18 kg/m^2 and female sex was associated with only 21% 1-year waiting-list survival without transplantation.[15] Many centers recommend aggressive nutritional support for undernourished patients during the pretransplant period to improve weight and lean body mass; however, studies reveal conflicting success with this approach. Earlier studies showed that it was possible to increase energy intake and/or weight by intensified nutritional support, including with gastrostomy tube feedings.[16,17] Conversely, other studies failed to show an increase in energy intake or weight gain by intensified nutritional support or with dietetic intervention with oral nutritional supplements, tube feeding, or both.[14,18] After transplantation, studies uniformly show that weight and nutritional status improves. However, unique transplant-related complications, such as osteoporosis and diabetes related to steroids, should be closely monitored.[14,19,20]

PATHOGENESIS OF DISORDERED NUTRITION IN CYSTIC FIBROSIS

Significant progress has been made in the nutritional status of both the pediatric and adult CF population since the 1980s. However, according to the latest CF Patient Registry Report, 45.3% of children and 52.6% of adults with CF have nutritional measures that decrease to less than the nutritional goals.

Undernutrition

Undernutrition in CF results from an imbalance between energy demand and energy intake. Unique complications of CF further aggravate the situation by increasing energy loss (**Fig. 1**).

Increased demand

There seems to be increased resting energy expenditure (REE) in children and adults with

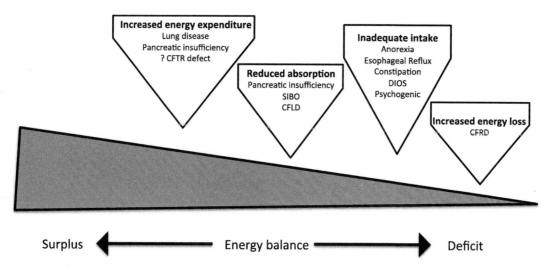

Fig. 1. Important mechanisms underlying the pathogenesis of disordered nutrition in CF. CFLD, CF-related liver disease; CFRD, CF-related diabetes; CFTR, CF transmembrane conductance regulator; DIOS, distal intestinal obstructive syndrome; SIBO, small intestinal bacterial overgrowth.

CF.[21–23] Studies suggest that this increase is greater for females than for males.[24–26] CF-related lung disease can partially explain the higher REE seen in CF; but other mechanisms, including pancreatic insufficiency and intrinsic CF transmembrane conductance regulator (CFTR) defect, have been considered.[27,28] Lung disease in CF increases energy demand in adults through several mechanisms. The continuous cycle of chronic inflammation, bacterial colonization, and recurrent infection causes a systemic hypermetabolic state with elaboration of proinflammatory cytokines, such as tumor necrosis factor, interleukin (IL)-1, and IL-6, that increase energy expenditure. Pulmonary disease also progresses during the second and third decades of life with increased airflow obstruction and hyperinflation, all of which increase the oxygen cost of ventilation.[23]

Reduced intake

A variety of factors limit nutritional intake in patients with CF. Anorexia, which is often associated with the use of antibiotics, can interfere with the amount and type of food ingested. In addition, inadequate airway clearance can lead to mucus production, which is then swallowed, and contributes to reduced appetite and increased satiety.[28] Gastroesophageal reflux, which can be accompanied by postprandial vomiting, is a common complication of CF. Constipation and distal intestinal obstructive syndrome cause symptoms that range from bloating to abdominal pain and bowel obstruction.[29] Patients with CF seem to be predisposed to bacterial overgrowth, which can directly interfere with absorption by competing for nutrients or indirectly by causing anorexia and abdominal symptoms.[30] Murine models demonstrate that intestinal motility is reduced in CF and mucous properties are altered, which interferes with clearance of adherent mucus from the epithelium promoting overgrowth of bacteria.[31,32]

Increased loss

Pancreatic insufficiency is present in 85% of patients with CF and causes macronutrient malabsorption, including severe fat malabsorption, which is not fully corrected even after adequate PERT.[33] Fat malabsorption is further compounded by bile acid precipitation in the acidic environment in the proximal intestine created by impaired pancreatic bicarbonate secretion. Furthermore, abnormal bile acid metabolism seen in CF-related liver disease (CFLD) seems to facilitate depletion of the total bile salt pool. Lastly, CF-related diabetes (CFRD), which is present in up to 2% of children, 19% of adolescents, and 50% of adults, contributes to energy loss through glycosuria.[34]

Overnutrition

CF is commonly associated with undernutrition; however, the proportion of overweight and obese individuals has been increasing. In one US pediatric CF center, 23% of patients with CF aged 2 to 18 years were found to have an average BMI percentile greater than 90. Surprisingly, 88% of the overweight patients and 69% of the obese patients had CFTR mutations associated with pancreatic insufficiency.[35] In a longitudinal cohort study that spanned from 1985 to 2011, the proportion of overweight or obese adults in a CF center in Toronto increased from 7% to 18%. In this study, the higher BMI was associated with better lung function; however, most of these patients were PS and possessed milder mutations.[2] Another cross-sectional study similarly showed that overweight adult subjects with CF were more likely to be PS and have milder mutations.[36] Although achieving weight gain in undernourished individuals has been shown to slow the rate of decline in lung function and prolong survival, the benefit of increasing one's BMI over the normal level seems to be small and improvements in lung function seem to be blunted for adults with BMI greater than 25.[2,37] Moreover, recent studies show higher proportions of obese individuals with CF have elevated triglycerides and total cholesterol.[36,38] Dietary recommendations for such patients should focus on a balanced diet and a healthy lifestyle with good exercise habits; however, published data are lacking.

Body Composition in Cystic Fibrosis

Several investigators caution that standard BMI screening may fail to detect depletion of FFM. FFM, derived from dual x-ray absorptiometry (DXA), is a measure of both muscle mass and bone mass, whereas lean body mass (LBM) refers to the muscle mass excluding bone mass. An important observation is that 25% to 38% of adults with CF with normal or elevated BMI have low levels of FFM. Studies suggest that the benefit of higher BMI in improving lung function may be derived from muscle mass and not fat mass. King and colleagues[39] showed that FFM depletion was associated with severe lung function independent of BMI level. Recently Sheik and colleagues[40] confirmed that LBM was more strongly associated with pulmonary function than BMI. Interestingly, this association was more prominent in undernourished children and adolescents. In a cross-sectional analysis of 77 pediatric patients with CF, Engelen and colleagues[41] assessed whether determination of FFM was a better screening method for nutritional failure than the currently recommended BMI alone. Only 52% of patients with FFM depletion were detected when using BMI criteria of less than 10%. Further analysis showed that those pediatric patients with FFM had reduced FEV_1 values (independent of BMI) and lower bone mineral densities. Those patients with a BMI lower than the 20th percentile showed a larger decrease in FFM and increased bone mineral loss. This finding suggests that, in children, a

BMI percentile of less than 20%, instead of 10%, may be a more sensitive marker to evaluate nutritional failure.[41] These findings indicate that body composition needs to be assessed in all overweight/obese, as well as underweight, patients with CF. In obese individuals, this can help identify sarcopenic obesity, which is a condition whereby fat mass accounts for the bulk of the weight in the face of severe FFM wasting. In underweight patients with CF, identification of LBM depletion can guide appropriate and targeted intervention. Nutritional recommendations in CF should be tailored according to the degree and type of malnutrition taking into account the severity of genetic mutations and the status of the lung function. Furthermore, strategies should be aimed at improving the muscle mass instead of focusing only on increasing body weight or BMI given the aforementioned information.

NUTRITIONAL ASSESSMENT

A thorough and comprehensive nutritional assessment performed by care providers at clinical visits is essential in the management of patients with CF (**Fig. 2**). Anthropometric data, including weight, height, and BMI, should be carefully followed at each clinic visit. Routine assessments of these parameters allow for early detection of problems and subsequent early interventions. The CF Foundation recommends that children and adults with CF have quarterly visits to CF care centers. For children, anthropometric data should be plotted on a standard Centers for Disease Control and Prevention growth chart at each clinic visit, whereas the weight, height, and BMI should be charted in adults. In addition, a thorough dietary history and evaluation for other comorbidities, such as bone disease, CFRD, and CF-related liver disease, should be assessed.[8] Routine laboratory evaluation is important to assess nutritional status. Patients with pancreatic insufficiency are at risk for fat-soluble vitamin deficiency. Vitamin D (25-hydroxyvitamin [25-OH] vitamin D), vitamin A (retinol), vitamin E (alpha-tocopherol), and vitamin K (proteins induced by vitamin K absence or antagonism [PIVKA-II] or prothrombin time) levels should be assessed at least yearly. Protein stores, specifically albumin and prealbumin, can be assessed yearly and more frequently in those patients with nutritional failure or those at risk for malnutrition. Evaluation of essential fatty acid status should be considered in patients with malnutrition. Yearly comprehensive metabolic profiles and complete blood counts allow monitoring for evidence of anemia, electrolyte abnormalities, and liver and kidney function.

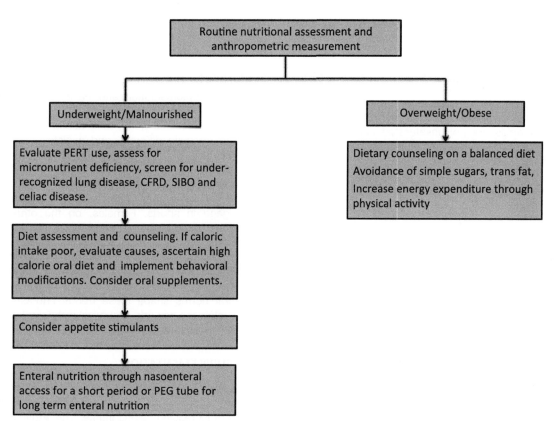

Fig. 2. Suggested algorithm for the nutritional management in CF. CFRD, CF-related diabetes; PEG, percutaneous endoscopic gastrostomy; SIBO, small intestinal bacterial overgrowth.

ENERGY INTAKE, VITAMIN AND MINERAL SUPPLEMENTATION

Adequate energy intake is essential in patients with CF, especially those with pancreatic insufficiency. The recommendation for caloric intake in individuals with CF ranges from 110% to 120% of the estimated average intake of which 35% to 40% is recommended to be from fat.[9] Several pediatric and adult studies indicate that most patients with CF do not achieve the recommended energy intake[41–46] despite having a higher absolute caloric intake compared with healthy individuals. In a study that compared the dietary intake of children with CF with healthy controls, the consumption of saturated fat was found to be well greater than 10% of the total energy intake in patients with CF.[46] This increased consumption of saturated fats may place patients at increased risk of hypercholesterolemia/hypertriglyceridemia and its subsequent comorbidities later in life.

Pancreatic Enzyme Replacement Therapy

PERT is essential to improve fat malabsorption in pancreatic-insufficient patients. Although individual dosing varies, attention should be made to clinical symptoms of steatorrhea, failure to gain weight, abdominal pain, and bloating. Current guidelines recommend that PERT dosing should be less than 2500 lipase units per kilogram per meal and less than 10,000 lipase units per kilogram per day to prevent occurrence of fibrosing colonopathy.[47,48]

Fat-Soluble Vitamins

Patients with CF, especially those with pancreatic insufficiency, are at risk for fat-soluble vitamin malabsorption. Up to 40% of patients with CF have been shown to be deficient in vitamin D. Vitamin E acts as an antioxidant and prevents cell membrane damage. Because of its antioxidant properties, deficiency in this enzyme may promote inflammation and further contribute to CF-related lung disease. Vitamin A plays an important role in vision, growth, and immune function and has been found to be deficient in up to 40% of patients with CF in cross-sectional studies.[49] Vitamin K deficiency can result in coagulation abnormalities, and stores can be assessed by a prothrombin time or international normalized ratio (INR); however,

PIVKA-II is a more sensitive measure of vitamin K stores. See **Table 1** for further information on fat-soluble vitamins.

Essential Fatty Acids

Essential fatty acid deficiency can be seen in both PS and insufficient patients with CF.[50] Essential fatty acids are polyunsaturated fats, which are metabolized to linoleic acid and alpha-linoleic acids.[9] Although some deficient patients are asymptomatic, others can have problems with alopecia, skin rashes, easy bruising, increased infections, and poor growth. Essential fatty acid deficiency should be considered when there is persistent poor weight gain and malnutrition. Essential fatty acids can be measured with a triene/tetraene ratio. However, serum linoleic acid concentration has been suggested to be a more clinically relevant biomarker of essential fatty acid status.[51] A Cochrane review in 2011 found that supplementation of omega-3 fatty acids in patients with CF may provide some antiinflammatory benefits that contribute to improved lung function.[52]

Sodium

Patients with CF are at increased risk for sodium depletion due to excessive salt losses through the skin. A high-salt diet is often recommended in children and adults, especially in summer months when sodium losses may be more significant. Serum sodium levels may not reflect the degree of sodium depletion because hypernatremia is insensitive and often a late manifestation. Measurement of urinary sodium and calculation of the fractional excretion of sodium were found to be more sensitive tests in a UK study that evaluated sodium requirements of infants with CF.[53]

Zinc

Zinc deficiency may present with poor weight gain, diarrhea, and dermatitis or may be asymptomatic. Plasma levels may not indicate adequate stores of zinc, and low zinc levels may influence vitamin A status in patients with CF.[54] In patients with persistent failure to thrive, an empiric trial of zinc supplementation for 6 months may be considered.[9]

BEHAVIORAL CONSIDERATION

In patients with malnutrition, and even those at risk for nutritional failure, intervention should be timely and closely monitored. In pediatrics, evaluation of mealtime behavior at all stages of development is important as problematic mealtime behavior can contribute to poor oral intake. Various behavioral

modifications and interventions, such as gradually increasing calories at an individual meal, negotiating with children regarding food choices, and identifying rewards for appropriate caloric intake, have improved dietary intake when paired with nutritional supplementation and have improved mealtime behaviors in children.[9] The challenges faced by adolescents and young adults are reported to be quite different, and a distinct sex gap exists at this stage. Males were reported to have poorer body images compared with females and strove to improve their weight and muscularity. Males were also more likely to exercise and engage in sports. Females, on the other hand, were found to be more content with their low body weight and were less likely to exercise.[55,56] There are also reports of intentional noncompliance with PERT by females to remain slender, and this could be expected with men. Sociocultural norms shape these trends and can partly explain the sex gap in survival with females at a survival disadvantage.[55]

ORAL SUPPLEMENTATION

For those patients in need of nutritional intervention, oral supplementation is the preferred initial method of increasing caloric intake. The addition of high-calorie supplements, such as oral protein energy drinks, to patients' current diets can be a starting point in an attempt to gain weight; however, they should not be considered essential. In a recent Cochrane meta-analysis, there was no significant difference between patients with CF receiving oral protein energy supplements or dietary advice alone in nutritional indices or lung function.[57]

APPETITE STIMULATION

Use of appetite stimulants may provide additional benefits in the short-term to help increase appetite and boost and/or maintain nutritional status in those patients with poor appetite. Cyproheptadine and megestrol have been shown to be effective in patients with CF with early satiety. Side effects associated with megestrol should be carefully considered before use.[58] A Cochrane Review in 2014 evaluating appetite stimulants for people with CF reported on 3 trials with a total of 47 patients comparing appetite stimulants with placebo. A meta-analysis of the trials showed that use of appetite stimulants resulted in a larger increase in weight z score compared with placebo (mean difference of 0.61 and a 95% confidence interval 0.29–0.93). There was no significant difference in FEV_1 between the study and placebo groups over

Table 1
Fat-soluble vitamins and micronutrients in CF

Vitamin/Mineral	Function	Deficiency	Laboratory Evaluation	Frequency of Evaluation	Additional Notes
Vitamin A	Vision, growth, immune regulation	Night blindness	Vitamin A level	Yearly Consider more frequent in liver disease	Treat it with the water-soluble form. Vitamin A can be an acute-phase reactant and falsely elevated during illness.
Vitamin D	Calcium absorption and bone growth	Osteopenia/osteoporosis	25-OH vitamin D level	Yearly Consider more frequent in liver disease	Treat it with cholecalciferol for levels <30 ng/mL. The minimum level should be at least 30 mg/mL.
Vitamin E	Antioxidant, prevents cell membrane damage	Hemolytic anemia, peripheral neuropathy, retinal changes	Alpha-tocopherol/ cholesterol ratio or alpha tocopherol/ total serum lipid ratio	Yearly Consider more frequent checks in liver disease	It can be affected by serum lipid levels.
Vitamin K	Key cofactor in coagulation pathway	Coagulopathy	PT/INR PIVKA-II level	Yearly Consider more frequent in liver disease	PIVKA-II is a more sensitive measure of vitamin K stores. It is important in bone health.
Calcium	Bone growth	Osteopenia Osteoporosis Bone fracture	Calcium level Ionized calcium	Yearly	It is not a sensitive indicator for calcium deficiency.
Zinc	Growth Immune function	Hypogeusia Can affect vitamin A status	Zinc level	Yearly Consider if FTT	Empirical trials of zinc can be considered in children younger than 2 y with unexplained FTT.
Sodium	Major cation in extracellular fluid	Hyponatremia	Sodium level	Yearly	It may require high-salt diets especially in summer months
Essential fatty acids	Antioxidant properties, immune function, growth	Failure to thrive in young infants	Triene/tetraene ratio Linoleic acid level	Consider in poor weight gain and malnutrition	It may have antiinflammatory properties that affect lung health.

Abbreviations: FTT, failure to thrive; PT, prothrombin time.

the course of the studies. Although short-term use of appetite stimulants in adults and children did improve weight and appetite in the patients studied, the conclusions were drawn from a small number of trials; therefore, use of appetite stimulants could not be conclusively recommended based on the findings of this Cochrane Review.[59]

ENTERAL SUPPLEMENTATION

When oral supplementation does not meet the necessary daily calorie requirements for adequate weight gain, use of enteral feedings should be considered. Introducing the idea of enteral feeds as a form of nutritional supplementation at an early age, before patients are nutritionally at risk, may help ease the transition to enteral feeds if the need becomes apparent. Standard formulas are usually well tolerated; however, hydrolyzed and elemental formulas may be an option in patients with gastrointestinal complaints such as diarrhea, abdominal pain, and bloating with standard formulas. Use of nocturnal feeds may help encourage better eating habits during the day. Although calorie goals are unique to each individual patient, it is common to start nocturnal feeds at 30% to 50% of the daily estimated energy requirements and then adjust formula intake based on patients' rate of growth.[9] It is important to monitor for complications when beginning enteral feeding regimens. Monitoring glucose tolerance and screening for glucosuria is important. Gastrostomy tubes are commonly used. Jejunostomy tubes are placed in patients with gastroparesis. Bolus feeds are problematic in patients with a jejunostomy tube. In cases whereby PERT has to be administered via an enteral tube, a larger-bore tube of at least 16F is recommended to avoid clogging.[60] Routine evaluation of the new gastrostomy tube site is important to check for leakage, skin breakdown, or infection. Use of PERT given orally before nocturnal feeds is recommended in the 2002 Consensus Report on Nutrition for Pediatric Patients. Additional doses may be required midway through and at the end of feeds.[9]

COMPLICATIONS OF CYSTIC FIBROSIS

CF directly or indirectly affects several organ systems causing disorders that range from bone disease, CFLD, pancreatic disorders, gastro-reflux disease, CFRD, and bacterial overgrowth. CFRD, CFLD, and bone health are briefly covered in this section.

Cystic Fibrosis–Related Diabetes

CFRD is one of the most common complications seen in CF, and it is reported in more than 30%

of patients with CF older than 18 years and 50% of patients older than 30 years.[61] A prediabetic state may exist before the onset of classic symptoms, and annual screening tests are recommended starting at 10 years of age using an oral glucose tolerance test. The pathophysiology underlying CFRD is distinct from that of type I and type II diabetes and seems to arise from progressive loss of islet cells due to pancreatic damage in addition to a component of insulin sensitivity. CFRD is associated with significantly increased morbidity and mortality in both children and adults, but early diagnosis and aggressive treatment over the past 15 years has resulted in significant reduction in mortality related to CFRD.[34,62] The onset of CFRD often correlates with a decline in pulmonary function, which may be related to the loss of the anabolic effects of insulin or due to the damaging effects of hyperglycemia.[63,64] Analysis from the CF Danish registry reveals that there is a decline in the weight and BMI of individuals with CF in the 4 years before the diagnosis of overt CFRD. This decline seems to be most prominent in adolescents 15 to 19 years of age.[65] Glucose intolerance that develops with gradual loss of the anabolic effects of insulin is thought to contribute to this decline,[65] which explains the improved nutritional status seen on initiation of insulin. However, pubertal growth and maximum height potential may not be achieved in children with CFRD even with early intensive insulin therapy.[66] Nutritional therapy is a crucial part of the management of patients with CF with CFRD. Caloric restriction normally recommended in diabetes is not an option for patients with CFRD who need to ingest sufficient protein and calories to maintain normal growth. In general, simple sugars should be avoided and substituted with complex carbohydrates in combination with fats and proteins. Not all patients with CFRD, however, are undernourished; dietary recommendations should be individualized. A recent study reported that among 115 adults with CFRD, 12.1% were overweight or obese.[67]

Bone Health

Bone disease is well documented in CF and is characterized by kyphosis, osteopenia, osteoporosis, and an increased rate of fractures. Studies reveal that 34% to 79% of patients with CF have a low bone mass density (BMD).[68,69] A recent study compared BMD between age-, race-, and sex-matched cohorts of young adults with CF in 2 time periods (1995–1999 and 2011–2013), 15 years apart. Despite improvements in clinical care and life expectancy, the study did not identify a significant difference in BMD measurements between the two cohorts.[70] Multiple risk factors, including malabsorption of calcium, hepatobiliary disease, and malnutrition, are involved in the pathogenesis of bone disease in CF. Furthermore, use of glucocorticoids and other medications, such as proton pump inhibitors, interfere with bone growth and development. Vitamin D functions to increase calcium absorption and, therefore, is important in bone growth. Up to 40% of patients with CF have been found to have vitamin D deficiency, which is probably an important contributor to bone disease in patients with CF. Those living in northern latitudes are at increased risk for further deficiency secondary to limited sunlight exposure. The CF Foundation recommends yearly determination of calcium, phosphorus, and 25-OH vitamin D starting at CF diagnosis. The desired range for 25-OH vitamin D levels is between 30 and 60 ng/mL. Those with levels less than 30 ng/mL should be supplemented orally with vitamin D3 (cholecalciferol).[71] Bone density should be assessed using DXA scanning starting at 18 years of age; however, if risk factors are present, screening should be performed starting as young as 8 years.

Cystic Fibrosis–Related Liver Disease

With increased life expectancy over the last 2 decades, hepatobiliary complications have become more common, with CFLD now being the third leading cause of death among patients with CF.[9] Impaired bile flow, cirrhosis, and hepatic dysfunction place patients at increased risk for malabsorption, fat-soluble vitamin deficiencies, and subsequent malnutrition. Patients with CFLD often require more frequent monitoring and higher doses of vitamins A, D, E, and K.[9]

SUMMARY

Patients with CF are at risk for malnutrition secondary to increased losses from malabsorption and increased energy demand from infections, chronic disease, and decreased oral intake. Complications including CFRD and CFLD place patients with CF at further risk for poor nutritional status. Optimizing growth and nutrition has a clear positive influence on lung health and overall survival. Comprehensive nutritional assessments at regular intervals are necessary to identify those at risk of nutritional failure even before malnutrition is manifested. Aggressive nutritional support should be implemented early, and patients should be monitored closely to ensure adequate growth and development.

REFERENCES

1. Peterson ML, Jacobs DR Jr, Milla CE. Longitudinal changes in growth parameters are correlated with changes in pulmonary function in children with cystic fibrosis. Pediatrics 2003;112:588–92.
2. Stephenson AL, Mannik LA, Walsh S, et al. Longitudinal trends in nutritional status and the relation between lung function and BMI in cystic fibrosis: a population-based cohort study. Am J Clin Nutr 2013;97:872–7.
3. Ledder O, Oliver MR, Heine RG, et al. Clinical audit results in earlier nutritional intervention in malnourished children with cystic fibrosis with improved outcome. J Paediatr Child Health 2015; 51(10):988–93.
4. Bronstein MN, Sokol RJ, Abman SH, et al. Pancreatic insufficiency, growth, and nutrition in infants identified by newborn screening as having cystic fibrosis. J Pediatr 1992;120:533–40.
5. Corey M, McLaughlin FJ, Williams M, et al. A comparison of survival, growth, and pulmonary function in patients with cystic fibrosis in Boston and Toronto. J Clin Epidemiol 1988;41:583–91.
6. Konstan MW, Butler SM, Wohl ME, et al. Growth and nutritional indexes in early life predict pulmonary function in cystic fibrosis. J Pediatr 2003; 142:624–30.
7. Yen EH, Quinton H, Borowitz D. Better nutritional status in early childhood is associated with improved clinical outcomes and survival in patients with cystic fibrosis. J Pediatr 2013;162:530–5.e1.
8. Stallings VA, Stark LJ, Robinson KA, et al. Evidence-based practice recommendations for nutrition-related management of children and adults with cystic fibrosis and pancreatic insufficiency: results of a systematic review. J Am Diet Assoc 2008;108: 832–9.
9. Borowitz D, Baker RD, Stallings V. Consensus report on nutrition for pediatric patients with cystic fibrosis. J Pediatr Gastroenterol Nutr 2002;35:246–59.
10. Steinkamp G, Wiedemann B. Relationship between nutritional status and lung function in cystic fibrosis: cross sectional and longitudinal analyses from the German CF Quality Assurance (CFQA) project. Thorax 2002;57:596–601.
11. Vandenbranden SL, McMullen A, Schechter MS, et al. Lung function decline from adolescence to young adulthood in cystic fibrosis. Pediatr Pulmonol 2012;47:135–43.
12. Hosenpud JD, Bennett LE, Keck BM, et al. Effect of diagnosis on survival benefit of lung transplantation for end-stage lung disease. Lancet 1998; 351:24–7.
13. Schwebel C, Pin I, Barnoud D, et al. Prevalence and consequences of nutritional depletion in lung transplant candidates. Eur Respir J 2000;16:1050–5.

14. Hollander FM, van Pierre DD, de Roos NM, et al. Effects of nutritional status and dietetic interventions on survival in cystic fibrosis patients before and after lung transplantation. J Cyst Fibros 2014;13:212–8.

15. Snell GI, Bennetts K, Bartolo J, et al. Body mass index as a predictor of survival in adults with cystic fibrosis referred for lung transplantation. J Heart Lung Transplant 1998;17:1097–103.

16. Forli L, Bjortuft O, Vatn M, et al. A study of intensified dietary support in underweight candidates for lung transplantation. Ann Nutr Metab 2001;45:159–68.

17. Fulton JA, Orenstein DM, Koehler AN, et al. Nutrition in the pediatric double lung transplant patient with cystic fibrosis. Nutr Clin Pract 1995;10:67–72.

18. Forli L, Pedersen JI, Bjortuft O, et al. Dietary support to underweight patients with end-stage pulmonary disease assessed for lung transplantation. Respiration 2001;68:51–7.

19. Madill J, Maurer JR, de Hoyos A. A comparison of preoperative and postoperative nutritional states of lung transplant recipients. Transplantation 1993;56:347–50.

20. Kalnins D, Pencharz PB, Grasemann H, et al. Energy expenditure and nutritional status in pediatric patients before and after lung transplantation. J Pediatr 2013;163:1500–2.

21. Magoffin A, Allen JR, McCauley J, et al. Longitudinal analysis of resting energy expenditure in patients with cystic fibrosis. J Pediatr 2008;152:703–8.

22. Thomson MA, Wilmott RW, Wainwright C, et al. Resting energy expenditure, pulmonary inflammation, and genotype in the early course of cystic fibrosis. J Pediatr 1996;129:367–73.

23. Moudiou T, Galli-Tsinopoulou A, Vamvakoudis E, et al. Resting energy expenditure in cystic fibrosis as an indicator of disease severity. J Cyst Fibros 2007;6:131–6.

24. Allen JR, McCauley JC, Selby AM, et al. Differences in resting energy expenditure between male and female children with cystic fibrosis. J Pediatr 2003;142:15–9.

25. Stallings VA, Tomezsko JL, Schall JI, et al. Adolescent development and energy expenditure in females with cystic fibrosis. Clin Nutr 2005;24:737–45.

26. Barclay A, Allen JR, Blyler E, et al. Resting energy expenditure in females with cystic fibrosis: is it affected by puberty? Eur J Clin Nutr 2007;61:1207–12.

27. Moudiou T, Galli-Tsinopoulou A, Nousia-Arvanitakis S. Effect of exocrine pancreatic function on resting energy expenditure in cystic fibrosis. Acta Paediatr 2007;96:1521–5.

28. Pencharz PB, Durie PR. Pathogenesis of malnutrition in cystic fibrosis, and its treatment. Clin Nutr 2000;19:387–94.

29. Lai HC, Kosorok MR, Laxova A, et al. Nutritional status of patients with cystic fibrosis with meconium ileus: a comparison with patients without meconium ileus and diagnosed early through neonatal screening. Pediatrics 2000;105:53–61.

30. Lisowska A, Wójtowicz J, Walkowiak J, et al. Small intestine bacterial overgrowth is frequent in cystic fibrosis: combined hydrogen and methane measurements are required for its detection. Acta Biochim Pol 2009;56:631–4.

31. De Lisle RC. Altered transit and bacterial overgrowth in the cystic fibrosis mouse small intestine. Am J Physiol Gastrointest Liver Physiol 2007;293:G104–11.

32. Ehre C, Ridley C, Thornton DJ. Cystic fibrosis: an inherited disease affecting mucin-producing organs. Int J Biochem Cell Biol 2014;52:136–45.

33. Murphy JL, Wootton SA, Bond SA, et al. Energy content of stools in normal healthy controls and patients with cystic fibrosis. Arch Dis Child 1991;66:495–500.

34. Moran A, Dunitz J, Nathan B, et al. Cystic fibrosis-related diabetes: current trends in prevalence, incidence, and mortality. Diabetes Care 2009;32:1626–31.

35. Hanna RM, Weiner DJ. Overweight and obesity in patients with cystic fibrosis: a center-based analysis. Pediatr Pulmonol 2015;50:35–41.

36. Coderre L, Fadainia C, Belson L, et al. LDL-cholesterol and insulin are independently associated with body mass index in adult cystic fibrosis patients. J Cyst Fibros 2012;11:393–7.

37. Kastner-Cole D, Palmer CN, Ogston SA, et al. Overweight and obesity in deltaF508 homozygous cystic fibrosis. J Pediatr 2005;147:402–4.

38. Rhodes B, Nash EF, Tullis E, et al. Prevalence of dyslipidemia in adults with cystic fibrosis. J Cyst Fibros 2010;9:24–8.

39. King SJ, Nyulasi IB, Strauss BJ, et al. Fat-free mass depletion in cystic fibrosis: associated with lung disease severity but poorly detected by body mass index. Nutrition 2010;26:753–9.

40. Sheikh S, Zemel BS, Stallings VA, et al. Body composition and pulmonary function in cystic fibrosis. Front Pediatr 2014;2:33.

41. Engelen MP, Schroder R, Van der Hoorn K, et al. Use of body mass index percentile to identify fat-free mass depletion in children with cystic fibrosis. Clin Nutr 2012;31:927–33.

42. Powers SW, Patton SR, Byars KC, et al. Caloric intake and eating behavior in infants and toddlers with cystic fibrosis. Pediatrics 2002;109:E75–85.

43. White H, Morton AM, Peckham DG, et al. Dietary intakes in adult patients with cystic fibrosis–do they achieve guidelines? J Cyst Fibros 2004;3:1–7.

44. Moen IE, Nilsson K, Andersson A, et al. Dietary intake and nutritional status in a Scandinavian adult cystic fibrosis-population compared with recommendations. Food Nutr Res 2011;55.

45. Sands D, Mielus M, Umławska W, et al. Dietary pattern and its relationship between bone mineral

density in girls and boys with cystic fibrosis - preliminary report. Dev Period Med 2015;19:105–13.

46. Woestenenk JW, Castelijns SJ, van der Ent CK, et al. Dietary intake in children and adolescents with cystic fibrosis. Clin Nutr 2014;33:528–32.

47. Borowitz DS, Grand RJ, Durie PR. Use of pancreatic enzyme supplements for patients with cystic fibrosis in the context of fibrosing colonopathy Consensus Committee. J Pediatr 1995;127:681–4.

48. FitzSimmons SC, Burkhart GA, Borowitz D, et al. High-dose pancreatic-enzyme supplements and fibrosing colonopathy in children with cystic fibrosis. N Engl J Med 1997;336:1283–9.

49. Palin D, Underwood BA, Denning CR. The effect of oral zinc supplementation on plasma levels of vitamin A and retinol-binding protein in cystic fibrosis. Am J Clin Nutr 1979;32:1253–9.

50. Christophe AB, Warwick WJ, Holman RT. Serum fatty acid profiles in cystic fibrosis patients and their parents. Lipids 1994;29:569–75.

51. Maqbool A, Schall JI, Garcia-Espana JF, et al. Serum linoleic acid status as a clinical indicator of essential fatty acid status in children with cystic fibrosis. J Pediatr Gastroenterol Nutr 2008;47:635–44.

52. Oliver C, Jahnke N. Omega-3 fatty acids for cystic fibrosis. Cochrane Database Syst Rev 2011;(8):CD002201.

53. Coates AJ, Crofton PM, Marshall T. Evaluation of salt supplementation in CF infants. J Cyst Fibros 2009;8:382–5.

54. Van Biervliet S, Van Biervliet JP, Vande Velde S, et al. Serum zinc concentrations in cystic fibrosis patients aged above 4 years: a cross-sectional evaluation. Biol Trace Elem Res 2007;119:19–26.

55. Tierney S. Body image and cystic fibrosis: a critical review. Body Image 2012;9:12–9.

56. Habib AR, Manji J, Wilcox PG, et al. A systematic review of factors associated with health-related quality of life in adolescents and adults with cystic fibrosis. Ann Am Thorac Soc 2015;12:420–8.

57. Smyth RL, Rayner O. Oral calorie supplements for cystic fibrosis. Cochrane Database Syst Rev 2014;(11):CD000406.

58. Nasr SZ, Drury D. Appetite stimulants use in cystic fibrosis. Pediatr Pulmonol 2008;43:209–19.

59. Chinuck R, Dewar J, Baldwin DR, et al. Appetite stimulants for people with cystic fibrosis. Cochrane Database Syst Rev 2014;(7):CD008190.

60. Shlieout G, Koerner A, Maffert M, et al. Administration of CREON(R) pancrelipase pellets via gastrostomy tube is feasible with no loss of gastric resistance or lipase activity: an in vitro study. Clin Drug Investig 2011;31:e1–7.

61. Cystic Fibrosis Foundation Patient Registry. 2013 annual data report to the center directors. Bethesda (MD): Cystic Fibrosis Foundation; 2014. Available at: https://www.cff.org/2013_CFF_Annual_Data_Report_to_the_Center_Directors.pdf.

62. Kelly A, Moran A. Update on cystic fibrosis-related diabetes. J Cyst Fibros 2013;12:318–31.

63. Leclercq A, Gauthier B, Rosner V, et al. Early assessment of glucose abnormalities during continuous glucose monitoring associated with lung function impairment in cystic fibrosis patients. J Cyst Fibros 2014;13:478–84.

64. Hameed S, Morton JR, Jaffé A, et al. Early glucose abnormalities in cystic fibrosis are preceded by poor weight gain. Diabetes care 2010;33:221–6.

65. Koch C, Cuppens H, Rainisio M, et al. European Epidemiologic Registry of Cystic Fibrosis (ERCF): comparison of major disease manifestations between patients with different classes of mutations. Pediatr Pulmonol 2001;31:1–12.

66. Bizzarri C, Montemitro E, Pedicelli S, et al. Glucose tolerance affects pubertal growth and final height of children with cystic fibrosis. Pediatr Pulmonol 2015;50:144–9.

67. Brennan AL, Beynon J. Clinical updates in cystic fibrosis-related diabetes. Semin Respir Crit Care Med 2015;36:236–50.

68. Sheikh S, Gemma S, Patel A. Factors associated with low bone mineral density in patients with cystic fibrosis. J Bone Miner Metab 2015;33:180–5.

69. Conway SP, Morton AM, Oldroyd B, et al. Osteoporosis and osteopenia in adults and adolescents with cystic fibrosis: prevalence and associated factors. Thorax 2000;55:798–804.

70. Putman MS, Baker JF, Uluer A, et al. Trends in bone mineral density in young adults with cystic fibrosis over a 15 year period. J Cyst Fibros 2015;14:526–32.

71. Tangpricha V, Kelly A, Stephenson A, et al. An update on the screening, diagnosis, management, and treatment of vitamin D deficiency in individuals with cystic fibrosis: evidence-based recommendations from the Cystic Fibrosis Foundation. J Clin Endocrinol Metab 2012;97:1082–93.

Gastrointestinal Disorders in Cystic Fibrosis

David N. Assis, MD[a],*, Steven D. Freedman, MD, PhD[b]

KEYWORDS

- Cystic fibrosis • Reflux • Pancreas insufficiency • Pancreatitis • Dysmotility
- Distal intestinal obstruction syndrome • Constipation • Gastrointestinal malignancy

KEY POINTS

- Gastrointestinal reflux is common in cystic fibrosis (CF) and has unique pathophysiology in this setting.
- Effective management of pancreatic complications, including pancreatic insufficiency and pancreatitis in those with pancreatic sufficiency, is a key element of high-quality CF care.
- Determination of small bowel intestinal overgrowth in CF requires careful exclusion of other causes followed by empirical antibiotic therapy.
- It is necessary to distinguish between symptoms of chronic constipation and distal intestinal obstruction syndrome in patients with CF.
- Patients with CF have an increased rate of luminal gastrointestinal malignancies, and strategies for effective cancer screening in this population are needed.

INTRODUCTION

Gastrointestinal (GI) abnormalities are integral to the clinical manifestations of cystic fibrosis (CF). Indeed, the very first publication of CF in 1938 reported pediatric steatorrhea with unexpected cystic lesions of the pancreas.[1] Subsequent studies revealed that the CF transmembrane conductance regulator (CFTR) protein is expressed in all epithelia, including the GI tract. Congruent with this finding, the spectrum of GI presentation and disease severity is extremely wide in CF, even among patients with the same CFTR mutation profile. The past 2 decades witnessed fundamental advances in multidisciplinary CF management with remarkable improvements in patient survival and quality of life.[2] Despite this, the clinical burden of GI disorders in CF continues to be high and affects patients of all ages. Innovative drugs targeting the underlying CFTR defect were recently approved by the Food and Drug Administration (FDA) with a focus on improving pulmonary manifestations.[3,4] However, whether this therapeutic advance will also translate to GI manifestations remains unstudied. Therefore, ongoing and careful attention to GI presentations is essential for high-quality care to improve morbidity and quality of life in CF. This article focuses on clinical insights and the approach to GI disorders in CF by addressing key areas of greatest impact. Hepatobiliary manifestations of CF have been recently reviewed elsewhere.[5,6]

Disclosures: None.

Funding: The work of author D.N. Assis is supported by a grant from the Cystic Fibrosis Foundation: Developing Innovative GastroEnterologic Specialty Training (DIGEST).

[a] Section of Digestive Diseases, Yale School of Medicine, 333 Cedar Street, 1080 LMP, New Haven, CT 06510, USA; [b] Harvard Medical School, 25 Shattuck Street, Boston, MA 02115, USA

* Corresponding author.

E-mail address: david.assis@yale.edu

chestmed.theclinics.com

GASTROESOPHAGEAL REFLUX DISEASE

The estimated prevalence of gastroesophageal reflux disease (GERD) in North America ranges from 18% to 28%.[7] By contrast, epidemiologic studies of GERD in CF consistently show a much higher prevalence, ranging from 30% to 85%.[8–11] In clinical practice, GERD is one of the most common and challenging symptoms in patients with CF and can affect both children and adults.

Recently it was reported that 90% of reflux episodes in adult patients with CF occur during transient lower esophageal sphincter relaxation (TLESR), though the actual frequency of TLESRs was similar to controls.[12] Interestingly, reflux episodes occurred most often during the inspiratory phase of the respiratory cycle. The mechanism seems to be an elevated inspiratory negative intrathoracic pressure, with resulting increased gastroesophageal pressure gradients (GEPG). By contrast, the elevated GEPG of non-CF GERD is caused by increased intra-abdominal pressure, commonly associated with obesity. Therefore, GERD in CF is mechanistically distinct and may be partially induced by concurrent respiratory disease. However, the finding of GERD in infants with CF before the onset of lung disease argues for additional risk factors. Other potential mechanisms for GERD in CF may include frequent coughing, lack of esophageal clearance of digestive contents, and gastric dysmotility (especially regarding duodenogastric reflux of bile acids).

Although respiratory disease contributes to GERD in CF, reflux itself negatively impacts respiratory function. Reflux of gastric and duodenal contents often reaches the proximal esophagus in CF,[12] resulting in aspiration events. Indeed, gastric contents were commonly found in bronchoalveolar lavage fluid (BAL) of patients with CF.[13] Bile acids were detected in the sputum of 56% adult patients with CF, resulting in elevated airway inflammatory markers (neutrophil elastase) and a negative correlation with forced expiratory volume in the first second of expiration (FEV$_1$).[14] Additional studies suggest a relationship between GERD and lung decline in adults and children with CF.[15,16] Finally, acid reflux and associated gastric aspiration can negatively affect respiratory function after lung transplant, leading to chronic rejection.[17] This finding was illustrated in one series whereby 60% of patients with CF who received a lung transplant had bile acids measured in BAL fluid.[13]

As a result, all patients with CF should be carefully interviewed with questions regarding GERD symptoms, which may go unreported. Patients with reflux symptoms should be given a trial of an acid-suppressing therapy, either a proton pump inhibitor (PPI) or a histamine 2 receptor (H2R) antagonist, and assessed for response within several weeks. Furthermore, patients with CF with unexplained decline in lung function may be considered for a trial of acid suppression, though invasive testing with pH impedance for asymptomatic patients may yield false-negative results and is, thus, not advised.[18]

Registry data suggest that at least 50% of patients with CF are treated with PPI therapy,[11] and the rate is nearly universal following lung transplant. Recent studies have raised concerns about PPI use, including a small increased risk of pneumonia and *Clostridium difficile* infections.[19] Although this has not been clearly demonstrated in the setting of CF, there should be ongoing assessment of the need for PPI in the clinic. A retrospective analysis of more than 200 pediatric patients with CF demonstrated that acid suppression slowed the rate of decline in lung function.[20] In contrast, a small, randomized 36-week study of esomeprazole for adults with CF and GERD did not demonstrate an impact on pulmonary exacerbations or an effect on FEV$_1$ compared with placebo.[21] Some patients with refractory GERD may respond to combination of PPI and H2R blocker therapy. The recently approved drug combination lumacaftor-ivacaftor may decrease the exposure and effectiveness of PPI therapy; thus, monitoring for increased GERD in these patients is warranted.[22]

Surgical fundoplication to prevent respiratory decline in CF-related GERD has produced mixed results in the literature. One pediatric study revealed no improvement in lung function and a recurrence rate of 48%.[23] By contrast, a study in 6 adults showed borderline significant improvement in FEV$_1$ after fundoplication.[24] Fundoplication in patients undergoing lung transplant has been more widely suggested as a method to prevent aspiration and chronic rejection (**Box 1**).

PANCREATIC INSUFFICIENCY AND PANCREATITIS

Exogenous pancreatic insufficiency (PI) in CF is almost exclusively diagnosed among patients with class I, II, or III CFTR mutations.[25] Therefore, PI is associated with a more severe CF phenotype and overall disease progression. On cross-sectional imaging of a patient with CF, the finding of pancreas atrophy with replacement by fatty tissue is synonymous with PI. It is critical to identify PI as early as possible in the course of CF; if untreated, this results in major health decline through nutritional impairment, growth delay, mineral bone and vitamin deficiency, and dysmotility.[26] Furthermore, malnutrition in CF is strongly linked to

---

Box 1
Reflux

- GERD is common in patients with CF of all ages.
- The mechanism of GERD in CF includes increased intrathoracic inspiratory pressure from respiratory disease.
- GERD with proximal esophageal reflux may contribute to respiratory decline through aspiration.
- Aggressive pharmacotherapy with PPI and/or H2R antagonists is essential to reduce symptoms.
- GERD should be considered in patients with signs of post–lung transplant rejection; fundoplication may reduce rate of decline.
- Lumacaftor-ivacaftor use may reduce PPI effectiveness, and changes in GERD symptoms should be assessed.

---

subsequent decline in lung function and overall survival.[27],[28] Clinical manifestations of PI include steatorrhea, fat-soluble vitamin deficiency, poor growth in children, weight loss, or nonspecific abdominal symptoms, such as bloating, flatulence, and diarrhea.

PI was previously diagnosed with a 72-hour quantitative fecal fat collection using a cutoff of 7 g/d. Currently, the diagnosis is typically made by measurement of fecal elastase, which quantifies the elastase-3B serine protease enzyme.[29] A cutoff value less than 100 μg/g had a sensitivity and specificity of 100% in a pediatric CF cohort with PI,[30] whereas values less than 200 μg/g are generally diagnostic of non-CF PI. A value between 100 and 200 μg/g in CF may be nonspecific and should be investigated further. Other tests include measurement of serum trypsinogen, with a value less than 20 ng/mL consistent with PI. Lastly, a robust response to an empirical trial of enzyme replacement is highly suggestive of PI. Patients who were not diagnosed with PI but remain at risk should have yearly fecal elastase measurements for longitudinal monitoring of the exocrine function.

At least 85% of patients in the CF Foundation Registry take pancreatic enzyme replacement therapy (PERT).[11] Although this demonstrates the common occurrence of PI in this disease, it also reflects current standardized screening for CF in newborns with subsequent PERT initiation for nearly all at diagnosis.[31] Indeed, most patients with CF will develop PI, particularly those who are Phe508del homozygous; 87% of a cohort of more than 1000 patients had confirmed PI.[32] However, a recent study showed that 18% of patients with normal fecal elastase in early infancy continued to have normal levels at 1 year.[33] Therefore, serial fecal elastase measurements may be a valuable stratification tool to prevent misdiagnosis of PI and unnecessary PERT dosing.

Patients with CF and diagnosed PI should receive indefinite treatment with PERT. Enzyme preparations should be taken at the moment of initiating each meal or snack and should include adequate hydration. A typical starting dose is 500 units of lipase per kilogram per meal with a maximum per-meal dose of 2500 units of lipase per kilogram of body weight, with half the full dose used for snacks.[34] Several formulations of PERT are available and meet current FDA standards that were enacted in 2010. Frequent reassessment and dose adjustment through a multidisciplinary team including a nutritionist is critical. Inadvertent underdosing may result in steatorrhea and malnutrition, whereas supratherapeutic doses can lead to fibrosing colonopathy, a permanent fibrotic disorder. To avoid the risk of fibrosing colonopathy, the recommended maximum daily dose should be 10,000 units of lipase per kilogram.[34] However, this guidance is not evidence based; a recent publication questioned if these limits may provide insufficient doses to infants with PI.[35]

Pancreatic lipase is inactive in the acidic environment. Most currently available PERT products have enteric coating with acid suppressing film to ensure bioactivity in the duodenum. In addition, older literature suggests that ensuring a neutral duodenal pH of 5.5 or greater through acid suppression can improve effectiveness of PERT in patients who have persistent steatorrhea despite PERT.[36] However, a recent retrospective analysis of PERT clinical trials with pancrelipase/pancreatin did not reveal a need for adding acid suppression,[37] a finding that stands in line with existing treatment guidelines for PERT in CF.[38] Treatment goals are to relieve GI symptoms from PI, improve digestion, and promote adequate growth and development. Failure to improve should prompt questions about adherence to PERT and review of feeding habits and fat content in meals. It is important to alleviate potential fears that a more solid stool consistency due to PERT will result in intestinal obstruction, because this has not been found in available studies.

Although most patients with CF will ultimately develop PI, approximately 10% remain pancreatic sufficient (PS). These patients typically have milder lung disease, are nutritionally intact, and often are diagnosed with CF in adolescence or adulthood.[32]

Nonetheless, up to 20% of this patient subpopulation will develop acute pancreatitis. It is important to realize that only patients with preserved pancreatic tissue can develop pancreatitis. Thus, a diagnosis of PI with pancreas atrophy on imaging rules out the possibility of acute pancreatitis. A seminal study by Ooi and colleagues[39] characterized patients with CF who develop pancreatitis, demonstrating that they are older (median age 14.9 vs 9.3 years at diagnosis) and have milder CFTR mutations compared with PS patients without pancreatitis.

A growing body of literature suggests that acute pancreatitis is a 2-hit phenomenon in which the CFTR mutation may serve as a key contributor (**Fig. 1**). Even in patients with CF with PS and preserved pancreatic mass, bicarbonate flow through the pancreatic ducts is reduced.[40] Therefore, a variety of second hits may subsequently lower the threshold for pancreatitis. A study from Bishop and colleagues[41] showed that 40% of patients with idiopathic recurrent acute or chronic pancreatitis had at least one CFTR variant/mutation based on exhaustive CFTR sequencing compared with 22% of healthy controls. Importantly, 10% of those patients met the CF consensus statement criteria for the diagnosis of CF. Similarly, a study from Germany revealed that CFTR mutant alleles were twice as frequent in patients with idiopathic pancreatitis compared with healthy controls.[42] This finding suggests that patients with recurrent idiopathic pancreatitis should receive CFTR mutation analysis in conjunction with other genetic testing and risk factor assessments. Another study showed that although the frequency of pancreas divisum is not higher in patients with pancreatitis versus controls, it was significantly higher in patients with CFTR mutations who developed pancreatitis.[43] Finally, a very recent study of patients with acute alcoholic pancreatitis revealed a significant decrease in CFTR expression and localization, thereby suggesting that CFTR dysfunction can play a role in alcoholic pancreatitis.[44] Other potential agents include tobacco and drugs/metabolites.

Patients with recurrent idiopathic pancreatitis in which CFTR mutations are identified should undergo sweat chloride testing to rule out CF disease. Additional risk factors for pancreatitis should be addressed, such as alcohol and tobacco abuse and hypertriglyceridemia (**Box 2**).

DYSMOTILITY AND SMALL INTESTINAL BACTERIAL OVERGROWTH

Patients with CF may have slow transit time through the small intestine. One research group evaluated adult patients with CF with a magnetic-based motility tracking system and found that the pill reached the cecum by 7 hours in only 20% of patients compared with 80% of controls.[45] Another group also reported recently that small intestinal transit time was delayed in CF.[46] Interestingly, motility through the rest of the GI tract was not prolonged compared with controls. This localized small intestinal dysmotility in the setting of CF may specifically predispose to small intestinal bacterial overgrowth (SIBO). Indeed, several investigators have reported that SIBO is more common in patients with CF,[47,48] including one study in which the frequency was 56% compared with 20% in controls.[49] A history of prior bowel surgery also increases the risk for SIBO. One report demonstrated that patients with CF with SIBO did not have elevated fecal calprotectin, which suggests that the mucosal inflammatory phenotype may be distinct from bacterial overgrowth.[48] Finally, extensive antacid use for GERD management impairs physiologic gastric acidification, which may contribute to SIBO by preventing killing of environmental bacteria in the upper GI tract.

SIBO leads to numerous complications that are exacerbated in the setting of CF, especially in patients with PI. These complications include malabsorption of nutrients and vitamins, mucosal inflammation, increased mucus formation, and steatorrhea despite adherence to PERT. Patients may present with abdominal pain, bloating, nausea, and watery diarrhea. The diagnosis of SIBO was historically made through culture of duodenal aspirates during endoscopy. More recently, the hydrogen breath test has become the clinical standard. However, in CF there is a

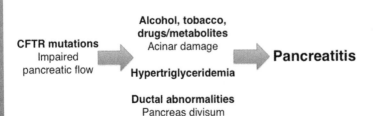

CFTR mutations
Impaired
pancreatic flow

**Alcohol, tobacco,
drugs/metabolites**
Acinar damage

Hypertriglyceridemia

Ductal abnormalities
Pancreas divisum

Pancreatitis

Fig. 1. Key contributors to pancreatitis in patients with CF.

Box 2
PI and pancreatitis

- PI affects nearly 90% of patients with CF.
- PI is associated with a more severe CF phenotype.
- Early detection and initiation of PERT can prevent complications (ie, malnutrition and decline in lung function).
- PS patients are older and have milder CFTR mutations and overall disease course.
- PS patients with CF have a 20% risk of pancreatitis.
- Patients with CF may develop pancreatitis from an additional trigger (ie, alcohol, drugs, hypertriglyceridemia), which should be minimized.
- Patients with idiopathic recurrent pancreatitis often have unrecognized CFTR mutations.

---

high baseline fasting hydrogen breath concentration, likely a sign of malabsorption and dysmotility from CF itself rather than a sign of SIBO.[50] Therefore, the standard breath test is considered to be highly inaccurate in the diagnosis of SIBO in CF. One study suggested that a combination of hydrogen glucose and methane breath testing could improve the chances of diagnosis.[51] Nonetheless, this is not considered a standard approach; most clinicians rely on clinical suspicion, empirical treatment, and assessment of response when dealing with suspected SIBO in CF.

A therapeutic trial of antibiotics for SIBO is most commonly initiated based on persistent symptoms of bloating, flatulence, new malabsorption, and diarrhea of unclear cause. It is necessary to first rule out uncontrolled PI as well as *C difficile* diarrhea. Empirical antibiotic use typically consists of oral metronidazole or rifaximin. Fortunately, these drugs do not interact with the antibiotic regimens used in respiratory tract infections and, thus, should not result in future resistance of airway pathogens. However, clinical trials demonstrating efficacy of these drugs for SIBO in CF are lacking. One small study of patients with CF with SIBO administered oral ciprofloxacin and reported improved fat absorption.[52]

Future treatment options for SIBO in CF might also include probiotic regimens. However, there is currently insufficient evidence to support the use of probiotics in the management of SIBO. One Spanish study gave *Lactobacillus rhamnosus* GG, 10^{11} colony-forming units to children with CF reporting a small improvement in symptoms as well as fecal content of undigested sugars and fat.[53] The rapidly growing literature on the positive effects of probiotics on intestinal inflammation[54–57] and respiratory tract in CF[58] should be highlighted, although these trials did not specifically evaluate patients with SIBO. Further investigation into the mechanistic differences between CF with and without SIBO is warranted (**Box 3**).

DISTAL INTESTINAL OBSTRUCTION SYNDROME AND CONSTIPATION

Distal intestinal obstruction (DIOS) is a specific and unique complication of CF. DIOS is defined as the acute onset of abdominal pain and/or distension, a fecal mass in the ileocecal area, and concurrent small bowel dilation with or without air-fluid levels on imaging.[59] A change in bowel movement frequency may or may not be present. On imaging, the fecal matter often has a bubbling appearance in the right lower quadrant with proximal dilation (**Fig. 2**). Patients with acute pain and a fecal mass in the ileocecum but without obstructive or dilated bowel may have impending DIOS. In pediatrics the incidence is estimated at 6.2 per 1000 patient-years and usually affects PI patients,

---

Box 3
Dysmotility and SIBO

- Patients with CF frequently have specific slow transit in the small intestine.
- SIBO is common in CF, and the relationship to intestinal inflammation is unclear.
- Risk factors for SIBO include dysmotility, PI, and prior bowel surgery.
- The hydrogen glucose breath test is inadequate for SIBO diagnosis in CF because of the elevated baseline levels from malabsorption.
- Empirical antibiotic trials of oral metronidazole or rifaximin is not evidence based in CF but may be effective.
- There is insufficient evidence for the use of probiotics in management of SIBO.

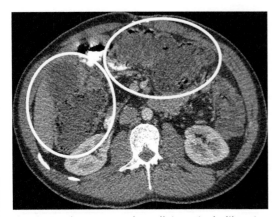

Fig. 2. Fecal matter and small intestinal dilatation seen on CT imaging.

although PS patients are also at risk.[59] Adults, however, are at a much higher risk of DIOS compared with children, with a reported incidence of 35.5 per 1000 patient-years.[60,61] The reason for this nearly 6-fold increase in incidence among adolescents and adults is unclear; one unproven speculation is that adherence to PERT may decrease over time.

The mechanism of DIOS is the accumulation of viscid luminal material, composed of mucus and undigested food contents, which strongly adheres to villi and crypts within the small intestine. This accumulation is worsened by decreased luminal water secretion due to impaired CFTR and exacerbated by dehydration. Gut dysmotility in the small intestine, and disruption of bile acid-induced terminal ileal secretion, have been proposed as additional mechanisms. Although one study reported that patients with DIOS have decreased lung function compared with controls, a mechanistic relationship has not been identified.[62] In addition to PERT nonadherence, other risk factors include history of meconium ileus at birth, prior history of DIOS, dehydration, mucosal inflammation, opiate use for pain control, and decreased absorption of dietary fat.

Suspicion for DIOS should lead to prompt medical assessment, imaging, and management to avoid complications and relieve the obstruction. Special care should be taken to prevent aspiration in obstructed patients who are vomiting. If there is imaging evidence of a complete obstruction, surgical evaluation should be requested. In most instances of partial obstruction, DIOS responds to aggressive medical management with intravenous hydration and oral laxatives containing polyethylene glycol 3350 (PEG). Lavage with PEG preparations can also be used. Lactulose is less optimal in this setting because of the frequent bloating and flatulence. Water-soluble contrast enemas based on sodium meglumine diatrizoate

have long been used when oral intake is held because of full obstruction in DIOS and can be given twice daily.[60] In large volumes, they effectively reflux into the terminal ileum and relieve the site of obstruction. In less than 5% of patients, emergent surgical intervention in the form of a cecotomy or small bowel resection is needed because of failure of medical measures or evidence of bowel ischemia. Long-term prevention of recurrent DIOS is critical and centers around efforts to maximize PERT dosing, increase fluid intake, and the addition of routine laxative preparations to counteract stool retention.

The main differential diagnosis of DIOS is discomfort from constipation. Chronic constipation in CF is characterized by frequent or ongoing abdominal pain, instead of abrupt symptoms, and by the absence of small bowel dilation on imaging. Further, imaging in patients with CF with chronic constipation often shows copious stool in the colon; however, it is diffuse rather than focal at the ileocecum. There is no evidence that constipation is more common in patients with CF than the general population. Many patients with chronic constipation may have daily bowel movements and may not require additional dietary fiber, as is the case in the non-CF population. Management of constipation in CF is based on regular intake of osmotic laxative solutions. One small short-term pilot study in adults with CF suggested symptomatic response to the type 2 chloride channel activating agent lubiprostone, which increases luminal water secretion.[63] However, this has not yet been studied sufficiently in children; no randomized studies have been conducted to date (**Box 4**).

Box 4
DIOS and constipation

- DIOS is the acute onset of abdominal pain, distension, a fecal mass in the ileocecum. and radiographic signs of distal small bowel distension or obstruction.

- Risk factors include nonadherence to PERT, dehydration, and opiate use.

- Prompt medical evaluation is required, including aggressive hydration and laxatives with PEG-based solutions.

- Patients with obstruction may benefit from meglumine diatrizoate enemas.

- Surgical intervention is rare but necessary if there is persistent obstruction or ischemia.

- Chronic constipation is clinically distinct from DIOS and should be managed with osmotic laxatives.

GASTROINTESTINAL MALIGNANCY

The overall cancer risk in CF is similar to that of the general population according to an analysis of more than 40,000 US patients.[64] However, the specific incidence of luminal GI malignancy was increased with a risk ratio of 3.5 (45.0 observed vs 26.8 expected). A disproportionate risk of GI cancers was also reported in a large study of patients with CF from both the United States and Europe.[65] The risk seems to be particularly increased in patients who receive transplantation, likely because of chronic immunosuppression use. Sites of GI malignancy include the esophagus, stomach, biliary tract, small bowel, and colon. Colon cancer is, for unclear reasons, the most frequent site by far, with a risk ratio of 6.2.[64]

The pathophysiology of malignancy in CF is not known but likely results from persistent inflammation generated or exacerbated by the CFTR absence in epithelial tissues. In fact, malignancies reported in CF originate in locations that normally have high CFTR expression. A very recent study of pediatric patients CF with PI revealed strong evidence of increased intestinal cell turnover, raising the possibility that this contributes to malignancy later in life.[66] However, the investigators did not find a relationship between a marker of cell turnover (M2-pyruvate kinase) and the inflammation marker fecal calprotectin. Although not conclusive, this suggests that these two purported mechanisms may act independently. Additional possible mechanisms include acid reflux (esophageal carcinomas), reduced mucin expression (lower GI tract carcinomas), and potentially the result of dysbiosis in the GI lumen.

Unfortunately, there is no evidence-based guideline at this time for GI cancer screening in patients with CF. This point is particularly important because patients with CF continue to live longer and, thus, cancer screening becomes increasingly relevant. Therefore, clinicians should maintain a high index of suspicion for any patient with CF with persistent or concerning manifestations of any GI disorder. Adults with refractory GERD or unexplained new upper GI symptoms should be considered for upper endoscopy to exclude Barrett esophagus. Furthermore, given the clear colon cancer risk, early screening colonoscopies may be appropriate for some subgroups, such as those older than 40 years or after transplantation. One recent single-center study of 45 patients with nontransplanted CF with a mean age of 47 years who underwent screening colonoscopy revealed an elevated number of adenomatous polyps, particularly in men with a median of 5 per positive examination.[67] However, when considering screening

---

Box 5
GI malignancies

- GI malignancy risk is increased in CF, especially after transplantation.
- Colon cancers are most frequent, but the entire GI tract is at risk.
- Mechanisms likely include persistent inflammation and high cell turnover as well as dysbiosis.
- A high index of suspicion is needed for new, concerning, or unresolved symptoms.
- There is an urgent need for GI cancer screening guidelines specific to CF.
- Pulmonary function should be carefully assessed before any endoscopic procedure.
- Additional bowel preparation may be needed for colonoscopies.

---

endoscopic procedures for pretransplant patients with advanced respiratory disease it is important to closely determine the risk of pulmonary decompensation during anesthesia and work closely with their CF providers. Furthermore, many patients with CF have difficulty achieving adequate bowel preparation due in part to dysmotility and PI. Therefore, standard protocols may be insufficient to achieve a good preparation and extended regimens may be necessary (**Box 5**).

SUMMARY AND FUTURE CONSIDERATIONS

In this new era of targeted therapy with improvements in respiratory disease, clear opportunities exist to study the effect of CFTR-modulating treatments for CF-related GI disorders. Before these efforts can be successfully undertaken, a fundamental knowledge of the clinical manifestations, disease spectrum, and management of relevant GI manifestations is critical. Only then will clinicians and researchers be positioned to appropriately select patients who are likely to benefit from CFTR-modulating therapies. Furthermore, there is a need to define and validate clinical surrogates and end points for GI disorders in CF by which to assess for meaningful clinical improvements. The challenge of determining this was discussed by a recent international working group.[68] Finally, close attention to epidemiology, presentation, and longitudinal therapy is essential for clinicians taking care of patients with CF. With increasing average survival of patients well past the fourth decade of life, adult GI providers will need to acquire increasing knowledge and experience in order to provide high-quality care to this community.

REFERENCES

1. Andersen D. Cystic fibrosis of the pancreas and its relation to celiac disease: a clinical and pathologic study. Am J Dis Child 1938;56(2):344–99.
2. MacKenzie T, Gifford AH, Sabadosa KA, et al. Longevity of patients with cystic fibrosis in 2000 to 2010 and beyond: survival analysis of the Cystic Fibrosis Foundation patient registry. Ann Intern Med 2014;161(4):233–41.
3. Ramsey BW, Davies J, McElvaney NG, et al. A CFTR potentiator in patients with cystic fibrosis and the G551D mutation. N Engl J Med 2011;365(18):1663–72.
4. Wainwright CE, Elborn JS, Ramsey BW, et al. Lumacaftor-ivacaftor in patients with cystic fibrosis homozygous for Phe508del CFTR. N Engl J Med 2015;373(3):220–31.
5. Flass T, Narkewicz MR. Cirrhosis and other liver disease in cystic fibrosis. J Cyst Fibros 2013;12(2):116–24.
6. Colombo C. Liver disease in cystic fibrosis. Curr Opin Pulm Med 2007;13(6):529–36.
7. El-Serag HB, Sweet S, Winchester CC, et al. Update on the epidemiology of gastro-oesophageal reflux disease: a systematic review. Gut 2014;63(6):871–80.
8. Sabati AA, Kempainen RR, Milla CE, et al. Characteristics of gastroesophageal reflux in adults with cystic fibrosis. J Cyst Fibros 2010;9(5):365–70.
9. Ledson MJ, Tran J, Walshaw MJ. Prevalence and mechanisms of gastro-oesophageal reflux in adult cystic fibrosis patients. J R Soc Med 1998;91(1):7–9.
10. Brodzicki J, Trawinska-Bartnicka M, Korzon M. Frequency, consequences and pharmacological treatment of gastroesophageal reflux in children with cystic fibrosis. Med Sci Monit 2002;8(7):CR529–37.
11. Foundation, CF. Patient registry, 2012 annual data report to the center directors. Bethesda (MD): Cystic Fibrosis Foundation; 2012.
12. Pauwels A, Blondeau K, Dupont LJ, et al. Mechanisms of increased gastroesophageal reflux in patients with cystic fibrosis. Am J Gastroenterol 2012;107(9):1346–53.
13. Blondeau K, Dupont LJ, Mertens V, et al. Gastro-oesophageal reflux and aspiration of gastric contents in adult patients with cystic fibrosis. Gut 2008;57(8):1049–55.
14. Pauwels A, Decraene A, Blondeau K, et al. Bile acids in sputum and increased airway inflammation in patients with cystic fibrosis. Chest 2012;141(6):1568–74.
15. Navarro J, Rainisio M, Harms HK, et al. Factors associated with poor pulmonary function: cross-sectional analysis of data from the ERCF. European Epidemiologic Registry of Cystic Fibrosis. Eur Respir J 2001;18(2):298–305.
16. Palm K, Sawicki G, Rosen R. The impact of reflux burden on Pseudomonas positivity in children with cystic fibrosis. Pediatr Pulmonol 2012;47(6):582–7.
17. Blondeau K, Mertens V, Vanaudenaerde BA, et al. Gastro-oesophageal reflux and gastric aspiration in lung transplant patients with or without chronic rejection. Eur Respir J 2008;31(4):707–13.
18. Robinson NB, DiMango E. Prevalence of gastro-esophageal reflux in cystic fibrosis and implications for lung disease. Ann Am Thorac Soc 2014;11(6):964–8.
19. Wilhelm SM, Rjater RG, Kale-Pradhan PB. Perils and pitfalls of long-term effects of proton pump inhibitors. Expert Rev Clin Pharmacol 2013;6(4):443–51.
20. van der Doef HP, Arets HG, Froeling SP, et al. Gastric acid inhibition for fat malabsorption or gastroesophageal reflux disease in cystic fibrosis: longitudinal effect on bacterial colonization and pulmonary function. J Pediatr 2009;155(5):629–33.
21. Dimango E, Walker P, Keating C, et al. Effect of esomeprazole versus placebo on pulmonary exacerbations in cystic fibrosis. BMC Pulm Med 2014;14:21.
22. Orkambi(R), Orkambi [package insert]. Boston: Vertex Pharmaceuticals; 2015.
23. Boesch RP, Acton JD. Outcomes of fundoplication in children with cystic fibrosis. J Pediatr Surg 2007;42(8):1341–4.
24. Fathi H, Moon T, Donaldson J, et al. Cough in adult cystic fibrosis: diagnosis and response to fundoplication. Cough 2009;5:1.
25. Ahmed N, Corey M, Forstner G, et al. Molecular consequences of cystic fibrosis transmembrane regulator (CFTR) gene mutations in the exocrine pancreas. Gut 2003;52(8):1159–64.
26. Baker SS, Borowitz D, Baker RD. Pancreatic exocrine function in patients with cystic fibrosis. Curr Gastroenterol Rep 2005;7(3):227–33.
27. Zemel BS, Jawad AF, FitzSimmons S, et al. Longitudinal relationship among growth, nutritional status, and pulmonary function in children with cystic fibrosis: analysis of the cystic fibrosis foundation national CF patient registry. J Pediatr 2000;137(3):374–80.
28. Konstan MW, Butler SM, Wohl ME, et al. Growth and nutritional indexes in early life predict pulmonary function in cystic fibrosis. J Pediatr 2003;142(6):624–30.
29. Borowitz D, Baker SS, Duffy L, et al. Use of fecal elastase-1 to classify pancreatic status in patients with cystic fibrosis. J Pediatr 2004;145(3):322–6.
30. Beharry S, Ellis L, Corey M, et al. How useful is fecal pancreatic elastase 1 as a marker of exocrine pancreatic disease? J Pediatr 2002;141(1):84–90.

31. Borowitz D, Gelfond D. Intestinal complications of cystic fibrosis. Curr Opin Pulm Med 2013;19(6): 676–80.

32. Durno C, Corey M, Zielenski J, et al. Genotype and phenotype correlations in patients with cystic fibrosis and pancreatitis. Gastroenterology 2002; 123(6):1857–64.

33. O'Sullivan BP, Baker D, Leung KG, et al. Evolution of pancreatic function during the first year in infants with cystic fibrosis. J Pediatr 2013;162(4): 808–12.e1.

34. FitzSimmons SC, Burkhart GA, Borowitz D, et al. High-dose pancreatic-enzyme supplements and fibrosing colonopathy in children with cystic fibrosis. N Engl J Med 1997;336(18):1283–9.

35. Borowitz D, Gelfond D, Maguiness K, et al. Maximal daily dose of pancreatic enzyme replacement therapy in infants with cystic fibrosis: a reconsideration. J Cyst Fibros 2013;12(6):784–5.

36. Tran TM, Van den Neucker A, Hendriks JJ, et al. Effects of a proton-pump inhibitor in cystic fibrosis. Acta Paediatr 1998;87(5):553–8.

37. Sander-Struckmeier S, Beckmann K, Janssen-van Solingen G, et al. Retrospective analysis to investigate the effect of concomitant use of gastric acid-suppressing drugs on the efficacy and safety of pancrelipase/pancreatin (CREON(R)) in patients with pancreatic exocrine insufficiency. Pancreas 2013;42(6):983–9.

38. Cystic Fibrosis Foundation, Borowitz D, Robinson KA, et al. Cystic fibrosis foundation evidence-based guidelines for management of infants with cystic fibrosis. J Pediatr 2009;155(6 Suppl):S73–93.

39. Ooi CY, Dorfman R, Cipolli M, et al. Type of CFTR mutation determines risk of pancreatitis in patients with cystic fibrosis. Gastroenterology 2011;140(1): 153–61.

40. Kopelman H, Forstner G, Durie P, et al. Origins of chloride and bicarbonate secretory defects in the cystic fibrosis pancreas, as suggested by pancreatic function studies on control and CF subjects with preserved pancreatic function. Clin Invest Med 1989;12(3):207–11.

41. Bishop MD, Freedman SD, Zielenski J, et al. The cystic fibrosis transmembrane conductance regulator gene and ion channel function in patients with idiopathic pancreatitis. Hum Genet 2005;118(3–4): 372–81.

42. Weiss FU, Simon P, Bogdanova N, et al. Complete cystic fibrosis transmembrane conductance regulator gene sequencing in patients with idiopathic chronic pancreatitis and controls. Gut 2005;54(10): 1456–60.

43. Bertin C, Pelletier AL, Vullierme MP, et al. Pancreas divisum is not a cause of pancreatitis by itself but acts as a partner of genetic mutations. Am J Gastroenterol 2012;107(2):311–7.

44. Maléth J, Balázs A, Pallagi P, et al. Alcohol disrupts levels and function of the cystic fibrosis transmembrane conductance regulator to promote development of pancreatitis. Gastroenterology 2015; 148(2):427–39.e16.

45. Hedsund C, Gregersen T, Joensson IM, et al. Gastrointestinal transit times and motility in patients with cystic fibrosis. Scand J Gastroenterol 2012; 47(8–9):920–6.

46. Gelfond D, Ma C, Semler J, et al. Intestinal pH and gastrointestinal transit profiles in cystic fibrosis patients measured by wireless motility capsule. Dig Dis Sci 2013;58(8):2275–81.

47. Lewindon PJ, Robb TA, Moore DJ, et al. Bowel dysfunction in cystic fibrosis: importance of breath testing. J Paediatr Child Health 1998;34(1):79–82.

48. Lisowska A, Madry E, Pogorzelski A, et al. Small intestine bacterial overgrowth does not correspond to intestinal inflammation in cystic fibrosis. Scand J Clin Lab Invest 2010;70(5):322–6.

49. Fridge JL, Conrad C, Gerson L, et al. Risk factors for small bowel bacterial overgrowth in cystic fibrosis. J Pediatr Gastroenterol Nutr 2007;44(2):212–8.

50. Schneider AR, Klueber S, Posselt HG, et al. Application of the glucose hydrogen breath test for the detection of bacterial overgrowth in patients with cystic fibrosis–a reliable method? Dig Dis Sci 2009;54(8):1730–5.

51. Lisowska A, Wojtowicz J, Walkowiak J. Small intestine bacterial overgrowth is frequent in cystic fibrosis: combined hydrogen and methane measurements are required for its detection. Acta Biochim Pol 2009;56(4):631–4.

52. Lisowska A, Pogorzelski A, Oracz G, et al. Oral antibiotic therapy improves fat absorption in cystic fibrosis patients with small intestine bacterial overgrowth. J Cyst Fibros 2011;10(6):418–21.

53. Infante Pina D, Redecillas Ferreiro S, Torrent Vernetta A, et al. Improvement of intestinal function in cystic fibrosis patients using probiotics [in Spanish]. An Pediatr (Barc) 2008;69(6):501–5.

54. Bruzzese E, Raia V, Gaudiello G, et al. Intestinal inflammation is a frequent feature of cystic fibrosis and is reduced by probiotic administration. Aliment Pharmacol Ther 2004;20(7):813–9.

55. Fallahi G, Motamed F, Yousefi A, et al. The effect of probiotics on fecal calprotectin in patients with cystic fibrosis. Turk J Pediatr 2013;55(5):475–8.

56. Bruzzese E, Callegari ML, Raia V, et al. Disrupted intestinal microbiota and intestinal inflammation in children with cystic fibrosis and its restoration with lactobacillus GG: a randomised clinical trial. PLoS One 2014;9(2):e87796.

57. del Campo R, Garriga M, Pérez-Aragón A, et al. Improvement of digestive health and reduction in proteobacterial populations in the gut microbiota of cystic fibrosis patients using a Lactobacillus reuteri

probiotic preparation: a double blind prospective study. J Cyst Fibros 2014;13(6):716–22.

58. Di Nardo G, Oliva S, Menichella A, et al. Lactobacillus reuteri ATCC55730 in cystic fibrosis. J Pediatr Gastroenterol Nutr 2014;58(1):81–6.

59. Houwen RH, van der Doef HP, Sermet I, et al. Defining DIOS and constipation in cystic fibrosis with a multicentre study on the incidence, characteristics, and treatment of DIOS. J Pediatr Gastroenterol Nutr 2010;50(1):38–42.

60. Colombo C, Ellemunter H, Houwen R, et al. Guidelines for the diagnosis and management of distal intestinal obstruction syndrome in cystic fibrosis patients. J Cyst Fibros 2011;10(Suppl 2):S24–8.

61. Andersen HO, Hjelt K, Waever E, et al. The age-related incidence of meconium ileus equivalent in a cystic fibrosis population: the impact of high-energy intake. J Pediatr Gastroenterol Nutr 1990; 11(3):356–60.

62. Dray X, Bienvenu T, Desmazes-Dufeu N, et al. Distal intestinal obstruction syndrome in adults with cystic fibrosis. Clin Gastroenterol Hepatol 2004;2(6):498–503.

63. O'Brien CE, Anderson PJ, Stowe CD. Lubiprostone for constipation in adults with cystic fibrosis: a pilot study. Ann Pharmacother 2011;45(9):1061–6.

64. Maisonneuve P, Marshall BC, Knapp EA, et al. Cancer risk in cystic fibrosis: a 20-year nationwide study from the United States. J Natl Cancer Inst 2013; 105(2):122–9.

65. Neglia JP, FitzSimmons SC, Maisonneuve P, et al. The risk of cancer among patients with cystic fibrosis. Cystic Fibrosis and Cancer Study Group. N Engl J Med 1995;332(8):494–9.

66. Pang T, Leach ST, Katz T, et al. Elevated fecal M2-pyruvate kinase in children with cystic fibrosis: a clue to the increased risk of intestinal malignancy in adulthood? J Gastroenterol Hepatol 2015;30(5): 866–71.

67. Billings JL, Dunitz JM, McAllister S, et al. Early colon screening of adult patients with cystic fibrosis reveals high incidence of adenomatous colon polyps. J Clin Gastroenterol 2014;48(9):e85–8.

68. Bodewes FA, Verkade HJ, Taminiau JA, et al. Cystic fibrosis and the role of gastrointestinal outcome measures in the new era of therapeutic CFTR modulation. J Cyst Fibros 2015;14(2):169–77.

Cystic Fibrosis Transitions of Care

Lessons Learned and Future Directions for Cystic Fibrosis

Megumi J. Okumura, MD, MAS[a,b,c],*, Mary Ellen Kleinhenz, MD[d]

KEYWORDS

- Cystic fibrosis • Adolescents • Young adults • Transition • Pediatric CF care • Adult CF care

KEY POINTS

- Youth with cystic fibrosis (CF) have an exceptional portfolio of resources through the CF Care Center Network to facilitate transition from pediatric to adult care.
- Collaboration between the pediatric and adult CF programs ensures a successful health care transition process and transfer to the adult program.
- Transition processes should start early with iterative evaluations of each patient for "transition readiness."
- Quality improvement efforts that address programmatic need and harmonize delivery of care between pediatric and adult programs may improve overall care delivery.
- Transition efforts can serve as valuable mechanisms to monitor self-care preparation, validate transition tools, and develop benchmarks for patients.

DEVELOPMENT AND IMPLEMENTATION OF A CYSTIC FIBROSIS CARE CENTER NETWORK TRANSITION POLICY

The growing population of adults with cystic fibrosis (CF) is not a chance occurrence. This exemplar of medical innovation and clinical success is the product of engaged, informed providers working in collaboration with multiple specialties and services. Survivorship is also attributed to the substantial investment in clinical research and basic science, as well as reliable, current data on health status and clinical outcomes, which has driven a culture of quality/process improvement.

In North America, specialized care of adults with CF dates to the 1970s. Adult CF care programs emerged at several academic medical centers participating in the CF Care Center Network. In 1993, these were the first 14 adult centers approved by the Cystic Fibrosis Foundation (CFF) through its accreditation body, the Center Committee. By 2000, the Center Committee required CF Centers with 40 or more adult patients to establish an Adult CF Program. By 2007, more

Disclosure: The authors have no financial disclosures to report.
[a] Division of General Pediatrics, University of California, San Francisco, 3333 California Street, Suite 245, San Francisco, CA 94118, USA; [b] Division of General Internal Medicine, University of California, San Francisco, 3333 California Street, Suite 245, San Francisco, CA 94118, USA; [c] Philip R. Lee Institute for Health Policy Studies, University of California, San Francisco, 3333 California Street, STE 265, San Francisco, CA 94118, USA; [d] Division of Pulmonary, Critical Care, Allergy and Sleep Medicine, Department of Internal Medicine, University of California, San Francisco, 400 Parnassus Avenue, San Francisco, CA 94143-0359, USA
* Corresponding author. Divisions of General Pediatrics and General Internal Medicine, University of California, San Francisco, 3333 California Street, Suite 245, San Francisco, CA 94118.
E-mail address: okumuram@peds.ucsf.edu

Clin Chest Med 37 (2016) 119–126
http://dx.doi.org/10.1016/j.ccm.2015.11.007
0272-5231/16/$ – see front matter © 2016 Elsevier Inc. All rights reserved.

than 96 adult CF programs were accredited by the center. In 2008, CFF introduced a requirement to transfer the majority of patients to adult care by 21 years of age. Currently, nearly all of the network's 113 centers in the United States offer care through an adult CF program.

Integration of adult CF care into the CF care model has been transformative and challenging. The CFF Center Committee expanded its membership to include clinicians experienced in the care of adults with CF. Annual grants to care centers from the CFF were increased with a supplement to support administration of adult CF care centers. Clinical practice guidelines for adult CF care were developed by the CFF to standardize adult-focused CF care.[1] The requirement for transition from pediatric to adult care, which was added in 2008, specified a process that included these elements: a formal plan of transition, annual meetings of pediatric and adult care teams, active transfer of patients to adult care to occur between the ages of 18 to 21 years, and a target goal that 90% of adult patients be transferred to the adult CF program by age 21 years.

CF centers were then left to individually develop mechanisms to implement health care transition without formal guidelines or well-tested tools. Fortunately, emerging evidence supports ways to improve transitions of care, with several centers evaluating, and subsequently developing, mechanisms to transition and transfer patients between pediatric and adult programs.[2,3] We review the current landscape for transition in the CF community and summarize current transition efforts and areas needing further work and research. To guide clinical practice, research, and policy, we then discuss the role of quality improvement initiatives as a means to improve transition of care for patients with CF.

What Has Transition From Pediatric to Adult Cystic Fibrosis Care Looked Like?

In 2008, fewer than one-half of CF centers in the United States and Canada reported formal programs to transition patients to adult care centers, although many had informal mechanisms to transition and transfer.[4,5] Several CF centers have published results of their experiences with transition improvement efforts.[6–9] Although these programs developed interventions unique to their centers, each program addressed both transition preparedness and assisting youth through the transfer to adult health care (eg, transition navigation). Some programs were patient focused, using transition readiness assessments, whereas others developed curricula as the basis for comprehensive programs.[2,9]

IMPROVING CYSTIC FIBROSIS TRANSITIONS

The literature describing transition from pediatric to adult health care reports a host of barriers encountered by aging children, and their families, with childhood-onset chronic diseases.[10] Some young CF adults have experienced adverse events as they transitioned to adult CF care, including hospitalization, new health morbidities, and disruption of care by patient nonadherence or loss of insurance. Although the morbidity associated with these events can be considerable, patients with CF, in fact, seem to fair better after transition than those with other chronic conditions, benefitting from the availability of dedicated CF health care systems.[11–13] Despite encouraging health outcomes for young adults with CF,[14] the need to improve transition services remains. Each CF center works from a different menu of potential transition resources (eg, availability of case management, available transition tools, overlapping institutional transition initiatives). Therefore, to allow adaptation to the unique needs of each program, the following sections are structured to address transition from the perspective of the patient, family, and provider.

The Patient

Part of the challenge in transition preparation derives from the complexity of CF therapy. Although a focus of transition programs for young adults with CF is to learn about their own health care needs and to become autonomous in managing CF care, the issues essential to "growing up" cannot be subordinated to health concerns. Work, relationships, reproductive health issues, and family planning emerge as important issues around the time of transition and transfer.[15] Concern regarding peer relationships may interfere with the execution of care regimens; for example, patients may avoid taking medications at school if they fear that doing so will make them seem "different" from other youth. Abstract thinking is poorly developed in these young adults, limiting the ability to plan and prepare for their medical needs.[16,17] Youth with CF share with their healthy peers a difficulty in anticipating the future consequences of current actions. The health consequences of avoiding intrusive care seem remote, and the pleasure of risky behaviors offset potential health consequences. Thus, assessing patient self-care readiness, medical regimen adherence, and mental health status are critical to the transition process.

Assessing patient readiness

Evidence suggests that the transition process should start early in youth to allow for the gradual acquisition of critical disease self-management skills.[18] Generic transition tools and measures such as GotTransition[19] have value in addressing school planning, housing, access to insurance and entitlements, and legal considerations[19] that are essential elements of the transition from youth to adulthood. Unfortunately, "developmental milestones" for CF self-care have not been established. Such benchmarks would guide progress in self-care, warn programs of deficiencies, and support remediation or contingency plans if the problem will persist after transfer of care. For example, developing criteria for when a child should be able to name medications, execute chest therapy, and/or report on symptoms would be important to standardize self-management skills and evaluate progress toward these milestones. Self-care scales to help monitor skill acquisition for patients with CF include the self-care Independence Scale[20] and the Transition Readiness Assessment Questionnaire.[21] These assessment tools provide potential mechanisms to evaluate how "prepared" a youth is to transition and to identify knowledge deficits that can be addressed. However, they do not replace the need for curriculum development and standardized education programs for CF adolescents and young adults in preparation for life as adults with CF.

Improving patient readiness

Resources for disease knowledge are available to families at CFF.org, but we currently lack transition preparedness curriculums for CF care. CF care is rigorous, time consuming, and complex.[22] It includes the setup and cleaning of devices, preparation of medications, administering multiple medications throughout the day (some with meals, some aerosols need to be in a specific sequence), and the potential for discomfort with some therapies. When unattended, the logistics and time burden of the daily regimen can overwhelm patients, prompting "burnout" and avoidance of treatment.[23] Therefore, having CF team members systematically monitor and address how a youth, rather than their parent, manages their complex CF treatment, and copes with the stressors that come with adherence to the medical program, is key through the transition period.

Mental health in young adults with cystic fibrosis

Depression is prevalent among adolescents as well as adults with CF.[24,25] In a recent study, symptoms of depression were found in 10% of adolescents and 19% of adults with CF. Anxiety afflicted 22% of adolescents, and 32% of adults with CF. Compared with the community, these conditions were 2 to 3 times more prevalent among CF patients. Among CF patients, depression increases hospital admission rates and associated costs by nearly 3-fold.[26] When depression and mental health burdens go unaddressed in patients with chronic illness and their families, self-management and adherence to adult care are neglected, leading to poorer health outcomes.[27,28] Therefore, annual screening of patients and families for depression and/or anxiety will be an important part of the transition process.[29,30] Existing team members can be trained to help patients and families navigate mental health issues and promote referral to mental health professionals when needed. To the extent that these mechanisms lead to improved self-management and care,[31,32] the negative effects of depression on adherence can be mitigated to promote long-term wellness in CF patients.

Adherence and burnout

Recent studies report fewer than one-half of CF patients consistently adhere to their full treatment regimen.[33] Older adolescents have a lesser adherence to medical regimens than younger children.[27] Poor adherence leads to increased hospitalizations and higher health care costs as compared with those with high adherence.[33] Numerous barriers to adherence are known: poor understanding of the consequences of nonadherence, depression, social stigma of having a chronic disease, forgetting to take medications, lack of time, lack of individual support, and poor family support.[34–37] Better measures of adherence and mechanisms to support reachable adherence goals are still necessary for young adults with CF.[38,39] Recognizing that problems with adherence are the norm for CF patients is an important first step toward a nonjudgmental approach from caregivers. Several options to improve adherence can be applied: screening adherence during visits,[40,41] adapting medication regimens to be less time consuming,[42] behavioral support through teleconferencing,[43] providing peer support,[44] building autonomy for youths from parents,[45] and/or improving family views of treatment. Development and testing of reliable mechanisms to address self-management and self-promoted adherence in young adults remains necessary if adherence is to become a lifelong practice for patients with CF.

Special populations: developmental disability

CF patients with developmental disabilities warrant special consideration relative to transition and transfer of care. Developmental disability superimposed on chronic disease adds a significant burden on families.[46] Patients with CF and developmental delay have multiple conditions that require case management and care coordination with specialists outside of CF centers. For such patients, the best approach seems to be nesting their CF-specific care plans within a broader framework that takes into account aging parents, potential residential care, and medical and social supervision.[47] Further work is required to understand how to assist families of aging children with developmental disabilities who also have CF. Regardless of developmental capacity, families need to be guided by individual patient needs with regard to conservatorship/guardianship, school transitions, and future home placement.[48]

The Family, Friends, and Significant Others

Establishing expectations that transition to adult care is the norm is especially important for parents nurturing a child with CF. Parental support is critical to ensure appropriate care delivery for children with CF; it demands knowledge, skill, time, and energy.[49] Standardization of patient self-care milestones would help CF centers to prepare parents in shifting their role from primary care givers to support figures. The early introduction of the transition plan and process within the CF Center reassures families that their extraordinary needs are anticipated and are addressed within the context of routine CF care. In addition, by including other persons who are important in a patient's life, such as significant others, friends, or roommates in the care plan, centers can improve patient disease management. Such partnerships provide the patient with emotional and medical support. By sharing responsibility for care with friends and significant others, the patient experience is improved.[44,50]

Cultural competency

CF transition care should accommodate the ethnic and cultural diversity of patients. The CFF has information in Spanish for Spanish-speaking patients with CF (www.cff.org/LivingWithCF/Espanol/). Family traditions and values may impact choices for CF patients. Concepts of family and expectations regarding how family members participate in health care delivery vary among cultural groups. Views of long term care (home care vs in-home support services), or reluctance to ask for family assistance may be rooted in cultural or ethnic norms.[51] Ensuring that families understand their options in caring for their adult children is as important as preparing the youth themselves.

The Provider

Historically, the dearth of adult-trained physicians knowledgeable about childhood-onset diseases was a barrier to CF care in age-appropriate settings by providers of adult health care. This asymmetry between pediatric and adult care has improved with incentives from the CFF to improve adult care provider capacity. For example, the Program for Adult Care Excellence Award inaugurated in 2008 provides 3 years of financial support, protected time, and mentorship for adult-focused providers to develop critical knowledge and skills needed for adult CF care.

Although provider capacity has improved, differences in approaches to care within pediatric and adult care models persist. Pediatrics follows a "family-centered," model whereas the adult health care model is more "patient centered." These differences can be jarring if, for example, parents are excluded from decision-making process and youth abruptly find they are expected to manage their decision making during transfer of care.[52] To avoid disruption of care related to these potential philosophic differences between pediatric and adult care, pediatric and adult providers must respect the difference in the culture of care and actively collaborate so the care can be seen as "seamless" by the patient and the family. Until a patient is successfully established within the adult CF program, assigning 1 member of the care team as "transition navigator" may be a helpful resource for the patient and providers.[53]

CLINICAL OUTCOMES: MEASURING SUCCESS IN TRANSITIONS

Measures of quality of life and patient/family experience of care now supplement the CFF Patient Registry's biometric and process data.[54,55] Even without a uniform transition process metric, capturing data from these instruments for patients and families preparing for transition (13–18 years), and in transfer (18–22 years), can be coupled with biometric (body mass index, percent forced expiratory volume predicted) and process measures (quarterly clinic attendance, hospitalizations) to capture a more comprehensive picture of how transition activities impacts patients and families. Metrics are needed to discriminate which children will succeed toward clinical independence and which youth risk failure. Tying together registry outcome data with current and future transition activities will be critical to understand what transition activities are related to the best clinical outcomes (**Box 1**).

TRANSITION AS A QUALITY IMPROVEMENT PROCESS

Centers that engage both pediatric and adult providers in the transition process have been able to

---

Box 1
Quality improvement: transition

1. Start the transition process early (age ≤11).

2. Ensure the youth has knowledge and understanding of his or her disease.

3. Ensure the youth knows how to manage his or her disease, and understands future contingencies for which he or she needs to prepare. This includes youth developing self-advocacy skills, learning to interact with adult health care providers, maintaining insurance, and planning on how the disease will affect future family planning, schooling, and vocational activities. For those with developmental disabilities, future planning will include designating who will be primarily responsible for the patient's health care needs. These activities can be operationalized through the development of a written transition plan.

4. Evaluate the transition preparedness of the youth. This can be done by assessing youths on their understanding of their diseases and their own self-efficacy in disease management, which can be facilitated through the use of available transition tools (www.gottransition.org).

5. Assess adherence, peer supports, and mental health.

6. Prepare youth and parents for the differences between pediatric and adult health care (in terms of expectations from patients as well as their providers). This includes discussion of the changing role of the parents during the transfer process. Activities such as developing "medical passports" or a "portable medical summary" can be helpful in this area. For those patients whose parents will need to be their primary caretakers, legal processes for power of attorney or medical proxy need to be discussed.

7. Ensure that the disease care and preparation during the transfer process is actively coordinated and discussed between the referring pediatric provider and the receiving adult provider. This may require a period where a patient is cared for by both pediatric and adult clinics.

8. Ensure transfer to adult care is completed. Clinics need to develop systems to monitor and follow up (either via case management or transition navigator) on failures to transfer. The goal is to attain a seamless transfer of care and proper follow-up with accountability by the medical teams.

---

sustain their work over the long term, improve their transition process, and decrease the stress perceived by patients as they transfer.[7,9] Although the CFF mandates a transition navigator, providers, case managers, social workers, nutritionists, and pharmacists individually and collectively have critical roles in preparing a family for transition. Patients vary in their need for overlapping of services from the pediatric and adult teams. Some patients benefit from latitude in returning to the pediatric clinic after episodes of treatment in adult care. Addressing transitions across pediatric and adult care programs is the opportunity to standardize expectations and care delivery.[6,56,57] Approaches to clinical problems can be harmonized across the center. This creates a perception of seamless care delivery for the patient and family.

Incorporating joint quality improvement efforts to address mental health care or adherence can help to resolve challenging issues for both pediatric and adult CF care teams. When quality improvement efforts are aligned, transition between pediatric and adult CF care is improved as an ancillary benefit.[41] The authors' CF center identified differences in the approach to nutrition

assessment and infection control as barriers to transition from pediatric to adult CF care.[9] By developing standardized approaches between pediatric and adult programs, we gave consistent messages to patients and families and we improved our center's rate of nutrition screening, created a pathway for glucose tolerance testing in the adult CF clinic, and facilitated implementation of the 2013 CF infection prevention and control guidelines.

FUTURE NEEDS AND CURRENT CAPACITY FOR MEASURING QUALITY IMPROVEMENT ACTIVITIES

CF-specific tools and guidelines to address transition still need to be developed and implemented. Consensus on developmentally based milestones for adolescents related to knowledge of CF and CF therapy and disease management skills would be a valuable shared resource for the care center network. Transition readiness should be tracked iteratively at developmentally appropriate intervals with a common, validated tool such as the Transition Readiness Assessment Questionnaire. Providing financial support for the center's transition navigation process would enhance commitment to the process and move centers toward standard transition approaches. Tracking self-care skills and transition readiness would underscore the normative nature of transition and provide for leverage for centers to address this developmental care process as a shared responsibility. Without a uniform approach to transition, it will not be possible to assess which mechanisms work and what are best practices of care. A selection of measures from the CF Patient Registry and the Experience of Care Survey are potential metrics for evaluation of system-wide patient outcomes as standards of care are implemented. Alternatively, standard approaches to transition and transfer could positively impact adherence, depression, and patient satisfaction measures. Standard transition models throughout the care center network would ensure that young adults with CF possess the life skills, motivation, and disease management tools necessary to sustain the improved health outcomes achieved in pediatric CF care.

SUMMARY

Over the course of 2 decades, the CF Care Center Network has developed adult CF programs to complement the pediatric programs in delivering life-long, disease-specific care to patients with CF. Engagement of pediatric and adult teams in the transition process, assessment of readiness for transition, development of transition curricula, and quality improvement approaches have helped individual care centers to improve the transition process. Standardization of the transition process represents a needed innovation in CF care. Although current clinical and research efforts have enabled our ability to improve transitions over the last 20 years, further work is required to understand how to ensure appropriate mental health services, transition services, and disease self-management and autonomy if we are to generate best practices in CF transitions of care and improve patient outcomes.[2,3]

ACKNOWLEDGMENTS

The authors thank Diana Dawson for her thoughtful insights to this article.

REFERENCES

1. Yankaskas JR, Marshall BC, Sufian B, et al. Cystic fibrosis adult care: consensus conference report. Chest 2004;125(Suppl 1):1S–39S.
2. Crowley R, Wolfe I, Lock K, et al. Improving the transition between paediatric and adult healthcare: a systematic review. Arch Dis Child 2011;96(6): 548–53.
3. McPheeters M, Davis AM, Taylor JL, et al. Transition care for children with special health needs. Technical Brief No. 15 (Prepared by the Vanderbilt University Evidence-based Practice Center under Contract No. 290-2012-00009- I). AHRQ Publication No.14-EHC027-EF. Rockville (MD): Agency for Healthcare Research and Quality; 2014.
4. Gravelle A, Davidson G, Chilvers M. Cystic fibrosis adolescent transition care in Canada: a snapshot of current practice. Paediatr Child Health 2012; 17(10):553–6.
5. McLaughlin SE, Diener-West M, Indurkhya A, et al. Improving transition from pediatric to adult cystic fibrosis care: lessons from a national survey of current practices. Pediatrics 2008;121(5):e1160–6.
6. Gravelle AM, Paone M, Davidson AG, et al. Evaluation of a multidimensional cystic fibrosis transition program: a quality improvement initiative. J Pediatr Nurs 2015;30(1):236–43.
7. Chaudhry SR, Keaton M, Nasr SZ. Evaluation of a cystic fibrosis transition program from pediatric to adult care. Pediatr Pulmonol 2012;48(7):658–65.
8. Steinkamp G, Ullrich G, Muller C, et al. Transition of adult patients with cystic fibrosis from paediatric to adult care—the patients' perspective before and after start-up of an adult clinic. Eur J Med Res 2001; 6(2):85–92.
9. Okumura MJ, Ong T, Dawson D, et al. Improving transition from paediatric to adult cystic fibrosis care: programme implementation and evaluation. BMJ Qual Saf 2014;23(Suppl 1):i64–72.
10. Lotstein DS, Inkelas M, Hays RD, et al. Access to care for youth with special health care needs in the transition to adulthood. J Adolesc Health 2008; 43(1):23–9.
11. Tuchman L, Schwartz M. Health outcomes associated with transition from pediatric to adult cystic fibrosis care. Pediatrics 2013;132(5):847–53.
12. McManus MA, Pollack LR, Cooley WC, et al. Current status of transition preparation among youth with special needs in the United States. Pediatrics 2013;131(6):1090–7.
13. Okumura MJ, Hersh AO, Hilton JF, et al. Change in health status and access to care in young adults with special health care needs: results from the 2007 national survey of adult transition and health. J Adolesc Health 2013;52(4):413–8.
14. Cystic fibrosis foundation patient registry annual data report 2013. 2013. Available at: www.cff.org/UploadedFiles/research/ClinicalResearch/PatientRegistryReport/2013_CFF_Annual_Data_Report_to_the_Center_Directors.pdf. Accessed June 20, 2015.
15. Frayman KB, Sawyer SM. Sexual and reproductive health in cystic fibrosis: a life-course perspective. Lancet Respir Med 2014;3(1):70–86.

16. Kazak AE, Alderfer MA, Streisand R, et al. Treatment of posttraumatic stress symptoms in adolescent survivors of childhood cancer and their families: a randomized clinical trial. J Fam Psychol 2004;18(3):493–504.

17. Suris JC, Michaud PA, Viner R. The adolescent with a chronic condition. Part I: developmental issues. Arch Dis Child 2004;89(10):938–42.

18. Tuchman LK, Slap GB, Britto MT. Transition to adult care: experiences and expectations of adolescents with a chronic illness. Child Care Health Dev 2008; 34(5):557–63.

19. The National Health Care Transition Center. Six core elements of health care transition. 2011. Available at: www.gottransition.org/UploadedFiles/Files/Six_core_Elements_PDF_Package1.pdf. Accessed April 1, 2015.

20. Patton SR, Graham JL, Varlotta L, et al. Measuring self-care independence in children with cystic fibrosis: the Self-Care Independence Scale (SCIS). Pediatr Pulmonol 2003;36(2):123–30.

21. Sawicki GS, Lukens-Bull K, Yin X, et al. Measuring the transition readiness of youth with special health-care needs: validation of the TRAQ–Transition Readiness Assessment Questionnaire. J Pediatr Psychol 2011;36(2):160–71.

22. Sawicki GS, Ren CL, Konstan MW, et al. Treatment complexity in cystic fibrosis: trends over time and associations with site-specific outcomes. J Cyst Fibros 2013;12(5):461–7.

23. Jamieson N, Fitzgerald D, Singh-Grewal D, et al. Children's experiences of cystic fibrosis: a systematic review of qualitative studies. Pediatrics 2014; 133(6):e1683–97.

24. Riekert KA, Bartlett SJ, Boyle MP, et al. The association between depression, lung function, and health-related quality of life among adults with cystic fibrosis. Chest 2007;132(1):231–7.

25. Quittner AL, Goldbeck L, Abbott J, et al. Prevalence of depression and anxiety in patients with cystic fibrosis and parent caregivers: results of the international depression epidemiological study across nine countries. Thorax 2014;69(12):1090–7.

26. Snell C, Fernandes S, Bujoreanu IS, et al. Depression, illness severity, and healthcare utilization in cystic fibrosis. Pediatr Pulmonol 2014;49(12):1177–81.

27. Logan D, Zelikovsky N, Labay L, et al. The illness management survey: identifying adolescents' perceptions of barriers to adherence. J Pediatr Psychol 2003;28(6):383–92.

28. Hilliard ME, Eakin MN, Borrelli B, et al. Medication beliefs mediate between depressive symptoms and medication adherence in cystic fibrosis. Health Psychol 2015;34(5):496–504.

29. Abbott J, Elborn JS, Georgiopoulos AM, et al. Cystic fibrosis foundation and European cystic fibrosis society survey of cystic fibrosis mental health care delivery. J Cyst Fibros 2015;14(4):533–9.

30. Nobili RM, Duff AJ, Ullrich G, et al. Guiding principles on how to manage relevant psychological aspects within a CF team: interdisciplinary approaches. J Cyst Fibros 2011;10(Suppl 2):S45–52.

31. Goldbeck L, Fidika A, Herle M, et al. Psychological interventions for individuals with cystic fibrosis and their families. Cochrane Database Syst Rev 2014;(6):CD003148.

32. Quittner AL, Barker DH, Snell C, et al. Prevalence and impact of depression in cystic fibrosis. Curr Opin Pulm Med 2008;14(6):582–8.

33. Quittner AL, Zhang J, Marynchenko M, et al. Pulmonary medication adherence and health-care use in cystic fibrosis. Chest 2014;146(1):142–51.

34. Koster ES, Philbert D, de Vries TW, et al. "I just forget to take it": asthma self-management needs and preferences in adolescents. J Asthma 2015;52(8):1–7.

35. Nagae M, Nakane H, Honda S, et al. Factors affecting medication adherence in children receiving outpatient pharmacotherapy and parental adherence. J Child Adolesc Psychiatr Nurs 2015; 28(2):109–17.

36. Santer M, Ring N, Yardley L, et al. Treatment non-adherence in pediatric long-term medical conditions: systematic review and synthesis of qualitative studies of caregivers' views. BMC Pediatr 2014;14:63.

37. Dziuban EJ, Saab-Abazeed L, Chaudhry SR, et al. Identifying barriers to treatment adherence and related attitudinal patterns in adolescents with cystic fibrosis. Pediatr Pulmonol 2010;45(5):450–8.

38. O'Donohoe R, Fullen BM. Adherence of subjects with cystic fibrosis to their home program: a systematic review. Respir Care 2014;59(11):1731–46.

39. Goodfellow NA, Hawwa AF, Reid AJ, et al. Adherence to treatment in children and adolescents with cystic fibrosis: a cross-sectional, multi-method study investigating the influence of beliefs about treatment and parental depressive symptoms. BMC Pulm Med 2015;15:43.

40. Riekert KA, Eakin MN, Bilderback A, et al. Opportunities for cystic fibrosis care teams to support treatment adherence. J Cyst Fibros 2015;14(1):142–8.

41. Wildman MJ, Hoo ZH. Moving cystic fibrosis care from rescue to prevention by embedding adherence measurement in routine care. Paediatr Respir Rev 2014;15(Suppl 1):16–8.

42. Mohamed AF, Johnson FR, Balp MM, et al. Preferences and stated adherence for antibiotic treatment of cystic fibrosis pseudomonas infections. Patient 2015. [Epub ahead of print].

43. Harris MA, Freeman KA, Duke DC. Seeing is believing: using Skype to improve diabetes outcomes in youth. Diabetes Care 2015;38(8): 1427–34.

44. Helms SW, Dellon EP, Prinstein MJ. Friendship quality and health-related outcomes among adolescents

with cystic fibrosis. J Pediatr Psychol 2015;40(3): 349–58.

45. Sawicki GS, Heller KS, Demars N, et al. Motivating adherence among adolescents with cystic fibrosis: youth and parent perspectives. Pediatr Pulmonol 2015;50(2):127–36.

46. Koehler AD, Fagnano M, Montes G, et al. Elevated burden for caregivers of children with persistent asthma and a developmental disability. Matern Child Health J 2014;18(9):2080–8.

47. Zakrajsek AG, Hammel J, Scazzero JA. Supporting people with intellectual and developmental disabilities to participate in their communities through support staff pilot intervention. J Appl Res Intellect Disabil 2014;27(2):154–62.

48. Shogren KA, Plotner AJ. Transition planning for students with intellectual disability, autism, or other disabilities: data from the National Longitudinal Transition Study-2. Intellect Dev Disabil 2012;50(1): 16–30.

49. Butcher JL, Nasr SZ. Direct observation of respiratory treatments in cystic fibrosis: parent-child interactions relate to medical regimen adherence. J Pediatr Psychol 2015;40(1):8–17.

50. Besier T, Schmitz TG, Goldbeck L. Life satisfaction of adolescents and adults with cystic fibrosis: impact of partnership and gender. J Cyst Fibros 2009;8(2):104–9.

51. McCubbin HI, Thompson EA, Thompson AI, et al. Culture, ethnicity, and the family: critical factors in childhood chronic illnesses and disabilities. Pediatrics 1993;91(5 Pt 2):1063–70.

52. Okumura M, Saunders M, Rehm R. The role of health advocacy in transitions from pediatric to adult care for children with special health care needs: bridging families, provider and community services. J Pediatr Nurs 2015;30(5):714–23.

53. Becher C, Regamey N, Spichiger E. Transition - how adolescents with cystic fibrosis their parents experience the change from paediatric to adult care [in German]. Pflege 2014;27(6):359–68.

54. Quittner AL, Sawicki GS, McMullen A, et al. Psychometric evaluation of the cystic fibrosis questionnaire-revised in a national sample. Qual Life Res 2012; 21(7):1267–78.

55. Hamilton IM, McCubbin MA, Patterson JM, et al. Coping health inventory for parents: an assessment of parental coping patterns in the care of the chronically ill child. J Marriage Fam 1983;45(2):359–70.

56. Nasr SZ, Campbell C, Howatt W. Transition program from pediatric to adult care for cystic fibrosis patients. J Adolesc Health 1992;13(8):682–5.

57. Nazareth D, Walshaw M. Coming of age in cystic fibrosis - transition from paediatric to adult care. Clin Med 2013;13(5):482–6.

Lung Transplantation for Cystic Fibrosis

Matthew R. Morrell, MD[a], Joseph M. Pilewski, MD[a,b],*

KEYWORDS

- Lung transplantation • Cystic fibrosis • Advanced lung disease • Respiratory failure
- *Burkholderia cepacia* • Nontuberculous mycobacteria

KEY POINTS

- Lung transplantation is a good option for many patients with advanced lung disease due to cystic fibrosis (CF), including patients with comorbidities, resistant pathogens, prior thoracic procedures, and liver disease.
- Early referral is critical for patient education and intervention for comorbidities, such as malnutrition, poorly controlled diabetes, and atypical infections that may increase the risk of posttransplant complications.
- Criteria for lung transplant for patients with CF vary significantly among transplant centers; thus, referral to multiple centers may be necessary to maximize opportunities for individual patients.
- Patients with CF and respiratory failure requiring mechanical support with ventilation and/or extracorporeal membrane oxygenation may remain viable candidates for transplant with outcomes comparable with other patients with CF.

BACKGROUND

Lung transplantation is a viable option for many patients with end-stage lung disease. Since inception, more than 47,000 adult lung transplantations have been performed worldwide, according to the most recent International Society of Heart and Lung Transplantation report.[1] Despite the development of newer cystic fibrosis (CF) therapies and improved delivery of care, which has resulted in improved median survival for patients with CF,[2] lung transplantation provides an additional management option for patients with end-stage pulmonary disease from CF. In 1983 the first lung transplant for CF was performed, and CF now accounts for almost 17% of all pretransplant diagnoses.[1,3] Despite refinements in lung allocation practices, a proportion of patients with CF die while waiting for lung transplantation. Historically, the forced expiratory volume in 1 second (FEV_1) has been the most often used functional variable to predict prognosis, with early reports of a FEV_1 less than 30% predicted being associated with a 2-year mortality of 50%.[4] Other variables associated with a high risk of death from CF are hypoxia, hypercapnia, pulmonary hypertension, reduced 6-minute walk distance, and female sex.[4,5] From these variables, a few predictive models of survival in patients with CF have been developed; however, predicting survival for patients with CF is imprecise at best.[6–8] The goal of lung transplantation in patients with CF is to not only extend survival but also to improve quality of life. In comparison with other patients with end-stage lung disease, individuals with CF

Disclosure statement: The authors have nothing to disclose relevant to this article.
a Lung Transplant Program, University of Pittsburgh Medical Center, NW628 MUH, 3459 Fifth Avenue, Pittsburgh, PA 15213, USA; b Adult Cystic Fibrosis Program, Children's Hospital of Pittsburgh of UPMC and University of Pittsburgh Medical Center, NW628 MUH, 3459 Fifth Avenue, Pittsburgh, PA 15213, USA
* Corresponding author.
E-mail address: pilewskijm@upmc.edu

Clin Chest Med 37 (2016) 127–138
http://dx.doi.org/10.1016/j.ccm.2015.11.008
0272-5231/16/$ – see front matter © 2016 Elsevier Inc. All rights reserved.

chestmed.theclinics.com

face unique challenges when considering lung transplantation, yet the median survival for individuals with CF after transplant exceeds those of individuals who underwent a transplant for other end-stage lung diseases.[1]

GUIDELINES FOR REFERRAL AND EVALUATION

Listing for lung transplantation should be considered at a time when survival from respiratory-related complications from CF is considered to be less than survival after lung transplantation. To date, there are no prospective, randomized, well-powered studies that define the optimal timing of transplant referral and listing. Early referral to a lung transplant center, before the anticipated need for listing, is highly encouraged to initiate patient and family education and to identify and correct potential barriers to lung transplantation (eg, malnutrition, substance abuse, poor psychosocial support). The decision to list patients with CF is complex and should take into account the rate of decline in pulmonary function, frequency of exacerbations, and the development of baseline hypercapnia and pulmonary hypertension. Current recommendations from the International Society of Heart and Lung Transplantation are based on small studies and expert opinion consensus (**Box 1**). To determine the severity of disease and appropriateness for lung transplantation, several studies are performed during the evaluation process (**Box 2**).

Box 1
Criteria for listing for lung transplantation in patients with CF

- FEV_1 less than 30% predicted or rapidly declining lung function
- Frequent exacerbations requiring antimicrobial therapy
- Recent exacerbation requiring mechanical ventilation
- Increasing oxygen requirements
- Recurrent hemoptysis despite embolization procedures
- Refractory or recurrent pneumothorax
- Baseline hypercapnia (Pco_2 >50 mm Hg)
- Pulmonary hypertension
- Ongoing weight loss despite aggressive nutritional supplementation

---

Box 2
Studies performed during lung transplant evaluation for CF

- Chest radiograph
- Computed tomography of the chest
- Complete pulmonary function tests
- 6-minute walk
- Quantitative ventilation/perfusion scan
- Barium swallow
- Electrocardiogram
- Transthoracic echocardiogram
- Right +/− left heart catheterization
- Bone densitometry
- Age-appropriate health maintenance examinations
- Complete blood count
- Renal function panel
- Hepatic function panel
- Arterial blood gas
- Sputum culture, including fungal and AFB
- 24-hour urine for creatinine clearance
- Thrombosis risk panel
- HLA molecular typing
- HLA antibody screen
- Blood group type
- Hemoglobin A1C
- Urinalysis
- PPD/Quantiferon Gold TB test
- Serologies
  - HIV
  - Hepatitis B
  - Hepatitis C
  - Syphilis
  - Herpes simplex virus
  - Varicella-zoster virus
  - Cytomegalovirus
  - Epstein-Barr virus
  - Toxoplasmosis

Abbreviations: AFB, acid fast bacilli; HIV, human immunodeficiency virus; PPD, purified protein derivative; TB, tuberculosis.

SELECTION OF CANDIDATES FOR LUNG TRANSPLANTATION

Lung transplantation should be considered for patients whose clinical status has progressively declined despite maximal medical therapy. Candidates should have a high risk of death from lung disease (>50%) within 2 years without lung transplantation and a high likelihood of 5-year posttransplant survival in the setting of acceptable graft function.[9] The ideal candidate should be free of significant extrapulmonary comorbidities; however, the other systemic manifestations of CF rarely preclude lung transplantation. The absolute and relative contraindications for lung transplantation are constantly in flux as surgical techniques and management of complications has improved over the past decade. In general, patients with CF should be free from the following: malignancy within the past 2 years; significant and untreatable heart, renal, or hepatic dysfunction; significant chest wall deformity; uncorrectable bleeding diathesis; and psychiatric conditions that may impede adherence to a complex medical regimen. Candidates should be historically compliant with medical therapies, have good insight and a reliable social support system, have a good potential for physical rehabilitation, and be free of any recent substance abuse or dependence.[9]

TYPE OF TRANSPLANTATION

Although the first lung transplantation for CF was actually a combined heart and lung transplantation, bilateral sequential lung transplantation became the preferred procedure in the early 1990s.[10,11] This procedure originally involved transection of the sternum in a clamshell procedure to fully expose the chest cavity. However, bilateral anterior thoracotomies are now preferred at some centers as a sternal-sparing procedure to avoid surgical complications, such as nonunion of the sternum and sternal osteomyelitis.[12,13] However, for cases in which surgical challenges are expected, the clamshell procedure remains ideal to fully expose all intrathoracic structures.

To combat the high mortality among patients with CF awaiting lung transplantation, and limited donor lung availability, living-donor lobar lung transplantation was implemented as an alternative to conventional cadaveric lung transplantation.[14] With this procedure, single lobes are removed from one or more living donors and implanted in the recipient. Despite reports of comparable short- and long-term outcomes compared with conventional lung transplantation, this procedure is rarely performed now because of occasional donor complications and the recent changes in the urgency/benefit allocation system for cadaveric lung transplantation in the United States.[15,16] Cadaveric lobar lung transplantation carries the benefit of reducing wait-list mortality for patients with small stature without imposing any risk to a living donor.

In this procedure, individual lobes from deceased donors with larger chest cavities are implanted in recipients with smaller chest cavities. In this decade, cadaveric lobar lung transplantation has been safely performed in patients with CF with encouraging short- and long-term outcomes.[17,18]

COMORBIDITIES IN CYSTIC FIBROSIS AND IMPACT ON TRANSPLANT CANDIDACY AND OUTCOMES

An important consideration for lung transplantation is the impact of pretransplant comorbidities on outcomes. Several reports of single-center outcomes for patients with CF have been published; however, to date, there are no predictive models that allow estimation of risk associated with multiple comorbidities. CF-specific comorbidities and their individual impact on survival are listed in **Table 1**. Candidacy for lung transplant is based largely on center experience and level of risk aversion, which varies widely among transplant programs. Typically higher-volume transplant centers will often offer transplant listing to patients previously declined at less experienced centers. For this reason, it is imperative that CF clinicians explore referral to multiple transplant centers if the local center declines.

Prior Thoracic Procedures

Historically, prior thoracic procedures were considered to be a major contraindication to lung transplantation. Pneumothoraces are a risk factor for mortality in patients with CF; for the transplant surgeon, less aggressive measures are preferred over chemical or surgical pleurodesis.[19] Many patients can be managed with prolonged chest tube drainage, often with a indwelling pleural catheter, to minimize the short- and long-term risk of pleurodesis. Nevertheless, although few studies have detailed the impact of pleural procedures on transplant outcomes, many centers have found that prior pleural procedures increase the complexity of recipient pneumonectomy and increase pleural bleeding. In one large single-center report, Meachery and colleagues[20] reported on outcomes for 176 patients with CF who underwent lung or heart-lung transplantation from 1989 to 2007. For the 12% who had prior pneumothorax (including 6 patients with pleurodesis), outcomes were no worse in patients with prior pneumothoraces and pleurodesis compared with the larger cohort. Thus, patients with prior pneumothoraces, including those treated by pleurodesis, can, in the care of an experienced transplant team, have comparable outcomes.

Table 1
Controversial comorbidities in CF and their impact on transplant outcomes

Comorbidity	Impact on Outcomes
Multiple-drug resistant *Pseudomonas aeruginosa*	None
Gram-negative CF pathogens other than *Burkholderia gladioli* and *Burkholderia cenocepacia*	None
Burkholderia cenocepacia	Approximately 40% decrease in 1 y survival; minimal effect on 5-y survival
Mycobacterium abscessus	Increase in perioperative morbidity; no appreciable effect on mortality
Aspergillus fumigatus	None
Cirrhosis	None with Child-Pugh A and perhaps B
Malnutrition	Debated but worst case estimate 10% lower survival at 3 and 5 y with BMI <18
Mechanical support with invasive ventilation or ECMO	Increase morbidity; no appreciable decrease in short-term survival and unknown impact on long-term survival

Abbreviations: BMI, body mass index; ECMO, extracorporeal membrane oxygenation.

CF Bacterial Pathogens

Some transplant centers consider pretransplant colonization with pan-resistant strains of *Pseudomonas aeruginosa* or *Burkholderia cepacia* as predictive of poor posttransplant outcomes and, therefore, a contraindication to transplantation. Beginning with studies in 1997, there has been some controversy over the impact of pan-resistant bacteria other than *Burkholderia cepacia* on outcomes from lung transplantation for CF. In one of the larger reviews, Hadjiliadis and colleagues[21] retrospectively reviewed the experience at 2 transplant centers with 99 patients who underwent a transplant between 1988 and 2001. Pan-resistant *Pseudomonas* was defined as those isolates having resistant or intermediate susceptibility to one antibiotic from each class of antibiotics against these bacteria (eg, antipseudomonal penicillins, cephalosporins, carbapenems, quinolones, and aminoglycosides). Patients in the group with pan-resistant *Pseudomonas* (n = 45) had worse outcomes by overall comparison of survival with those with sensitive organisms (n = 58). The difference in survival was appreciable up until 2 years after transplant, after which the survival curves were comparable. In addition, patients in the pan-resistant *Pseudomonas* group tended to have infection as a more common cause of death than the sensitive *Pseudomonas* group; however, pan-resistant *Pseudomonas* was directly responsible for death in only 3 of the 45 patients in this group.[21] Patients in the pan-resistant group comprised almost half the study population, highlighting the frequency of highly resistant *Pseudomonas* in the CF population with end-stage lung disease. Although the investigators' conclusion that patients with pan-resistant *Pseudomonas* have a statistically worse outcome than those with sensitive *Pseudomonas* seems substantiated, outcomes in the pan-resistant group were comparable with those in the United Network of Organ Sharing (UNOS) registry. Thus, a corollary point is that patients with sensitive *Pseudomonas* seem to have better outcomes than other patients with CF undergoing transplantation. Nevertheless, as the investigators propose, both groups had very good outcomes, leading to the conclusion that patients with more resistant *Pseudomonas* species should not be excluded from consideration for transplantation.

There remains considerable debate regarding whether patients infected with *Burkholderia* species are appropriate candidates for lung transplantation. Studies in the 1990s indicated that patients infected with *B cepacia* had a high risk of posttransplant mortality; over time, fewer and fewer transplant centers have offered transplant evaluation and listing for patients infected with *B cepacia*.[22] Over the last decade or more, LiPuma and colleagues[23,24] have contributed immensely to understanding the microbiology of *Burkholderia*, first by distinguishing this group of pathogens from *Pseudomonas* and then more recently by identifying genotypically distinct species that seem to impact differently on transplant outcomes. Using 2 large databases (the CF Foundation patient registry and the Scientific Registry of Transplant Recipients) to identify cohorts of more than 1000 transplant candidates and more than 500 recipients, and the data available from the *Burkholderia* Research Laboratory and Repository, Murray and colleagues[23] were able to assess the mortality risk of different *Burkholderia* species. *Burkholderia* infection significantly impacted posttransplant survival in several ways: (1) patients infected with *B gladioli* had a significantly higher posttransplant mortality than uninfected recipients and recipients infected with *B multivorans*; (2) recipients infected with *B multivorans* before transplant had no appreciable difference in mortality compared with uninfected patients; (3) overall, transplant recipients infected with *B cenocepacia* (n = 31) before transplant did not have an overall worse 1- and 5-year survival compared with uninfected patients; (4) in contrast, subgroup analysis revealed that patients infected with nonepidemic *B cenocepacia* strains (eg, strains other than the two epidemic strains in this dataset: the Midwest and PHDC clones) before transplant had a significantly higher risk of mortality compared with uninfected recipients or recipients infected with *B multivorans*. The excess mortality associated with *B gladioli* and nonepidemic strains of *B cenocepacia* occurred in the first 6 months after transplant.

Other investigators have reported comparative analyses of transplant outcomes for patients with CF infected with *B cepacia* complex (Bcc) who underwent a transplant between 1990 and 2006. Survival rates for patients infected with *B cenocepacia* were significantly lower than for patients infected with other species, and patients with *B cenocepacia* were 6 times more likely to die in the first year after the transplantation (1-year survival 89%–92% for non-*Burkholderia* and Bcc species other than *cenocepacia* vs 29% for *B cenocepacia*–infected patients).[24] Similarly, in a study from France, patients infected with *B cenocepacia* before transplant had higher mortality rates than patients infected with other *Burkholderia* species, whereas patients infected with strains other than *cenocepacia* did not have a statistically higher mortality risk compared with patients not infected with Bcc species. Three of the 6 deaths in patients with *cenocepacia* occurred in the postoperative period and were directly attributable to *cenocepacia* infection.[25] These cumulative data suggest that more aggressive, or alternative, antibiotic regimens targeted at preventing early infection may improve outcomes. In addition, further correlation of molecularly characterized species with outcomes are needed to fully resolve subtype

differences and to determine definitively whether it is ethically appropriate to exclude all patients with *B cenocepacia* from lung transplantation.

The impact of other less frequent gram-negative CF pathogens is not well defined. *Stenotrophomonas* and *Achromobacter* species do not seem to pose an increased risk for early mortality.[26] Several studies have demonstrated a negative impact of infection with methicillin-resistant *Staphylococcus aureus* (MRSA) in patients with CF, but the impact of pretransplant MRSA on posttransplant outcomes is unclear.[27]

Fungal Pathogens

Aspergillus and other fungi are found in respiratory cultures from a significant fraction of patients with CF but, with few exceptions, do not seem to adversely impact transplant outcomes. Up to 70% of adults with CF harbor *Aspergillus fumigatus*, and allergic bronchopulmonary aspergillosis may occur in up to 10% of patients over the course of their disease. Mycetomas are much less common, and true invasive aspergillosis has rarely been reported. In one recent single-center study, 70% of patients who underwent a transplant for CF had *Aspergillus* before transplant and almost 40% had fungus in explanted lung cultures. The risk of invasive *Aspergillus* after transplant was high (22%) and often temporally related to the treatment of acute cellular rejection; however, preoperative *Aspergillus* did not appreciably increase the risk for early mortality after transplant.[28] Particularly with the availability of newer azole antifungals and inhaled amphotericin, *Aspergillus* species are not considered a contraindication to lung transplant. Other fungal pathogens, such as *Scedosporium* species are seen much less frequently and should be considered carefully given case reports of early mortality attributable to these fungi.[29]

Nontuberculous Mycobacteria

Atypical mycobacteria seem to be an increasing challenge for patients with CF and, as a result, significantly impact lung transplant candidacy. Prevalence studies at many US CF centers more than a decade ago demonstrated that approximately 13% of patients older than 10 had respiratory cultures with nontuberculous mycobacteria (NTM), with 72% being *M avium* and 16% *Mycobacterium abscessus*.[30] Although decline in lung function was not appreciably different between NTM-positive and NTM-negative patients, a subset of patients with multiple positive cultures had progressive computed tomography changes suggestive of progressive disease.[31] Differentiating colonization from infection is often difficult; however, what is clear is that patients with *M abscessus* who undergo a transplant are at risk for disseminated, or more frequently, localized infections (eg, at wounds or in pleural space). Consequently, patients with CF and NTM colonization or infection are often deemed to be unsuitable for transplant because of infectious complications. Data to support any NTM as an absolute contraindication for transplant are lacking; data for the more virulent and antibiotic resistant *M abscessus* are generally poor, but most single-center and small case series support lung transplantation in this CF population.

In one study, almost 20% of transplant referrals with CF had a history of NTM; of the 18 patients who had NTM before transplant, 7 were culture positive after transplant.[32] However, only 4 of these had NTM disease, including 2 wound infections among 8 patients who had *M abscessus* before transplant. Six of 8 patients with pretransplant *M abscessus* had negative airway cultures after transplant. There were no deaths attributable to NTM, and median survival among the NTM-positive and NTM-negative cohorts was not appreciably different. A more recent update reported 6 patients with *M abscessus* disease before transplant, with 3 posttransplant mycobacterial infections, all of which were controlled with therapy and were not associated with worse survival.[33] Similar conclusions resulted from a review of 4 patients with pretransplant *M abscessus*; 3 developed wound infections or cutaneous abscesses, and all resolved with debridement and prolonged mycobacterial therapy.[34] A similarly high frequency of postoperative infections in patients with pretransplant *M abscessus* was reported by others, supporting the conclusion that patients with pretransplant *M abscessus* have increased infectious risk and higher morbidity, without excess mortality.[35] With the emergence of alternative agents for NTM, most transplant centers and infectious disease clinicians currently take a conservative approach that potentially pathogenic NTM, particularly *M abscessus*, be controlled with a tolerable NTM regimen before transplantation to minimize the posttransplant risk. Patients with CF should be educated in detail about the risk and burden of prolonged posttransplant NTM therapy when NTM are isolated within the year before transplant.

Gastrointestinal Comorbidities

Several gastrointestinal (GI) complications of CF potentially impact transplant candidacy and outcomes, including liver dysfunction, exocrine pancreatic insufficiency, and malnutrition. Early autopsy studies reported almost uniform focal biliary cirrhosis among adults with CF, whereas more recent reviews report cholestasis by laboratory testing in more than a quarter of adults with CF. A very small proportion of patients with CF (<5%) manifest cirrhosis and portal hypertension, with the majority recognized before adulthood. Although the natural history of cirrhosis in CF seems to be relatively indolent, perhaps because of aggressive use of ursodeoxycholic acid for cholestasis in CF, most patients with cirrhosis complicating CF can be managed medically and/or endoscopically and do not require liver transplantation.[36,37] Several adult patients with CF are known to have cirrhosis and/or portal hypertension before referral for lung transplantation, or are found to have varying degrees of liver dysfunction during the evaluation process. Patients with liver disease limited to cholestasis are generally deemed low risk for perioperative liver decompensation. However, patients with cirrhosis are more controversial, as many are deemed unsuitable for isolated lung transplantation.

Data on the impact of cirrhosis are limited to small case series, making evidence-based decisions regarding lung transplantation in patients with CF liver disease difficult. A recent case control series strongly suggested that selected patients with CF and advanced liver disease can undergo uneventful lung transplantation without concomitant liver transplantation. Six patients with CF and liver cirrhosis, defined as esophageal varices, imaging evidence of cirrhosis, and/or splenomegaly or diagnostic histology, underwent isolated lung transplantation, with no appreciable difference in perioperative complications or survival compared with a matched control group.[38] Notably, none of the 6 patients with cirrhosis, with Model for End-Stage Liver Disease scores ranging from 27 to 34 and Child-Pugh scores of 5 to 8, exhibited decompensation of liver disease in the first 4 years after lung transplantation.[38] This single-center experience at a high-volume lung transplant program demonstrates the feasibility of isolated lung transplant in patients with CF and cirrhosis. Experience at the authors' institution is similar. For at least 6 patients with CF and Child A or B cirrhosis who underwent isolated lung transplantation, there was no perioperative mortality. The published and anecdotal experiences at high-volume transplant centers indicate that concomitant lung liver transplant is likely only necessary for patients with hepatocellular dysfunction and uncontrolled manifestations of CF liver disease. Therefore, most patients with CF and mild cirrhosis should not be declined for lung transplant because of liver disease. Because it is often challenging to obtain lung and liver en bloc in the United States unless both lung and liver allocation scores are very high, it is critical to better define the severity of CF liver disease that precludes isolated lung transplantation.

Pancreatic insufficiency and malnutrition are more common GI complications of CF. Pancreatic insufficiency affects greater than 85% of adults with CF; thus, lung transplantation for pancreatic-sufficient patients is relatively uncommon. Surprisingly, one recent review demonstrated that pancreatic-sufficient patients have a higher risk of mortality than pancreatic-insufficient patients and malnutrition (body mass index [BMI] <18.5) was not associated with worse outcomes.[39] The latter contradicts the conclusion of an earlier study using a larger registry cohort that demonstrated an approximately 10% lower 5-year survival for patients with CF who had a BMI less than 18.5 compared with a cohort with normal pretransplant BMI.[40] As survival was not appreciably different in the first 2 years after transplant, the mechanism for this observation is unclear. One possibility is suggested by an association of vitamin D deficiency with a higher risk of rejection after lung transplantation for CF; however, further studies that examine both nutritional status as assessed by BMI and by markers of protein and fat-soluble vitamin deficiency are necessary.[41] Although many US transplant centers will not offer lung transplant to patients with a BMI less than 18, most view this as a relative contraindication and an example of an often-modifiable risk factor for poorer outcomes after lung transplantation. In addition, achievement and maintenance of adequate nutrition is an intervention that can often be instituted early by the primary CF care team using enteral nutrition via feeding tubes, thereby improving transplant outcome and mitigating risk if a patient has a rapid decline in lung function and has an urgent need for transplantation.

Sinus Disease

Sinus disease, manifesting as chronic sinusitis with or without nasal polyposis, is nearly ubiquitous in patients with CF, particularly those with advanced lung disease. Very few studies have attempted to determine the impact of CF sinus disease on transplant outcomes. It can be assumed that the sinuses in patients with CF provide a reservoir for bacterial pathogens that predisposes patients to lower airway colonization or infection and thereby contribute to allograft dysfunction and worse post-transplant outcomes. In a recent study, cultures of the sinuses of patients with CF after transplantation were compared with lower airway cultures; there was significant concordance in isolates from sinus aspirates and bronchoscopic cultures,[42] which is consistent with the reservoir hypothesis. Moreover, patients who underwent sinus surgery followed by routine nasal douches had a higher incidence of negative sinus and lower airway Pseudomonas colonization after transplantation and improved survival and freedom from higher-grade bronchiolitis obliterans syndrome/chronic rejection. These findings corroborate earlier reports that patients with CF and Pseudomonas colonization after transplantation had worse outcomes compared with a Pseudomonas-negative cohort.[43,44] This finding suggests that outcomes after transplant in patients with CF may be improved by preventive measures against lower airway infection, particularly with management of sinus disease, and perhaps routine mucosal antibiotics to prevent lower airway colonization.

Osteoporosis

Osteoporosis is common in patients with advanced lung disease, and osteoporosis with fractures has long been considered a relative contraindication to lung transplantation. In adult patients with CF, osteoporosis is very common, with mean average bone mineral densities 2 standard deviations below an age-matched control population.[45] Patients with CF had increased fracture rates, particularly vertebral-compression and rib fractures, and a surprisingly high incidence of kyphosis associated with loss of height. Although the possible mechanisms for this high rate of severe bone disease in a young population are not fully defined, vitamin D deficiency, malnutrition, early puberty, glucocorticoid exposure, and chronic inflammation are favored mechanisms. The implication of this for transplantation in adults with CF is that the fracture risk is often high before transplant and may increase further with the required immunosuppressive regimen following transplantation. More recent studies have demonstrated safety and efficacy for bisphosphonates in conjunction with vitamin D and calcium supplementation to improve bone mineral density in adults with CF.[46,47] Thus, for most transplant centers, osteoporosis is perceived as a remediable comorbidity in patients with CF, and only uncontrolled pain related to fractures is considered a contraindication to lung transplantation.

Diabetes

Cystic fibrosis–related diabetes (CFRD) is the most common comorbidity in patients with CF, occurring in approximately 20% of adolescents and 40% to 50% of adults.[48] CFRD is associated with worse lung function, more chest infections, overall poorer nutrition, and increased mortality irrespective of lung transplantation.[49] New-onset diabetes occurs in approximately 38% of patients without preexisting CFRD following lung transplantation. Patients with CF should be counseled about the risk of developing diabetes following lung transplantation. In one study, both de novo and preexisting diabetes was associated with an increased risk of death following lung transplantation.[50] However, a more recent analysis did not demonstrate an impact of diabetes on transplant outcomes for patients with CF.[39] Poorly controlled diabetes is considered by many to be a relative contraindication for lung transplantation, as this may be a surrogate for patients' regimen adherence. Aggressive treatment of diabetes is strongly recommended before and following lung transplantation. However, further studies evaluating the impact that tight glycemic control has on overall survival after transplant are warranted.

MECHANICAL SUPPORT AS A BRIDGE TO LUNG TRANSPLANTATION

Historically, the requirement of mechanical ventilation had been considered to be a relative contraindication to lung transplantation as mechanical ventilation before lung transplantation was associated with a 1.5 times increased risk of mortality in the first year after lung transplantation.[1] However, in patients with CF, the risk attributed to mechanical ventilation has been controversial, with some reports suggesting that mechanical ventilation may be associated with a longer intensive care unit stay and longer need for mechanical ventilation after lung transplantation, although this did not change overall survival.[51,52] Noninvasive ventilation is useful to control respiratory acidosis and has been helpful to support patients with CF while waiting for lung transplantation. Noninvasive ventilation in patients with CF before lung transplantation is not associated with any adverse outcomes after lung transplantion.[53,54] More recently, extracorporeal membrane oxygenation (ECMO) has been used as a bridge to lung transplantation with comparable post–lung transplantation short-term and midterm outcomes as well as low mortality.[55,56] Newer ECMO strategies, including the use of a dual-lumen single cannula, which allows for ambulatory venovenous ECMO, can be done in awake, spontaneously breathing patients and allow for oral intake and participation in physical therapy.[57] In general, mechanical support can be efficacious as a bridge to lung transplantation in experienced centers with adequate resources.

SURVIVAL AND QUALITY OF LIFE CONCERNS

The median survival from lung transplantation in the international registry for patients with CF is 8.3 years, which is significantly better than patients who underwent a transplant in earlier eras or for other diseases, such as chronic obstructive pulmonary disease and pulmonary fibrosis.[1] Patients with CF who survive beyond the first year have a median survival of 10.5 years.[1] This survival may reflect the overall younger age and less cardiac and renal comorbidity of CF recipients, in comparison to other lung transplant recipients. The major causes of death within the first year following lung transplantation, irrespective of pretransplant lung disease, involve technical problems, primary graft dysfunction ultimately resulting in graft failure, and acute infections. Infections account for approximately 35% of deaths between 1 month and 1 year following lung transplantation.[1] After the first year, bronchiolitis obliterans syndrome/chronic rejection, and infections other than Cytomegalovirus account for 67% of deaths.[1]

The overall survival benefit from lung transplantation in patients with CF has been controversial. In 2005, an analysis involving data from the UNOS and the CF Foundation Patient Registry found that youth, the presence of B cepacia, and CF-related arthropathy were associated with a higher hazard of death.[58] Adult patients with CF with a 5-year predicted survival of less than 50%, without B cepacia or arthropathy, had improved survival compared with control patients with CF who did not undergo lung transplantation.[58] As pediatric lung transplantation is now uncommon for CF, some have questioned whether the prior studies associating younger age with poor survival are valid. Liou and colleagues[59] subsequently performed proportional hazards analysis on a cohort of patients with CF to identify variables that were associated with change in survival. In addition to transplantation, 4 variables were identified that impacted survival: B cepacia infection, diabetes, infection with S aureus, and age. B cepacia infection was associated with shortened survival with or without transplantation, whereas diabetes was associated with shorter pretransplant survival. Age and S aureus infection were also associated with shorter posttransplant survival. Using these variables as covariates, the investigators estimated the benefit or harm of transplant; of the 514 children on the waiting list during the analysis period of 1992 to 2002, the analysis estimated a clear survival advantage for only 5 patients, risk of harm for 315 patients, and neither benefit nor harm for 194 patients. The investigators concluded that benefit from lung transplantation cannot be assumed for children with CF.[59]

Several critiques of these findings included the investigators' utilization of covariates obtained more than 2 years before transplantation, thus leading to a potential bias against transplantation. In addition, many covariates that are known to predict survival in patients with CF, such as the need for mechanical ventilation, use of supplemental oxygen, and change in pulmonary function over time, were neglected from the study. Furthermore, the study was performed in an era before initiation of the US Lung Allocation Score (LAS) and may not be applicable to current practice.[60] Thus, only an analysis of outcomes with LAS will determine the relative benefit of lung transplantation for children.

A strong association between LAS and lung transplantation was identified, in that the higher the LAS at the time of transplantation, the greater the survival benefit of lung transplantation.[61] Overall, survival in CF is determined by multiple interactive factors involving the respiratory system; lung transplantation remains an appropriate option for patients with CF who have a high risk of short-term mortality.

Prior studies have documented worsening health-related quality of life in patients with CF as lung function declines.[62,63] Patients with CF are younger, spend more days on the waiting list, and are more likely to be working or going to school in comparison with other patients on the lung transplant waiting list.[64] However, in comparison with other patients with other end-stage lung diseases, patients with CF waiting for lung transplantation have lower levels of anxiety, higher levels of social support, and use more functional coping strategies.[65] Following lung transplantation, patients with CF report better quality of life, including physical and social functioning, treatment burden, and chest symptoms.[66,67] In addition, energy level and sleep quality are also significantly improved following lung transplantation.[64] In general, patients with CF have the same improvements in overall quality of life in comparison with patients with other solid organ transplants.[68]

OPPORTUNITIES FOR IMPROVED TRANSPLANT OUTCOMES

Despite improvements in surgical techniques that have reduced early mortality after lung transplantation, long-term survival remains poor relative to other solid organ transplants, with 5- and 10-year survivals estimated at 65% and 50%, respectively, based on registries.[1,39] Improvements in 1-year survival have not translated to improved long-term survival because of the high frequency of chronic lung allograft dysfunction that is most commonly manifest as bronchiolitis obliterans pathologically and progressive obstructive lung disease physiologically. Potential explanations for the lack of progress in preventing this common complication are infrequent patient follow-up with physicians trained in transplantation, resulting in late recognition of chronic rejection; lack of available biomarkers for early allograft dysfunction; wide variability in transplant center experience with transplant for CF; poor insight to the pathophysiology of chronic rejection; and lack of a defined optimal immunosuppressive regimen to prevent chronic rejection. The observation that there are differences in transplant outcomes between US centers[1] and across national boundaries[39,69] suggests that benchmarking to identify best practices and creation of a detailed registry of transplant outcomes, akin to the CF patient registry that has facilitated comparative effectiveness research and helped transform routine CF care, may provide critical observations that could improve the quality of posttransplant care, establish standard therapies that will facilitate multicenter clinical trials of new interventions, and ultimately improve the long-term survival for lung transplant recipients with CF.

SUMMARY

Lung transplantation remains a viable option for patients with CF and end-stage lung disease. Despite comorbidities, including infections with multidrug-resistant organisms, diabetes, and GI complications, patients with CF benefit from lung transplantation in terms of quantity and quality of life. Further studies are needed to optimize candidate selection and further improve outcomes following lung transplantation. Additional opportunities for research and discussion include mechanisms to prevent allograft colonization with CF pathogens, immune responses of transplant recipients with CF, and the effect that socioeconomic status and health care systems influence access to lung transplantation and outcomes.[39,69,70]

REFERENCES

1. Yusen RD, Edwards LB, Kucheryavaya AY, et al. The registry of the International Society for Heart and Lung Transplantation: thirty-first adult lung and heart-lung transplant report–2014; focus theme:

retransplantation. J Heart Lung Transplant 2014;33: 1009–24.

2. MacKenzie T, Gifford AH, Sabadosa KA, et al. Longevity of patients with cystic fibrosis in 2000 to 2010 and beyond: survival analysis of the Cystic Fibrosis Foundation patient registry. Ann Intern Med 2014;161:233–41.

3. Yacoub MH, Banner NR, Khaghani A, et al. Heart-lung transplantation for cystic fibrosis and subsequent domino heart transplantation. J Heart Transplant 1990;9:459–66 [discussion: 466–7].

4. Kerem E, Reisman J, Corey M, et al. Prediction of mortality in patients with cystic fibrosis. N Engl J Med 1992;326:1187–91.

5. Venuta F, Rendina EA, De Giacomo T, et al. Timing and priorities for cystic fibrosis patients candidates to lung transplantation. Eur J Pediatr Surg 1998;8:274–7.

6. Mayer-Hamblett N, Rosenfeld M, Emerson J, et al. Developing cystic fibrosis lung transplant referral criteria using predictors of 2-year mortality. Am J Respir Crit Care Med 2002;166:1550–5.

7. Augarten A, Akons H, Aviram M, et al. Prediction of mortality and timing of referral for lung transplantation in cystic fibrosis patients. Pediatr Transplant 2001;5:339–42.

8. Liou TG, Adler FR, Cahill BC, et al. Survival effect of lung transplantation among patients with cystic fibrosis. JAMA 2001;286:2683–9.

9. Weill D, Benden C, Corris PA, et al. A consensus document for the selection of lung transplant candidates: 2014–an update from the Pulmonary Transplantation Council of the International Society for Heart and Lung Transplantation. J Heart Lung Transplant 2015;34:1–15.

10. Mendeloff EN, Huddleston CB, Mallory GB, et al. Pediatric and adult lung transplantation for cystic fibrosis. J Thorac Cardiovasc Surg 1998;115: 404–13 [discussion: 413–4].

11. Shennib H, Noirclerc M, Ernst P, et al. Double-lung transplantation for cystic fibrosis. The cystic fibrosis transplant study group. Ann Thorac Surg 1992;54: 27–31 [discussion: 31–2].

12. Venuta F, Diso D, Anile M, et al. Evolving techniques and perspectives in lung transplantation. Transplant Proc 2005;37:2682–3.

13. Meyers BF, Sundaresan RS, Guthrie T, et al. Bilateral sequential lung transplantation without sternal division eliminates posttransplantation sternal complications. J Thorac Cardiovasc Surg 1999;117:358–64.

14. Cohen RG, Barr ML, Schenkel FA, et al. Living-related donor lobectomy for bilateral lobar transplantation in patients with cystic fibrosis. Ann Thorac Surg 1994;57:1423–7 [discussion: 1428].

15. Date H, Sato M, Aoyama A, et al. Living-donor lobar lung transplantation provides similar survival to cadaveric lung transplantation even for very ill patients. Eur J Cardiothorac Surg 2015;47:967–73.

16. Battafarano RJ, Anderson RC, Meyers BF, et al. Perioperative complications after living donor lobectomy. J Thorac Cardiovasc Surg 2000;120:909–15.

17. Shigemura N, D'Cunha J, Bhama JK, et al. Lobar lung transplantation: a relevant surgical option in the current era of lung allocation score. Ann Thorac Surg 2013;96:451–6.

18. Stanzi A, Decaluwe H, Coosemans W, et al. Lobar lung transplantation from deceased donors: a valid option for small-sized patients with cystic fibrosis. Transplant Proc 2014;46:3154–9.

19. Flume PA, Strange C, Ye X, et al. Pneumothorax in cystic fibrosis. Chest 2005;128:720–8.

20. Meachery G, De Soyza A, Nicholson A, et al. Outcomes of lung transplantation for cystic fibrosis in a large UK cohort. Thorax 2008;63:725–31.

21. Hadjiliadis D, Steele MP, Chaparro C, et al. Survival of lung transplant patients with cystic fibrosis harboring panresistant bacteria other than Burkholderia cepacia, compared with patients harboring sensitive bacteria. J Heart Lung Transplant 2007; 26:834–8.

22. Aris RM, Gilligan PH, Neuringer IP, et al. The effects of panresistant bacteria in cystic fibrosis patients on lung transplant outcome. Am J Respir Crit Care Med 1997;155:1699–704.

23. Murray S, Charbeneau J, Marshall BC, et al. Impact of Burkholderia infection on lung transplantation in cystic fibrosis. Am J Respir Crit Care Med 2008; 178:363–71.

24. Alexander BD, Petzold EW, Reller LB, et al. Survival after lung transplantation of cystic fibrosis patients infected with Burkholderia cepacia complex. Am J Transplant 2008;8:1025–30.

25. Boussaud V, Guillemain R, Grenet D, et al. Clinical outcome following lung transplantation in patients with cystic fibrosis colonised with Burkholderia cepacia complex: results from two French centres. Thorax 2008;63:732–7.

26. Lobo LJ, Tulu Z, Aris RM, et al. Pan-resistant Achromobacter xylosoxidans and Stenotrophomonas maltophilia infection in cystic fibrosis does not reduce survival after lung transplantation. Transplantation 2015;99(10):2196–202.

27. Dasenbrook EC, Checkley W, Merlo CA, et al. Association between respiratory tract methicillin-resistant Staphylococcus aureus and survival in cystic fibrosis. JAMA 2010;303:2386–92.

28. Luong ML, Chaparro C, Stephenson A, et al. Pretransplant Aspergillus colonization of cystic fibrosis patients and the incidence of post-lung transplant invasive aspergillosis. Transplantation 2014;97: 351–7.

29. Symoens F, Knoop C, Schrooyen M, et al. Disseminated Scedosporium apiospermum infection in a cystic fibrosis patient after double-lung transplantation. J Heart Lung Transplant 2006;25:603–7.

30. Olivier KN, Weber DJ, Wallace RJ Jr, et al. Nontuberculous mycobacteria. I: multicenter prevalence study in cystic fibrosis. Am J Respir Crit Care Med 2003;167:828–34.

31. Olivier KN, Weber DJ, Lee JH, et al. Nontuberculous mycobacteria. II: nested-cohort study of impact on cystic fibrosis lung disease. Am J Respir Crit Care Med 2003;167:835–40.

32. Chalermskulrat W, Sood N, Neuringer IP, et al. Non-tuberculous mycobacteria in end stage cystic fibrosis: implications for lung transplantation. Thorax 2006;61:507–13.

33. Lobo LJ, Chang LC, Esther CR Jr, et al. Lung transplant outcomes in cystic fibrosis patients with pre-operative Mycobacterium abscessus respiratory infections. Clin Transplant 2013;27:523–9.

34. Gilljam M, Schersten H, Silverborn M, et al. Lung transplantation in patients with cystic fibrosis and Mycobacterium abscessus infection. J Cyst Fibros 2010;9:272–6.

35. Qvist T, Pressler T, Thomsen VO, et al. Nontuberculous mycobacterial disease is not a contraindication to lung transplantation in patients with cystic fibrosis: a retrospective analysis in a Danish patient population. Transplant Proc 2013;45:342–5.

36. Nash KL, Allison ME, McKeon D, et al. A single centre experience of liver disease in adults with cystic fibrosis 1995-2006. J Cyst Fibros 2008;7:252–7.

37. Rowland M, Gallagher CG, O'Laoide R, et al. Outcome in cystic fibrosis liver disease. Am J Gastroenterol 2011;106:104–9.

38. Nash EF, Volling C, Gutierrez CA, et al. Outcomes of patients with cystic fibrosis undergoing lung transplantation with and without cystic fibrosis-associated liver cirrhosis. Clin Transplant 2012;26:34–41.

39. Stephenson AL, Sykes J, Berthiaume Y, et al. Clinical and demographic factors associated with post-lung transplantation survival in individuals with cystic fibrosis. J Heart Lung Transplant 2015;34(9):1139–45.

40. Lederer DJ, Wilt JS, D'Ovidio F, et al. Obesity and underweight are associated with an increased risk of death after lung transplantation. Am J Respir Crit Care Med 2009;180:887–95.

41. Lowery EM, Bemiss B, Cascino T, et al. Low vitamin D levels are associated with increased rejection and infections after lung transplantation. J Heart Lung Transplant 2012;31:700–7.

42. Vital D, Hofer M, Benden C, et al. Impact of sinus surgery on pseudomonal airway colonization, bronchiolitis obliterans syndrome and survival in cystic fibrosis lung transplant recipients. Respiration 2013;86:25–31.

43. Vos R, Vanaudenaerde BM, Geudens N, et al. Pseudomonal airway colonisation: risk factor for bronchiolitis obliterans syndrome after lung transplantation? Eur Respir J 2008;31:1037–45.

44. Botha P, Archer L, Anderson RL, et al. Pseudomonas aeruginosa colonization of the allograft after lung transplantation and the risk of bronchiolitis obliterans syndrome. Transplantation 2008;85:771–4.

45. Aris RM, Renner JB, Winders AD, et al. Increased rate of fractures and severe kyphosis: sequelae of living into adulthood with cystic fibrosis. Ann Intorn Med 1998;128:186–93.

46. Aris RM, Lester GE, Renner JB, et al. Efficacy of pamidronate for osteoporosis in patients with cystic fibrosis following lung transplantation. Am J Respir Crit Care Med 2000;162:941–6.

47. Aris RM, Lester GE, Caminiti M, et al. Efficacy of alendronate in adults with cystic fibrosis with low bone density. Am J Respir Crit Care Med 2004;169:77–82.

48. Moran A, Dunitz J, Nathan B, et al. Cystic fibrosis-related diabetes: current trends in prevalence, incidence, and mortality. Diabetes Care 2009;32:1626–31.

49. Brennan AL, Geddes DM, Gyi KM, et al. Clinical importance of cystic fibrosis-related diabetes. J Cyst Fibros 2004;3:209–22.

50. Hackman KL, Bailey MJ, Snell GI, et al. Diabetes is a major risk factor for mortality after lung transplantation. Am J Transplant 2014;14:438–45.

51. Bartz RR, Love RB, Leverson GE, et al. Pre-transplant mechanical ventilation and outcome in patients with cystic fibrosis. J Heart Lung Transplant 2003;22:433–8.

52. Vermeijden JW, Zijlstra JG, Erasmus ME, et al. Lung transplantation for ventilator-dependent respiratory failure. J Heart Lung Transplant 2009;28:347–51.

53. Spahr JE, Love RB, Francois M, et al. Lung transplantation for cystic fibrosis: current concepts and one center's experience. J Cyst Fibros 2007;6:334–50.

54. Moran F, Bradley JM, Piper AJ. Non-invasive ventilation for cystic fibrosis. Cochrane Database Syst Rev 2013;(4):CD002769.

55. Bermudez CA, Rocha RV, Zaldonis D, et al. Extracorporeal membrane oxygenation as a bridge to lung transplant: midterm outcomes. Ann Thorac Surg 2011;92:1226–31 [discussion: 1231–2].

56. Toyoda Y, Bhama JK, Shigemura N, et al. Efficacy of extracorporeal membrane oxygenation as a bridge to lung transplantation. J Thorac Cardiovasc Surg 2013;145:1065–70 [discussion: 1070–1].

57. Hayes D Jr, Kukreja J, Tobias JD, et al. Ambulatory venovenous extracorporeal respiratory support as a bridge for cystic fibrosis patients to emergent lung transplantation. J Cyst Fibros 2012;11:40–5.

58. Liou TG, Adler FR, Huang D. Use of lung transplantation survival models to refine patient selection in cystic fibrosis. Am J Respir Crit Care Med 2005;171:1053–9.

59. Liou TG, Adler FR, Cox DR, et al. Lung transplantation and survival in children with cystic fibrosis. N Engl J Med 2007;357:2143–52.

60. Sweet SC, Aurora P, Benden C, et al. Lung transplantation and survival in children with cystic fibrosis: solid statistics–flawed interpretation. Pediatr Transplant 2008;12:129–36.

61. Thabut G, Christie JD, Mal H, et al. Survival benefit of lung transplant for cystic fibrosis since lung allocation score implementation. Am J Respir Crit Care Med 2013;187:1335–40.

62. Gee L, Abbott J, Conway SP, et al. Validation of the SF-36 for the assessment of quality of life in adolescents and adults with cystic fibrosis. J Cyst Fibros 2002;1:137–45.

63. Gee L, Abbott J, Conway SP, et al. Quality of life in cystic fibrosis: the impact of gender, general health perceptions and disease severity. J Cyst Fibros 2003;2:206–13.

64. Vermeulen KM, van der Bij W, Erasmus ME, et al. Improved quality of life after lung transplantation in individuals with cystic fibrosis. Pediatr Pulmonol 2004;37:419–26.

65. Burker EJ, Carels RA, Thompson LF, et al. Quality of life in patients awaiting lung transplant: cystic fibrosis versus other end-stage lung diseases. Pediatr Pulmonol 2000;30:453–60.

66. Gee L, Abbott J, Hart A, et al. Associations between clinical variables and quality of life in adults with cystic fibrosis. J Cyst Fibros 2005;4:59–66.

67. Singer LG, Chowdhury NA, Faughnan ME, et al. Effects of recipient age and diagnosis on health-related quality of life benefit of lung transplantation. Am J Respir Crit Care Med 2015;192(8):965–73.

68. Busschbach JJ, Horikx PE, van den Bosch JM, et al. Measuring the quality of life before and after bilateral lung transplantation in patients with cystic fibrosis. Chest 1994;105:911–7.

69. Quon BS, Psoter K, Mayer-Hamblett N, et al. Disparities in access to lung transplantation for patients with cystic fibrosis by socioeconomic status. Am J Respir Crit Care Med 2012;186:1008–13.

70. Merlo CA, Clark SC, Arnaoutakis GJ, et al. National healthcare delivery systems influence lung transplant outcomes for cystic fibrosis. Am J Transplant 2015;15:1948–57.

Using Cystic Fibrosis Therapies for Non–Cystic Fibrosis Bronchiectasis

Wael ElMaraachli, MD[a], Douglas J. Conrad, MD[a,*],
Angela C.C. Wang, MD[b]

KEYWORDS

- Bronchiectasis • Cystic fibrosis • Non–cystic fibrosis • Chest medicine • Treatment

KEY POINTS

- Non–cystic fibrosis bronchiectasis is a significant cause of morbidity and mortality and its prevalence is increasing.
- A work-up must be initiated to determine the cause of the bronchiectasis but the etiology remains unknown in a significant percentage of cases.
- Unlike CF, adult non-CF bronchiectasis is a heterogeneous disease in regards to its cause, disease progression, and response to therapy.
- Hence, despite similarities in signs and symptoms, management of adult non-CF bronchiectasis cannot be routinely extrapolated from studies performed in patients with CF.

INTRODUCTION

Non–cystic fibrosis bronchiectasis (NCFB) is an increasingly prevalent disease in the United States and Europe. Its incidence increases with age, and peaks at ages 75 to 84.[1,2] NCFB is associated with longer hospital stays, more frequent clinic visits, more antibiotic use, and more extensive medical therapy than matched control subjects.[3] A review of 30 US health plans estimates that NCFB results in medical care expenditures of $630 million annually (2001 US dollars). Mortality is also increased, with an estimate of 10.6% in patients with NCFB over a 3.5-year observation period in a single study.[4] Many therapies used to treat cystic fibrosis (CF) are also used for patients with NCFB, with varying success. Unlike CF, however, NCFB is a heterogeneous disease, with a variety of predisposing factors and disease mechanisms implicated in its pathogenesis. This article explores the evidence for which therapeutic strategies used to treat CF have been translated into the care of NCFB. We conclude that therapies for adult NCFB cannot be simply extrapolated from CF clinical trials, and in some instances, doing so may actually result in harm.

PATHOPHYSIOLOGY

The "vicious cycle" hypothesis proposed by Cole[5] is the generally accepted explanation for the evolution of bronchiectasis. It is thought that airway damage resulting from a neutrophilic-dominant inflammatory response to infection, or tissue injury, leads to mucus stasis and predisposes to persistent infections thus perpetuating a "vicious cycle" of inflammation and damage.[5,6] Alternatively, endogenous innate immune deficiencies including ciliary dysfunction or immunoglobulin deficiencies, among many others, may initiate mucus stasis or

Disclosure Statement: The authors have nothing to disclose.
[a] Division of Pulmonary, Critical Care and Sleep Medicine, University of California, San Diego, 200 West Arbor Drive, MC 8372, San Diego, CA 92013, USA; [b] Division of Chest and Critical Care Medicine, Scripps Clinic, 10666 North Torrey Pines Road, W203, San Diego, CA 92037, USA
* Corresponding author.
E-mail address: dconrad@ucsd.edu

Clin Chest Med 37 (2016) 139–146
http://dx.doi.org/10.1016/j.ccm.2015.11.005
0272-5231/16/$ – see front matter © 2016 Elsevier Inc. All rights reserved.

changes in the airway microbiome. Airway bacterial colonization is facilitated by impaired neutrophil opsonophagocytic killing. Neutrophil elastase, released by activated neutrophils, can impair bacterial clearance by slowing ciliary beat frequency and promoting mucus hypersecretion.[7,8]

PATIENT EVALUATION

Causes of NCFB range from postinfectious to immune dysregulation (**Box 1**). The British Thoracic Society published guidelines for the evaluation of NCFB[9] (**Box 2**). However, the cause remains unknown in 10% to 53% of cases even after extensive evaluation.[10–12]

PHARMACOLOGIC TREATMENT OPTIONS

Pharmacologic and nonpharmacologic therapies are used in CF and NCFB with varying success. The differences in efficacy likely result from

---

Box 1
Etiologies of NCFB

Autoimmune disease
  Rheumatoid arthritis
  Sjögren syndrome
Primary ciliary dyskinesia
Connective tissue disease
  Tracheobronchomegaly   (Mounier-Kuhn syndrome)
  Marfan syndrome
  Cartilage   deficiency   (Williams-Campbell syndrome)
Allergic bronchopulmonary aspergillosis
Immune deficiency
  Human immunodeficiency virus
  Immunoglobulin deficiency
  Hyper-IgE syndrome
Inflammatory bowel disease
Previous infections
Aspiration
Smoke inhalation
Malignancy
  Chronic lymphocytic leukemia
  Stem cell transplantation, graft-versus-host disease
Obstruction (tumor, foreign body)
α_1-Antitrypsin syndrome

Box 2
Historical and diagnostic evaluation of NCFB

Historical
Neonatal symptoms
Infertility
Previous pneumonia
Gastric aspiration
Asthma
Connective tissue
Autoimmune symptoms

Diagnostic
Sputum culture; bacteria/mycobacteria
Pulmonary function testing
IgA, IgE, IgG, and IgM
Pneumococcal vaccine titers
Sweat chloride test
CFTR genetic analysis
ANA, RF, aCCP, SSA, SSB antibodies
α_1-Antitrypsin
Ciliary ultrastructure

---

differences in pathophysiology and patient demographics. The major areas of therapy used in CF and their utility in NCFB are reviewed next.

Bronchodilators

There is no definitive evidence that β-adrenergic or anticholinergic agents significantly improve outcomes in CF or NCFB.[13] Although bronchodilator therapies can potentially improve lung physiology and patient symptoms by improving mucociliary clearance, relieving bronchospasm, and reducing air-trapping, there is insufficient evidence to recommend regularly prescribing short-acting β_2-adrenergic agonists or anticholinergics for patients with CF or NCFB. These medications may be used safely if there is evidence of bronchospasm or air-trapping on pulmonary function testing, and continued if there is evidence for clinical improvement.[14,15]

Anti-inflammatory Therapy

The goal of anti-inflammatory therapy is to mitigate the airway remodeling, gas exchange abnormalities, and symptoms driven by inflammation without exacerbating airway infection or causing serious toxicity.

Corticosteroids
Theoretically, inhaled corticosteroids (ICS) may decrease airway inflammation without the increased

side effects of systemic steroids. Currently, however, ICS is not recommended for routine use in CF.[16] In one study of NCFB, high-dose ICS reduced sputum volume and inflammatory markers but did not affect lung function or frequency of exacerbations.[17] Martí-nez-García and colleagues[15] compared medium-dose budesonide (640 mg) plus formoterol with high-dose budesonide (1600 mg) in patients with NCFB in a 12-month randomized, double-blind, parallel-group trial. Patients receiving medium-dose budesonide plus formoterol experienced less dyspnea, required fewer rescue β-agonist inhalations, had an increase in cough-free days, and improved health-related quality of life scores compared with the high-dose budesonide group. However, lung function, exacerbation frequency, and chronic bacterial colonization were not different between the two study groups. In addition, the long-term use of high-dose ICS is associated with cataracts and osteoporosis. Therefore, the routine use of ICS in NCFB is not recommended except when there is airflow reversibility or allergic bronchopulmonary aspergillosis.

Systemic corticosteroids can benefit patients with CF and NCFB through incompletely understood anti-inflammatory effects. However, the chronic use of corticosteroids in NCFB and CF is associated with substantial side effects that are believed to outweigh potential benefits.[18,19] Therefore, except in cases of allergic bronchopulmonary aspergillosis or concomitant asthma, in which short courses are reasonable, long-term administration of systemic corticosteroids is not recommended in either CF or NCFB.

Nonsteroidal anti-inflammatory therapy

The use of nonsteroidal anti-inflammatory drugs in CF has been found to decrease the rate of lung function decline, particularly in the pediatric population.[20,21] In contrast, the use of inhaled or systemic nonsteroidal anti-inflammatory drugs is not established in NCFB and routine use is not recommended without further evidence.[22]

Macrolides

Macrolides possess several properties of potential benefit to patients with NCFB and CF. These include anti-infective effects on susceptible bacterial populations, anti-inflammatory properties, and their ability to alter bacterial virulence.[23,24] Long-term azithromycin is widely used in patients with CF and is recommended for use in patients with and without *Pseudomonas aeruginosa* (PA) infection.[25]

Three multicenter, randomized trials (EMBRACE, BAT, and BLESS trials) using different doses of azithromycin (500 mg three times weekly in EMBRACE[26]; 250 mg daily in BAT[27]) or erythromycin (400 mg twice daily in BLESS[28]) have shown reduced rates of exacerbations with use of a macrolide as compared with placebo in patients with NCFB. The trials are small but consistently show a reduction in exacerbations.[26–28] Therefore, maintenance macrolide use may be considered to reduce exacerbation frequency in NCFB.

The benefits of macrolide therapy in CF and NCFB must be balanced against its potential cardiovascular toxicity and ototoxicity, both of which require regular monitoring. In addition, the development of resistant strains of mycobacteria remains a major concern. In CF and NCFB, infection with nontuberculous mycobacteria must be ruled out before initiating chronic macrolide therapy.

Antibiotics

The use of antibiotics in patients with NCFB is driven mostly by studies in patients with CF, which are limited by their reliance on traditional sampling methods and culture techniques. Studies of the airway microbiome in CF and NCFB using culture-independent assessments are beginning to provide critical insights into taxonomy, dynamics, and metabolism of the airway microbial community that have the potential to provide new pathophysiologic insights and identify novel therapies targeting the ecologic dependencies of the bacterial, viral, and fungal populations. For instance, microbial community diversity in NCFB correlates positively with clinical health measurements.[29–32] These early microbiome studies in NCFB suggest that anaerobic bacterial populations may serve as an important therapeutic target.

Systemic antibiotics

In patients with CF, *Pseudomonas* spp, *Staphylococcus aureus*, *Stenotrophomonas maltophilia*, *Achromobacter* spp, and mycobacteria are frequently isolated from airway secretions. In NCFB, the most common pathogen is also PA, followed by *S aureus*, *Moraxella catarrhalis*, and *Haemophilus influenza*.[33] In CF and NCFB, exacerbation frequency, lung function, and disease extent are worse in patients infected with PA.[34]

Aggressive treatment of initial colonization by PA can result in eradication of the organism and prevent, or delay, colonization. In addition, PA eradication therapy has been demonstrated to reduce exacerbation frequency in NCFB.[35] Therefore, as in CF, eradication of PA in NFCB should be attempted, especially following initial colonization. Oral fluoroquinolones, such as ciprofloxacin, or intravenous aminoglycosides in combination with inhaled antibiotics are frequently used.

The treatment of acute exacerbations of NCFB should be guided by a patient's prior sputum cultures. Although no strong evidence is available to dictate duration of therapy, a 2-week course is currently recommended.[9] The use of higher doses of ciprofloxacin may be required to treat PA infection in NFCB.[36] This has been directly extrapolated from the CF literature. However, this higher dose must be used with caution in older patients given the higher incidence of side effects, such as *Clostridium difficile* colitis and tendinopathy. The use of inhaled tobramycin in combination with high-dose ciprofloxacin has also been studied.[37] Although the combination was found to be more effective than placebo at eradicating PA, no additional clinical benefit was demonstrated, possibly because of the increased wheezing caused by inhaled tobramycin.[37]

Inhaled antibiotics

Inhaled antibiotics offer significant advantages compared with oral therapies by delivering higher concentrations of drug to the airway with less systemic absorption and fewer side effects. Inhaled antibiotics reduce airway bacterial load and associated airway inflammation in NCFB.[38] In the CF population, inhaled antibiotics have been shown to reduce exacerbations and hospital admissions.[39] Older studies demonstrated no differences in exacerbation frequency.[40–42]

A single-blind randomized controlled trial of nebulized gentamicin for 12 months in NFCB reported significant benefits.[43] The study enrolled patients with chronic bacterial colonization (three positive sputum cultures in the past 12 months), two exacerbations in the previous year, and a forced expiratory volume in 1 second (FEV_1) greater than 30%, and excluded smokers and patients receiving other long-term antibiotics. A total of 27 patients were randomized to gentamicin, 80 mg twice daily, and 30 patients to 0.9% saline twice daily. After 12 months, in the gentamicin group, there was a significant reduction in bacterial density and improvement in the quality of life and exacerbation frequency. There was still a significant rate of bronchospasm at 21.9%, but only two patients were withdrawn from the study for this reason. No nephrotoxicity or ototoxicity was reported.

A recent, large phase III trial of inhaled colistin has been completed.[44] This trial recruited 144 patients with chronic PA colonization in the United Kingdom, Russia, and Ukraine. The study failed to meet the primary outcome of a difference in time to first exacerbation (colistin group 165 days vs placebo 111 days; $P = .11$). However, in the secondary end points, a significant improvement

in quality of life using the St. George's Respiratory Questionnaire was noted (mean difference, 10.5 points; $P = .006$).

Inhaled aztreonam therapy is used frequently in CF. Two recent randomized trials in patients with NCFB compared aztreonam with placebo for two 28-day cycles separated by 28 days off.[45] The primary outcome of improvement in quality of life was not reached, and there was a high rate of intolerance with up to 20% of patients discontinuing aztreonam therapy compared with 3% with placebo treatment.

A dry powder inhaled formulation of ciprofloxacin has the potential to significantly reduce treatment burden in patients with NCFB. In a phase II study (N = 60 patients for ciprofloxacin and N = 64 patients for placebo) ciprofloxacin was associated with a significant reduction in bacterial load during a 28-day treatment period, without any significant differences in exacerbations.[46]

The dual-release liposomal ciprofloxacin preparation seeks to improve drug tolerance by decreasing the amount of free drug in contact with the pulmonary epithelium. Slow release of the drug from liposomes allows for once-daily dosing, which may also aid compliance.[47] The phase II study demonstrated a significant reduction in PA CFU·mL−1 in the treatment arm over 24 weeks. There was also a reduction in time to next exacerbation (median, 134 days vs 58 days; $P = .046$ in the per protocol population). In contrast to previous experience with aminoglycosides and aztreonam, the dry powder and liposomal ciprofloxacin preparations were well tolerated. There are currently phase III trials for each of these preparations actively recruiting patients. The primary outcome for both of these trials is time to first exacerbation.[48,49]

Hyperosmolar and Mucolytic Therapy

Nebulized hypertonic saline, inhaled mannitol, and N-acetylcysteine seek to improve airway clearance by increasing hydration, decreasing viscosity, and improving mucus rheology by disrupting disulfide bond formation.[50,51] Inhaled DNase, however, was found to be potentially harmful in NCFB.

Nebulized hypertonic saline

Hypertonic saline benefits patients with CF older than 6 years of age by improving quality of life and reducing pulmonary exacerbations. In adults, hypertonic saline has been found to improve lung function.[52,53] The evidence for the use of hypertonic saline in NCFB is mixed. The studies are small and provide conflicting results. In one study of patients with NCFB, the use of 7% nebulized hypertonic saline improved lung function, quality of life, and health care use through changes in mucus rheology, increased ciliary motility, and enhanced cough clearance.[54] However, another study, which compared daily hypertonic saline (6%) with daily isotonic saline for 12 months, found no difference in exacerbation rates, quality of life, FEV_1, or sputum colonization.[55] Although there are no strong recommendations for routine use of hypertonic saline in NCFB, some patients seem to clearly benefit from this therapy.

Inhaled mannitol
In a recent international, multicenter, randomized, controlled trial, patients were treated with either inhaled mannitol, 400 mg, or low-dose mannitol control twice daily.[56] Although exacerbation rates were not affected, there were significant improvements in time to first exacerbation and quality of life as measured by the St. George's Respiratory Questionnaire.[56] Inhaled mannitol is not currently approved for use in the United States.

Inhaled DNase
Aerosolized dornase alpha reduces mucus viscosity, improves lung function, and reduces hospitalizations in patients with CF.[57] Dornase alpha was initially viewed as a potentially beneficial therapy in NCFB but eventually was found to cause greater reductions in FEV_1.[58] Its use is therefore not recommended in patients with bronchiectasis without CF.

NONPHARMACOLOGIC TREATMENT OPTIONS
Exercise

Exercise in patients with CF and NCFB improves cardiac conditioning and mobilization of airway secretions. Patients with NCFB who participate in regular exercise programs demonstrate significant improvement in exertional tolerance and health-related quality of life scores, and experience fewer respiratory exacerbations.[59–61]

Airway Clearance Therapy

Airway clearance therapy (ACT) is an integral component of CF care. It is recommended for all patients with CF with a grade B recommendation using the United States Preventive Services Task Force grading scheme.[62] There is insufficient evidence to recommend one particular method of ACT over another. The prescription of ACT in CF should be individualized based on such factors as age, patient preference, and adverse events, among others.[63] ACTs include active cycle of breathing techniques, postural drainage, oscillatory positive expiratory pressure, autogenic drainage, and high-frequency chest wall oscillation.

Studies examining the benefits of ACT in NCFB are small, uncontrolled, and use different comparators. Many of these studies do not have patient-important end points and use different outcome efficacy measures to assess the specific therapy.[64–71] Despite these shortcomings, it is still recommended that ACT be taught to all patients with bronchiectasis.[9] As in CF, the particular ACT to be used should be individualized.

SURGICAL TREATMENT OPTIONS

Although surgical options for CF, other than transplantation, are rare given the diffuse nature of lung disease, surgical evaluation for a lobectomy or segmentectomy in NFCB can be considered for patients with localized disease, or massive hemoptysis, who have failed medical management.[72–75]

EXPERIMENTAL THERAPIES

Experimental therapies currently under investigation for patients with CF include antiproteases (eg, α_1-antitrypsin supplementation, and neutrophil elastase inhibition) and mucolytics, such as N-acetylcysteine. Specific studies of these therapies in NCFB remain lacking.[76–78]

SUMMARY/DISCUSSION

Many aspects of the management of bronchiectasis in patients with no CF have been based on the experience gained from and the more extensive research studies performed in CF. However, therapies for NCFB cannot simply be extrapolated from CF, and some treatments, such as the use of inhaled DNase, may even be harmful. Clinical studies that specifically target patients with NCFB are sorely needed.

REFERENCES

1. Ringshausen FC, de Roux A, Pletz MW, et al. Bronchiectasis-associated hospitalizations in Germany, 2005-2011: a population-based study of disease burden and trends. PLoS One 2013;8:e71109.
2. Seitz AE, Olivier KN, Adjemian J, et al. Trends in bronchiectasis among Medicare beneficiaries in the United States, 2000 to 2007. Chest 2012;142:432–9.
3. Weycker D, Edelsberg J, Oster G, et al. Prevalence and economic burden of bronchiectasis. Clin Pulm Med 2005;12:205–9.
4. Goeminne PC, Scheers H, Decraene A, et al. Risk factors for morbidity and death in non-cystic fibrosis

bronchiectasis: a retrospective cross-sectional analysis of CT diagnosed bronchiectatic patients. Respir Res 2012;13:21.

5. Cole PJ. Inflammation: a two-edged sword–the model of bronchiectasis. Eur J Respir Dis Suppl 1986;147:6–15.

6. Fuschillo S, De Felice A, Balzano G. Mucosal inflammation in idiopathic bronchiectasis: cellular and molecular mechanisms. Eur Respir J 2008;31:396–406.

7. Amitani R, Wilson R, Rutman A, et al. Effects of human neutrophil elastase and *Pseudomonas aeruginosa* proteinases on human respiratory epithelium. Am J Respir Cell Mol Biol 1991;4:26–32.

8. Voynow JA, Young LR, Wang Y, et al. Neutrophil elastase increases MUC5AC mRNA and protein expression in respiratory epithelial cells. Am J Physiol 1999;276:L835–43.

9. Pasteur MC, Bilton D, Hill AT. British thoracic society non-CF bronchiectasis guideline group. British Thoracic Society guideline for non-CF bronchiectasis. Thorax 2010;65:577.

10. McShane PJ, Naureckas ET, Strek ME. Bronchiectasis in a diverse us population: effects of ethnicity on etiology and sputum culture. Chest 2012;142:159–67.

11. Pasteur MC, Helliwell SM, Houghton SJ, et al. An investigation into causative factors in patients with bronchiectasis. Am J Respir Crit Care Med 2000;162:1277–84.

12. Shoemark A, Ozerovitch L, Wilson R. Aetiology in adult patients with bronchiectasis. Respir Med 2007;101:1163–70.

13. Restrepo RD. Inhaled adrenergics and anticholinergics in obstructive lung disease: do they enhance mucociliary clearance? Respir Care 2007;52:1159–73 [discussion: 1173–5].

14. Eggleston PA, Rosenstein BJ, Stackhouse CM, et al. A controlled trial of long-term bronchodilator therapy in cystic fibrosis. Chest 1991;99:1088–92.

15. Martínez-García MÁ, Soler-Cataluña JJ, Catalán-Serra P, et al. Clinical efficacy and safety of budesonide-formoterol in non-cystic fibrosis bronchiectasis. Chest 2012;141:461–8.

16. Mogayzel PJ, Naureckas ET, Robinson KA, et al, Pulmonary Clinical Practice Guidelines Committee. Cystic fibrosis pulmonary guidelines. Chronic medications for maintenance of lung health. Am J Respir Crit Care Med 2013;187:680–9.

17. King P. Is there a role for inhaled corticosteroids and macrolide therapy in bronchiectasis? Drugs 2007;67:965–74.

18. Martínez-García MA, Soler-Cataluña J-J, Perpiñá-Tordera M, et al. Factors associated with lung function decline in adult patients with stable non-cystic fibrosis bronchiectasis. Chest 2007;132:1565–72.

19. Lai HC, FitzSimmons SC, Allen DB, et al. Risk of persistent growth impairment after alternate-day prednisone treatment in children with cystic fibrosis. N Engl J Med 2000;342:851–9.

20. Konstan MW, Byard PJ, Hoppel CL, et al. Effect of high-dose ibuprofen in patients with cystic fibrosis. N Engl J Med 1995;332:848–54.

21. Lands LC, Milner R, Cantin AM, et al. High-dose ibuprofen in cystic fibrosis: Canadian Safety and Effectiveness Trial. J Pediatr 2007;151:249–54.

22. Pizzutto SJ, Upham JW, Yerkovich ST, et al. Inhaled non-steroid anti-inflammatories for children and adults with bronchiectasis. Cochrane Database Syst Rev 2010;(4):CD007525.

23. Crosbie PA, Woodhead MA. Long-term macrolide therapy in chronic inflammatory airway diseases. Eur Respir J 2009;33:171–81.

24. Nguyen D, Emond MJ, Mayer-Hamblett N, et al. Clinical response to azithromycin in cystic fibrosis correlates with in vitro effects on *Pseudomonas aeruginosa* phenotypes. Pediatr Pulmonol 2007;42:533–41.

25. Mogayzel PJ, Naureckas ET, Robinson KA, et al. Cystic Fibrosis Foundation pulmonary guideline. Pharmacologic approaches to prevention and eradication of initial *Pseudomonas aeruginosa* infection. Ann Am Thorac Soc 2014;11:1640–50.

26. Altenburg J, de Graaff CS, Stienstra Y, et al. Effect of azithromycin maintenance treatment on infectious exacerbations among patients with non-cystic fibrosis bronchiectasis: the BAT randomized controlled trial. JAMA 2013;309:1251–9.

27. Serisier DJ, Martin ML, McGuckin MA, et al. Effect of long-term, low-dose erythromycin on pulmonary exacerbations among patients with non-cystic fibrosis bronchiectasis: the BLESS randomized controlled trial. JAMA 2013;309:1260–7.

28. Wong C, Jayaram L, Karalus N, et al. Azithromycin for prevention of exacerbations in non-cystic fibrosis bronchiectasis (EMBRACE): a randomised, double-blind, placebo-controlled trial. Lancet (London England) 2012;380:660–7.

29. Rogers GB, van der Gast CJ, Serisier DJ. Predominant pathogen competition and core microbiota divergence in chronic airway infection. ISME J 2015;9:217–25.

30. Rogers GB, Shaw D, Marsh RL, et al. Respiratory microbiota: addressing clinical questions, informing clinical practice. Thorax 2015;70:74–81.

31. Rogers GB, van der Gast CJ, Cuthbertson L, et al. Clinical measures of disease in adult non-CF bronchiectasis correlate with airway microbiota composition. Thorax 2013;68:731–7.

32. Segal LN, Rom WN, Weiden MD. Lung microbiome for clinicians. New discoveries about bugs in healthy and diseased lungs. Ann Am Thorac Soc 2014;11:108–16.

33. Chawla K, Vishwanath S, Manu MK, et al. Influence of *Pseudomonas aeruginosa* on exacerbation in

patients with bronchiectasis. J Glob Infect Dis 2015; 7:18–22.

34. King PT, Holdsworth SR, Freezer NJ, et al. Microbiologic follow-up study in adult bronchiectasis. Respir Med 2007;101:1633–8.

35. White L, Mirrani G, Grover M, et al. Outcomes of *Pseudomonas* eradication therapy in patients with non-cystic fibrosis bronchiectasis. Respir Med 2012;106:356–60.

36. Montgomery MJ, Beringer PM, Aminimanizani A, et al. Population pharmacokinetics and use of Monte Carlo simulation to evaluate currently recommended dosing regimens of ciprofloxacin in adult patients with cystic fibrosis. Antimicrob Agents Chemother 2001;45:3468–73.

37. Bilton D, Henig N, Morrissey B, et al. Addition of inhaled tobramycin to ciprofloxacin for acute exacerbations of *Pseudomonas aeruginosa* infection in adult bronchiectasis. Chest 2006;130:1503–10.

38. Chalmers JD, Smith MP, McHugh BJ, et al. Short- and long-term antibiotic treatment reduces airway and systemic inflammation in non–cystic fibrosis bronchiectasis. Am J Respir Crit Care Med 2012; 186:657–65.

39. Littlewood KJ, Higashi K, Jansen JP, et al. A network meta-analysis of the efficacy of inhaled antibiotics for chronic *Pseudomonas* infections in cystic fibrosis. J Cyst Fibros 2012;11:419–26.

40. Barker AF, Couch L, Fiel SB, et al. Tobramycin solution for inhalation reduces sputum *Pseudomonas aeruginosa* density in bronchiectasis. Am J Respir Crit Care Med 2000;162:481–5.

41. Couch LA. Treatment with tobramycin solution for inhalation in bronchiectasis patients with *Pseudomonas aeruginosa*. Chest 2001;120:114S–7S.

42. Drobnic ME, Suñé P, Montoro JB, et al. Inhaled tobramycin in non-cystic fibrosis patients with bronchiectasis and chronic bronchial infection with *Pseudomonas aeruginosa*. Ann Pharmacother 2005;39: 39–44.

43. Murray MP, Govan JRW, Doherty CJ, et al. A randomized controlled trial of nebulized gentamicin in non-cystic fibrosis bronchiectasis. Am J Respir Crit Care Med 2011;183:491–9.

44. Haworth CS, Foweraker JE, Wilkinson P, et al. Inhaled colistin in patients with bronchiectasis and chronic *Pseudomonas aeruginosa* infection. Am J Respir Crit Care Med 2014;189:975–82.

45. Barker AF, O'Donnell AE, Flume P, et al. Aztreonam for inhalation solution in patients with non-cystic fibrosis bronchiectasis (AIR-BX1 and AIR-BX2): two randomised double-blind, placebo-controlled phase 3 trials. Lancet Respir Med 2014;2:738–49.

46. Wilson R, Welte T, Polverino E, et al. Ciprofloxacin dry powder for inhalation in non-cystic fibrosis bronchiectasis: a phase II randomised study. Eur Respir J 2013;41:1107–15.

47. Serisier DJ, Bilton D, De Soyza A, et al. Inhaled, dual release liposomal ciprofloxacin in non-cystic fibrosis bronchiectasis (ORBIT-2): a randomised, double-blind, placebo-controlled trial. Thorax 2013;68: 812–7.

48. Aradigm Corporation. A multicenter, randomized, double-blind, placebo-controlled study to evaluate the safety and efficacy of pulmaquin in the management of chronic lung infections with *Pseudomonas aeruginosa* in patients with non-cystic fibrosis bronchiectasis, including 28 day open-label extension. ClinicalTrials.gov. [Internet]. NLM identifier: NCT02104245. Available at: https://clinicaltrials.gov/ct2/show/record/NCT02104245. Accessed July 11, 2015.

49. Bayer. Randomized, double-blind, placebo-controlled, multicenter study comparing ciprofloxacin DPI 32.5 mg BID (twice a day) intermittently administered for 28 days on/28 days off or 14 days on/14 days off versus placebo to evaluate the time to first pulmonary exacerbation and frequency of exacerbations in subjects with non-cystic fibrosis bronchiectasis. ClinicalTrials.gov. [Internet]. NLM identifier: NCT02106832. Available at: https://clinicaltrials.gov/ct2/show/record/NCT02106832. Accessed July 11, 2015.

50. Daviskas E, Robinson M, Anderson SD, et al. Osmotic stimuli increase clearance of mucus in patients with mucociliary dysfunction. J Aerosol Med 2002;15:331–41.

51. Shibuya Y, Wills PJ, Cole PJ. Effect of osmolality on mucociliary transportability and rheology of cystic fibrosis and bronchiectasis sputum. Respirology 2003;8:181–5.

52. Elkins MR, Robinson M, Rose BR, et al. A controlled trial of long-term inhaled hypertonic saline in patients with cystic fibrosis. N Engl J Med 2006;354: 229–40.

53. Wark P, McDonald VM. Nebulised hypertonic saline for cystic fibrosis. Cochrane Database Syst Rev 2009;(2):CD001506.

54. Kellett F, Robert NM. Nebulised 7% hypertonic saline improves lung function and quality of life in bronchiectasis. Respir Med 2011;105:1831–5.

55. Nicolson CHH, Stirling RG, Borg BM, et al. The long-term effect of inhaled hypertonic saline 6% in non-cystic fibrosis bronchiectasis. Respir Med 2012; 106:661–7.

56. Bilton D, Tino G, Barker AF, et al. Inhaled mannitol for non-cystic fibrosis bronchiectasis: a randomised, controlled trial. Thorax 2014;69:1073–9.

57. Fuchs HJ, Borowitz DS, Christiansen DH, et al. Effect of aerosolized recombinant human DNase on exacerbations of respiratory symptoms and on pulmonary function in patients with cystic fibrosis. The Pulmozyme Study Group. N Engl J Med 1994;331: 637–42.

58. O'Donnell AE, Barker AF, Ilowite JS, et al. Treatment of idiopathic bronchiectasis with aerosolized recombinant human DNase I. rhDNase Study Group. Chest 1998;113:1329–34.

59. Lee AL, Hill CJ, Cecins N, et al. The short and long term effects of exercise training in non-cystic fibrosis bronchiectasis: a randomised controlled trial. Respir Res 2014;15:44.

60. Mandal P, Sidhu MK, Kope L, et al. A pilot study of pulmonary rehabilitation and chest physiotherapy versus chest physiotherapy alone in bronchiectasis. Respir Med 2012;106:1647–54.

61. Newall C, Stockley RA, Hill SL. Exercise training and inspiratory muscle training in patients with bronchiectasis. Thorax 2005;60:943–8.

62. Harris RP, Helfand M, Woolf SH, et al. Current methods of the US Preventive Services Task Force: a review of the process. Am J Prev Med 2001;20: 21–35.

63. Flume PA, Robinson KA, O'Sullivan BP, et al. Cystic fibrosis pulmonary guidelines: airway clearance therapies. Respir Care 2009;54:522–37.

64. Eaton T, Young P, Zeng I, et al. A randomized evaluation of the acute efficacy, acceptability and tolerability of flutter and active cycle of breathing with and without postural drainage in non-cystic fibrosis bronchiectasis. Chron Respir Dis 2007;4:23–30.

65. Fink JB. Forced expiratory technique, directed cough, and autogenic drainage. Respir Care 2007; 52:1210–21 [discussion: 1221–3].

66. Murray MP, Pentland JL, Hill AT. A randomised crossover trial of chest physiotherapy in non-cystic fibrosis bronchiectasis. Eur Respir J 2009;34: 1086–92.

67. Nicolini A, Cardini F, Landucci N, et al. Effectiveness of treatment with high-frequency chest wall oscillation in patients with bronchiectasis. BMC Pulm Med 2013;13:21.

68. Patterson JE, Bradley JM, Elborn JS. Airway clearance in bronchiectasis: a randomized crossover trial of active cycle of breathing techniques (incorporating postural drainage and vibration) versus test of incremental respiratory endurance. Chron Respir Dis 2004;1:127–30.

69. Patterson JE, Bradley JM, Hewitt O, et al. Airway clearance in bronchiectasis: a randomized crossover trial of active cycle of breathing techniques versus Acapella. Respiration 2005;72:239–42.

70. Thompson CS, Harrison S, Ashley J, et al. Randomised crossover study of the Flutter device and the active cycle of breathing technique in noncystic fibrosis bronchiectasis. Thorax 2002;57: 446–8.

71. Tsang SMH, Jones AYM. Postural drainage or flutter device in conjunction with breathing and coughing compared to breathing and coughing alone in improving secretion removal and lung function in patients with acute exacerbation of bronchiectasis: a pilot study. Hong Kong Physiother J 2003;21:29–36.

72. Mitchell JD, Yu JA, Bishop A, et al. Thoracoscopic lobectomy and segmentectomy for infectious lung disease. Ann Thorac Surg 2012;93:1033–9 [discussion: 1039–40].

73. Vallilo CC, Terra RM, de Albuquerque ALP, et al. Lung resection improves the quality of life of patients with symptomatic bronchiectasis. Ann Thorac Surg 2014;98:1034–41.

74. Weber A, Stammberger U, Inci I, et al. Thoracoscopic lobectomy for benign disease: a single centre study on 64 cases. Eur J Cardiothorac Surg 2001;20:443–8.

75. Zhang P, Zhang F, Jiang S, et al. Video-assisted thoracic surgery for bronchiectasis. Ann Thorac Surg 2011;91:239–43.

76. Quinn DJ, Weldon S, Taggart CC. Antiproteases as therapeutics to target inflammation in cystic fibrosis. Open Respir Med J 2010;4:20–31.

77. Stockley R, De Soyza A, Gunawardena K, et al. Phase II study of a neutrophil elastase inhibitor (AZD9668) in patients with bronchiectasis. Respir Med 2013;107:524–33.

78. Tirouvanziam R, Conrad CK, Bottiglieri T, et al. High-dose oral N-acetylcysteine, a glutathione prodrug, modulates inflammation in cystic fibrosis. Proc Natl Acad Sci U S A 2006;103:4628–33.

Acquired Cystic Fibrosis Transmembrane Conductance Regulator Dysfunction in Chronic Bronchitis and Other Diseases of Mucus Clearance

S. Vamsee Raju, BPharm, PhD[a,b,1],
George M. Solomon, MD[a,1], Mark T. Dransfield, MD[c],
Steven M. Rowe, MD, MSPH[a,b,d],*

KEYWORDS

- Chronic obstructive pulmonary disease • Cystic fibrosis transmembrane conductance regulator
- Chronic bronchitis • Mucociliary clearance

KEY POINTS

- There is a considerable overlap in the clinical phenotypic features of patients with cystic fibrosis (CF) and chronic obstructive pulmonary disease (COPD) (chronic bronchitis phenotype), and to a lesser extent neutrophil-dominated asthma.
- CF, chronic bronchitis, and asthma are all associated with impaired mucociliary clearance and mucus hypersecretion, leading to chronic airway disease.
- Cigarette smoking, along with many other environmental exposures, results in acquired CF transmembrane conductance regulator (CFTR) dysfunction through a variety of molecular pathways, including reduced CFTR messenger RNA expression, diminished protein levels through accelerated degradation, and altered channel gating.
- Cigarette smokers and patients with COPD develop a clinical phenotype similar to mild CF that may be related to acquired CFTR dysfunction despite normal genetics; this is associated with the presence of chronic bronchitis.
- The role of CFTR dysfunction in asthma is unknown, but may be distinct across various allergic or inflammatory phenotypes.

Disclosures: None.
Funding and Conflicts of interest: See last page of article.
[a] Department of Medicine, Gregory Fleming James Cystic Fibrosis Research Center, University of Alabama at Birmingham, Birmingham, AL, USA; [b] Department of Cell Developmental and Integrative Biology, The Gregory Fleming James Cystic Fibrosis Research Center, University of Alabama at Birmingham, Birmingham, AL, USA; [c] Department of Medicine, The UAB Lung Health Center, University of Alabama at Birmingham, Birmingham, AL, USA; [d] Department of Pediatrics, The Gregory Fleming James Cystic Fibrosis Research Center, University of Alabama at Birmingham, Birmingham, AL, USA
[1] Authors contributed equally.
* Corresponding author. MCLM 706, 1918 University Boulevard, Birmingham, AL 35294-0006.
E-mail address: smrowe@uab.edu

Clin Chest Med 37 (2016) 147–158
http://dx.doi.org/10.1016/j.ccm.2015.11.003
0272-5231/16/$ – see front matter © 2016 Elsevier Inc. All rights reserved.

INTRODUCTION

New therapies are needed for the treatment of chronic obstructive pulmonary disease (COPD), which accounts for more than $30 billion in annual health care costs,[1] and recently surpassed stroke as the third leading cause of death in the United States.[2] Although smoking cessation is essential to slow the progression of disease, no current pharmaceuticals alter the natural history of the disease or improve the mucus retention that is characteristic of COPD, persists even in ex-smokers, and is independently associated with forced expiratory volume in 1 second FEV1 decline and death.[3–5] The chronic bronchitis phenotype of the disease is particularly problematic, because, more than 60% of patients with COPD show chronic mucus hypersecretion, which is independently associated with rate of lung function decline and death, and is without effective treatment.[3–5] Published data from multiple laboratories strongly indicate that exposure to cigarette smoke inhibits cystic fibrosis (CF) transmembrane conductance regulator (CFTR), the causative protein in CF,[6–10] leading to delayed mucociliary transport and mucus stasis.[6] Recent in vivo studies in mice[11] and humans[6,11,12] further show the presence of acquired CFTR dysfunction in patients with COPD and that the defect can persist in both the lung and periphery despite smoking cessation, and also that it is associated with chronic bronchitis severity. Similar pathways may also be involved in other diseases in which neutrophilic inflammation and mucus stasis are present, such as status asthmaticus. The development of efficacious modulators of CFTR anion transport has created the possibility that pharmacologic enhancement of CFTR activity may confer clinical benefit to this population, even in the absence of congenital CFTR mutations.[6,12,13] The concept that CFTR abnormalities may contribute to diseases beyond CF has captured the interest of prominent editorials,[14–16] and has the potential to elucidate a novel mechanism that could also apply to other diseases of mucus clearance, such as asthma and acute bronchitis. This article examines the latest data suggesting that acquired CFTR dysfunction can occur in smoking-related lung diseases and other related disorders of mucus clearance, and reviews the latest evidence suggesting that this may be a therapeutic target.

Disease States Associated with CFTR Dysfunction

An improved understanding of the role of CFTR in the maintenance of normal epithelial function has revealed that reduced CFTR activity plays a causative role in several diseases in addition to CF. For example, CFTR mutations that confer mild abnormalities are present in ~30% of individuals with recurrent idiopathic pancreatitis,[17,18] and similar associations have been established in congenital bilateral absence of the vas deferens,[19] allergic bronchopulmonary aspergillosis,[20] chronic sinusitis,[21] and idiopathic bronchiectasis.[22,23] The genetic basis of these diseases shows that mild CFTR dysfunction can contribute to substantial disorder.[24] With the recent discovery and clinical validation of potent modulators of CFTR ion channel activity, there is considerable scientific interest from academic and commercial laboratories to examine the effects of CFTR stimulation for diseases in which CFTR plays a pathogenic role, including COPD.[6–10,25]

Pathologic Resemblance of Cystic Fibrosis and Chronic Bronchitis

Like CF, the defining feature of COPD is airflow limitation, although it is recognized that the disease shows heterogeneous pathologic features in the lung.[26–30] Of the 2 classically defined COPD phenotypes, emphysema and chronic bronchitis,[28,31] the latter shows pathologic features similar to CF, including mucin hyperexpression, mucus accumulation, and goblet cell hyperplasia, and affects nearly two-thirds of patients with COPD.[27,31–33] A high incidence of bronchiectasis has also been reported in COPD.[34] These abnormalities lead to impaired airway clearance, chronic bacterial colonization, and persistent neutrophilic inflammation similar to CF lung disease.[26,29,32,35–39] Although these changes are usually less pronounced in patients with COPD, mucus obstruction is observed in the airways and is accompanied by delayed mucus clearance as judged by impaired tracheal mucus velocity and delayed elimination of inhaled radionuclear particles.[40–42] Furthermore, mucus obstruction also occurs in the small airways of patients with COPD and is associated with excess morbidity and mortality.[3,5,43] Based on the pronounced CFTR suppression caused by tobacco smoke exposure,[6–10] neutrophilic inflammation,[44,45] and hypoxia,[46] and also supported by several other laboratories,[6–8,10,12,13,45–48] there is now a large body of evidence strongly indicating that CFTR dysfunction may contribute to COPD pathogenesis, particularly among individuals with chronic bronchitis. A robust association between smoking and decreased CFTR activity was observed in 4 independent studies, each of which evaluated distinct CFTR readouts (eg, nasal potential difference [NPD],[6] lower airway potential difference,[12] sweat chloride,[47,49] and sweat rate[49]); all were associated with chronic bronchitis and/or cough severity, implicating the clinical significance of these findings.

Clinical Subphenotype in Chronic Obstructive Pulmonary Disease

Patients with COPD have historically been grouped into 2 categories: individuals showing emphysema (characterized by alveolar destruction and abnormally increased lung compliance), and those with chronic bronchitis (defined by chronic mucus production and characterized by goblet cell hyperplasia and mucus hypersecretion).[50] More recent data have established additional characteristics that contribute to patient phenotypes. These characteristics include the propensity to develop frequent exacerbations, cachexia, and airway hyperresponsiveness.[50–53] Moreover, new technology enabling quantification of emphysema and airways disease by computed tomography have emerged, enabling improved subphenotyping.[54] The need for a more targeted approach that identifies specific COPD subpopulations with discrete clinical or molecular characteristics has been emphasized at recent meetings of the American Thoracic Society, and is currently being examined by observational studies intended to define specific COPD subphenotypes. If successful, this may improve patient selection for targeted therapies, including the use of ion transport agonists that affect some, but not all, individuals with COPD (discussed later).

EXPERIMENTAL DATA SHOWING ACQUIRED CYSTIC FIBROSIS TRANSMEMBRANE CONDUCTANCE REGULATOR DYSFUNCTION FROM SMOKING
Cigarette Smoke Blockade of Cystic Fibrosis Transmembrane Conductance Regulator Function

Data generated in vitro have indicated that cigarette smoke exposure results in CFTR dysfunction. This finding is longstanding, beginning when Welsh[55] reported that cigarette smoke decreases Cl^- secretion across canine airway epithelium with minimal effect on sodium absorption.[55] This finding complemented in vitro studies in normal epithelial monolayers by Kreindler and colleagues,[8] who showed that cigarette smoke or cigarette smoke extract (CSE) reduced CFTR messenger RNA (mRNA) levels, protein expression, and ion channel function in airway epithelial cells grown in culture, a finding that led to ion transport discovery programs led by Novartis.[7,10] Dr Tarran's group confirmed these findings, and showed that cigarette smoke decreased airway surface liquid depth by partial internalization of

CFTR.[9] CSE effects on CFTR were not limited to airways alone; similar effects were also observed in T84 cells, an intestinal epithelial cell line, and sinonasal epithelia.[7,56]

To better understand these effects in the context of COPD, our laboratory defined the magnitude and dose dependence using well-differentiated primary epithelial cells derived from non-CF (CFTR wild type) donors. Incubation of CSE on the apical surface of primary airway epithelial cell monolayers resulted in dose-dependent reductions in CFTR-mediated Cl^- transport[6]; we also confirmed this with various whole cigarette smoke (WCS) exposure intensities.[48] Our group confirmed CFTR inhibition in vivo using a murine model by showing that WCS exposure causes a decrement in CFTR activity as determined by NPD, short circuit current of excised trachea, and intestinal current measurements.[47]

Current understanding of the effects of cigarette smoke, and its interaction with CFTR, continues to expand.[6,7,9] Single-channel conductance studies showed the deleterious effect of CSE on CFTR open-channel probability.[57] CSE exposure also reduced mature, fully glycosylated (the post-endoplasmic reticulum [ER] glycoform) CFTR C-band by Western blot, and was accompanied by reductions in CFTR mRNA expression by real-time reverse transcription polymerase chain reaction.[6] These findings are concordant with the results seen in Calu-3 pulmonary glandular monolayers with high-level wild-type CFTR expression.[6] Rasmussen and colleagues,[58] reported that cigarette smoke removes CFTR from the plasma membrane by increased cytoplasmic Ca^{2+}, depositing these channels into aggresomelike perinuclear compartments other than the lysosome. Further linking cytoplasmic Ca^{2+} as a pathway relevant to CFTR homeostasis. Maouche and colleagues[59] showed that chronic nicotine reduces alpha-7 nicotinic acetylcholine receptor expression, affecting Ca^{2+} entry and cyclic AMP–dependent CFTR activation. Combined with the effects of tobacco smoke on other ion channels, including basolateral K^+ conductance,[10] and results from other studies of WCS,[10] CSE,[7,8] and cigarette smoke in vivo,[7] the data establish specific and clinically meaningful reductions in CFTR-dependent ion transport caused by cigarette smoke exposure. The levels of reduced CFTR activity caused by smoke exposure are similar to the severity of CFTR reductions observed in vivo among individuals with nonclassic CF,[60] a phenotype that frequently presents with adult-onset chronic bronchitis or bronchiectasis.[24] These findings can persist even in culture, suggesting the potential for epigenetic influences to maintain these abnormalities.

Given the deleterious effects of cigarette smoke on CFTR-dependent anion conductance, we also examined the impact of smoke exposure on mucus expression and transport in vitro, pathways severely affected in COPD. CSE generated a pronounced increase in mucus expression measured by in vitro staining,[6] which was also observed in human smokers.[61] To establish whether the potent effects of CSE also result in downstream alterations of mucus propulsion, we monitored transport of fluorescent particles placed on the apical surface of primary human airway epithelial cells following exposure to CSE. Mucus transport was severely reduced by CSE at 24 hours. Note that a large proportion of particles following CSE exposure were static because of entrapment in thick mucus (75% with CSE vs 11% with control; P<.05), a finding that is consistent with mucus expression studies and prior observations of enhanced mucus secretion caused by CSE exposure.[8] Combined with the observation that tobacco smoke reduces cilia beat frequency and ciliogenesis,[56,62,63] we hypothesize that reduced CFTR-mediated anion secretion, together with stimulated mucin expression, results in a mucus to fluid secretion imbalance, thus severely inhibiting mucus transport.

ACQUIRED CYSTIC FIBROSIS TRANSMEMBRANE CONDUCTANCE REGULATOR DYSFUNCTION IN PATIENTS WITH CHRONIC OBSTRUCTIVE PULMONARY DISEASE

Patients with Chronic Obstructive Pulmonary Disease Show Reduced Cystic Fibrosis Transmembrane Conductance Regulator Activity in the Upper and Lower Airways

Cantin and colleagues[7] were the first to describe that healthy cigarette smokers (confirmed to be wild-type CFTR homozygotes) show decreased CFTR activity. They documented a ~40% reduction in chloride transport in vivo by NPD (Fig. 1A). Acute reductions in chloride transport by NPD were also observed in healthy smokers immediately after smoke insufflation of the nares.[9] Others have shown reduced mucociliary clearance in the nose of smokers, and posited that this may be caused by acquired CFTR abnormalities. We established that individuals with smoking-related COPD show reduced CFTR expression (mRNA levels) and activity (~50% decrement) measured by NPD.[6] The defect in chloride conductance in smokers with and without COPD was not attributable to changes in mucosal integrity and seemed to be specific to CFTR, because no significant difference in potential difference was observed

following adenosine triphosphate perfusion, which stimulates activity of Cl^- channels other than CFTR. Reduced CFTR activity measured by NPD was also predictive of the severity of bronchitis symptoms as determined by the Breathless Cough and Sputum Score, even when controlled for cigarette smoking, indicating a significant association with the chronic bronchitis phenotype. Furthermore, individuals with a history of COPD exacerbations during the past year showed 35% less CFTR function than those without a history of exacerbations, a result that points to important clinical consequences associated with acquired defects in CFTR activity.[6]

To confirm whether these findings were also present in the lung, we conducted the first lower airway potential difference measurements performed under conscious sedation in patients with COPD. Results showed marked reductions in CFTR activity among affected subjects compared with controls (CFTR function ~50% of normal in patients with COPD and smokers; Fig. 1B).[12] Like NPD, CFTR decrements in lower airway potential difference were associated with chronic bronchitis as well as dyspnea. These results indicate that clinically relevant CFTR dysfunction is present in the lung and detectable with in vivo markers of CFTR activity. In addition to cigarette smoking, increased levels of neutrophil elastase may also play a role, because neutrophil elastase can induce CFTR degradation and is found in high levels in the COPD airway.[44]

Sustained and Systemic Cystic Fibrosis Transmembrane Receptor Defects in Chronic Obstructive Pulmonary Disease

Because COPD is known as a systemic disease with several nonpulmonary manifestations,[64,65] we studied patients using sweat chloride analysis (the hallmark diagnostic test for CF) in patients who did not harbor an asymptomatic CFTR mutation. Sweat chloride levels showed that the sweat gland, a site that is sensitive to CFTR function and representative of peripheral CFTR activity, was affected by cigarette smoking and COPD. This evidence included a sustained decrement after smoking cessation (Fig. 1C).[47] In light of the established nonlinear relationship between sweat chloride and CFTR activity,[60] the severity of CFTR dysfunction in the sweat duct was similar to that observed in the airway in individuals with CFTR-related disorders and other clinical manifestations of CFTR deficiency (ie, ~50% decrement, similar to the NPD studies; Fig. 1D). As in other studies in patients with COPD, CFTR dysfunction in the sweat gland was associated with chronic bronchitis (as measured by Breathless Cough and Sputum Score score), an effect that persisted even when smoking, COPD status, and body mass index were included in a multivariate regression model.[47] Sweat chloride increase greater than or equal to 35 mEq/L also indicated disease severity, because it was associated with more severe airflow limitation (ie, COPD GOLD stage [The Global Initiative for Chronic Obstructive Lung Disease]).[47] Confirmatory studies in human intestine were consistent with an acquired extrapulmonary CFTR deficit in smokers (60% decrement in CFTR activity[47]). To corroborate these findings, β-adrenergic sweat rate, an assay that is well suited to detect modest CFTR abnormalities,[66] was used to show reduced CFTR function in COPD (**Fig. 1**E) and was associated with dyspnea severity.[49] In addition, sweat rate steadily improved in healthy smokers following smoking cessation, suggesting causality. These results indicate that CFTR abnormalities in smoking-related COPD can occur at sites remote from direct inhalation even in individuals who no longer smoke, and correlate with symptoms of bronchitis and COPD severity.[14,15] These data also suggest that CFTR dysfunction may be transmitted systemically, and point to a potential mechanism underlying the increased incidence of systemic disorders attributed to smoking that are also strongly associated with CFTR abnormality, including idiopathic pancreatitis,[67] diabetes mellitus,[68–70] and male infertility.[71]

MEDIATORS OF CYSTIC FIBROSIS TRANSMEMBRANE CONDUCTANCE REGULATOR DYSFUNCTION IN CIGARETTE SMOKE

The systemic nature of CFTR dysfunction in patients with COPD suggests the presence of toxic agents derived from tobacco that affect CFTR in extrapulmonary tissues. Initial testing suggested that nicotine and cotinine did not affect CFTR function in vitro.[47] Acrolein is a highly reactive component of cigarette smoke known to cause deleterious effects by reacting with biological nucleophiles in proteins and DNA and forming adducts within the lungs.[72–75] Free acrolein levels in the serum of smokers with and without COPD determined by mass spectroscopy were increased compared with controls.[47] Serum proteins showed acrolein modifications in smokers, which is evidence that acrolein could induce post-translational modifications. Acrolein exposure caused acute and dose-dependent reductions in CFTR function in vitro and in vivo.[47] In addition, single-channel studies showed that acrolein

greatly reduced the open probability of CFTR, akin to cigarette smoke.[47] These data provide evidence that acrolein is an important contributor to CFTR dysfunction caused by smoking and may systemically transmit these defects beyond respiratory tissues. The rapid effect of acrolein on CFTR channel gating suggests that direct modification of nucleophilic amino acid residues on CFTR protein that are critical for channel opening may be occurring.

Cigarette smoking is also associated with chronic accumulation of cadmium and arsenic.[76] Cadmium has been shown to reduce CFTR expression via a microRNA-dependent pathway, reducing channel function. Moreover, cadmium levels in lung were correlated with COPD disease severity independent of the duration of cigarette smoking.[77,78] The level of arsenic, another highly toxic contaminant, is increased in smokers and reduces CFTR surface expression by enhancing its ubiquitination.[79] Note that environmental arsenic exposure, even in the absence of smoking, in Bangladeshi workers revealed significant reductions in CFTR function as detected by sweat chloride analysis and measures of pulmonary function.[80] Thus, cigarette smoke can affect CFTR expression and function via more than 1 mechanism, in addition to indirect effects such as oxidative stress, unfolded protein response, and ER stress that can adversely affect CFTR homeostasis.[28,81,82]

SECONDHAND SMOKING

Exposure to secondhand smoke (SHS) is associated with several respiratory diseases, including COPD.[83] Exposure to SHS causes delayed mucociliary clearance in never-smokers, and may contribute to chronic bronchitis.[84,85] Savitsky and colleagues,[10] showed that exposure to SHS, like mainstream smoke, significantly suppressed CFTR ion transport in vitro, which may explain delayed mucociliary clearance. Note that circulatory acrolein is highly enriched in SHS and may be present in even greater amounts than mainstream smoke, suggesting causality. Ni and colleagues[86] showed that SHS significantly reduces phagocytic clearance of pathogenic bacteria by affecting CFTR function in macrophages, extending potential manifestations beyond the airway. The detrimental effects of SHS warrant further investigation into the mechanistic basis and physiologic significance underlying airway epithelial dysfunction in passive smokers, including its potential to contribute to COPD and respiratory infections, such as acute bronchitis or otitis media in the young.[87,88]

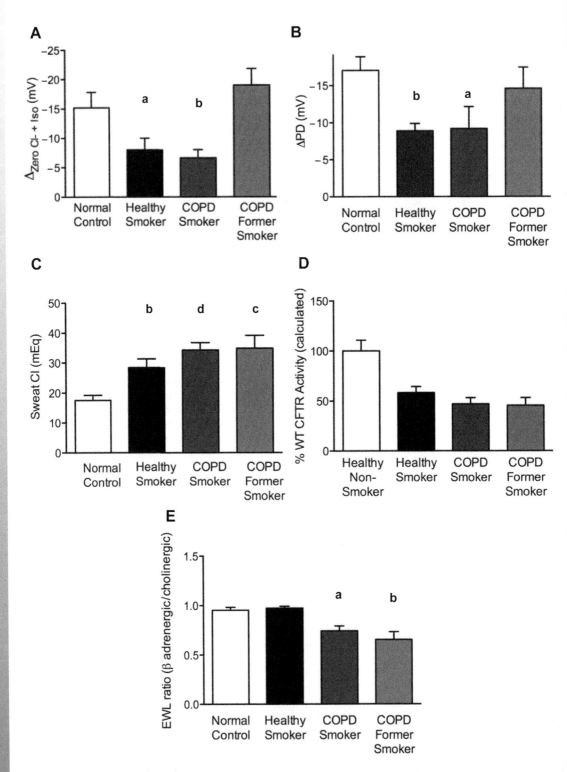

ACQUIRED CYSTIC FIBROSIS TRANSMEMBRANE RECEPTOR DYSFUNCTION AND ASTHMA

Asthma is an episodic airways disease[89] characterized by airway recruitment of eosinophils and CD4+ lymphocytes[89] that secrete an array of $T_{H}2$ (T helper 2) cytokines with varying phenotypes.[90,91] Predominant among these are interleukin (IL)-13, IL-4, and IL-5,[92] which have individually been targeted to treat severe asthma.[89] Persistence of this inflammatory process drives epithelial surface and glandular mucus metaplasia that characterizes the airways remodeling present in asthmatics.[93,94] The resultant mucus is pathologically distinct from that of normal people, particularly during status asthmaticus.[95] The abnormal mucus in asthmatics shares properties of CF mucus, including increased mucin density, high plasma protein concentration, and distinctly high protease levels (eg, neutrophil elastase).[94,95] Many of these features are present in patients with clinically severe asthma at the onset of neutrophil-associated inflammation.[96]

In asthma, airway metaplasia and pathologic alteration of mucus are associated with airway plugging[97] caused by impaired mucus clearance.[98,99] In addition, epithelial abnormalities may cause inherent ciliary dysmotility in severe asthmatics.[100] These processes cause episodic mucous plugging during acute exacerbations that complicate severe asthma.[97] In its most severe and chronic form, asthma that is affected by bronchiectasis has particularly poor outcomes, including increased infectious burden, exacerbation frequency, and poor treatment response, and is reminiscent of a mild form of CF.[101]

A large body of literature has examined the link between genetic abnormalities of the CFTR gene and the propensity for asthma.[102] Schroeder and colleagues[103] initially reported protection against bronchial asthma in patients heterozygous for Phe508del (also known as F508del), the most common CFTR mutation, although a larger Danish study, by Dahl and colleagues,[104] refuted this finding and noted an association with more severe airway obstruction in Phe508del heterozygotes.[104,105] This body of literature is inconclusive to determine whether the general population of patients with asthma has CFTR dysfunction.[106,107] However, more recent evidence suggesting a link

between neutrophilic bronchitis-type asthma and Phe508del heterozygosity[102,108] suggests a need to further phenotype patients with asthma to determine the populations most at risk for CFTR dysfunction.

In addition to the role of CFTR, non-CFTR anion channels have been implicated in modifying the mucus properties in murine asthma models. SLC26A9 and TMEM16A knockout mice show impaired mucociliary clearance, enhanced mucin production, and airway remodeling in response to induction of allergic asthma.[109,110] These findings provide further support that the ion transport environment is key to initiating and perpetuating asthma.

Because of the central role of CFTR in airway diseases, recent studies evaluated whether asthmatic inflammation may induce altered CFTR function in the absence of genetic mutations. In vitro studies by Skowron-zwarg and colleagues[111] showed that IL-13 exposure caused reduced mature protein levels at the plasma membrane surface in human airway epithelial cells, at least when cells were exposed to IL-13 before differentiation at the air-liquid interface. In contrast, chronic IL-13 exposure in mature human airway monolayers enhanced CFTR and Ca^{2+}-dependent chloride conductance, and reduced epithelial sodium channel (ENaC) activity.[112] Perhaps through a common signaling pathway, chronic IL-4 exposure had similar effects on CFTR and ENaC channels.[113] In vivo studies showed that CFTR activity in excised trachea of mice following intratracheal exposure of IL-13 was increased, complementing these more recent studies.[114] These findings were confirmed in a fungal exposure mouse model.[114] Although these models suggest increased, rather than reduced, CFTR currents with IL-13 and IL-4 exposures, these models have focused on pathways related primarily to allergic

---

Fig. 1. Acquired CFTR dysfunction in smokers and patients with COPD. (*A*) Reduced CFTR activity in smokers with and without COPD as measured by NPD (change in Cl^--free solution plus isoproterenol [Δ_{zero} Cl^- + Iso]). (*B*) Reduced CFTR activity in smokers with and without COPD measured by lower airway potential difference (PD) (change in Cl^--free solution plus isoproterenol). (*C*) Increased sweat chloride levels, a measure of CFTR activity, in smokers and patients with COPD. (*D*) Normalized CFTR activity estimated using sweat chloride values and corrected for the nonlinear relationship between sweat chloride level and CFTR function. (*E*) Reduced CFTR-dependent, β-adrenergic–stimulated sweat secretion measured by evaporative water loss (EWL) in patients with COPD. [a] $P<.05$, [b] $P<.01$, [c] $P<.001$, [d] $P<.0001$. % WT, mass percentage. (*Data from* [A] Sloane PA, Shastry S, Wilhelm A, et al. A pharmacologic approach to acquired cystic fibrosis transmembrane conductance regulator dysfunction in smoking related lung disease. PLoS One 2012;7:e39809; and [B] Dransfield MT, Wilhelm AM, Flanagan B, et al. Acquired cystic fibrosis transmembrane conductance regulator dysfunction in the lower airways in COPD. Chest 2013;144:498–506; and [C, D] Raju SV, Jackson PL, Courville CA, et al. Cigarette smoke induces systemic defects in cystic fibrosis transmembrane conductance regulator function. Am J Respir Crit Care Med 2013;188:1321–30; and [E] Courville CA, Tidwell S, Liu B, et al. Acquired defects in CFTR-dependent β-adrenergic sweat secretion in chronic obstructive pulmonary disease. Respir Res 2014;15:25.)

asthma. Whether these are relevant to severe, recalcitrant asthma, or during acute exacerbations, which tend to show neutrophil-dominated inflammation and more closely resemble CF and chronic bronchitis, remains an open question.

THERAPEUTIC APPROACHES

Because CF and COPD share phenotypic and pathophysiologic mechanisms, therapies initially directed toward CF have potential as treatments for COPD and other airways diseases. Although CF-specific mucolytic therapies for COPD have yielded marginal benefits,[115–117] as well as in non-CF bronchiectasis,[118] other mucolytic therapies show potential, including hypertonic saline.[119] To target the underlying common mechanism between chronic bronchitis, CF, and potentially specific phenotypes of asthma, an approach that addresses acquired CFTR dysfunction has been proposed, initially to study in patients with chronic bronchitis,[120] based on the concept that potentiation of wild-type CFTR may be beneficial in this population.[6] In addition, this approach with a systemically active agent may overcome the limitations of aerosolized therapies, which may show poor drug delivery to obstructed airways. Similarly, therapies that inhibit ENaC to address airway dehydration are under development.[6,121]

SUMMARY

Airway obstruction caused by mucus stasis is a consistent feature of many chronic airway diseases, including CF, COPD, and asthma. Their shared manifestations suggest that similarities in underlying pathologic mechanisms may be present. However, heterogeneity between phenotypes remains a challenge in defining common mechanisms. Emerging data regarding the physiologic role of CFTR, even in the absence of congenital CFTR mutations, indicate that acquired CFTR dysfunction may significantly contribute, particularly to phenotypes characterized by chronic bronchitis. Clear evidence in vitro indicates that cigarette smoking induces acquired CFTR dysfunction by several distinct mechanisms, including reduced expression, aberrant internalization, and disordered gating; these processes contribute to a partial deficiency of CFTR function, and, when accompanied by increased mucus expression, induce delayed mucociliary clearance. This evidence is supported by clinical evidence of CFTR functional decrements observed in smokers with and without COPD, and a consistent association with chronic bronchitis. Similar features may be present in neutrophilic asthma, although

eosinophil-dominated asthma seems to be protected to some extent from these maladaptive responses. Future work should focus on the therapeutic potential of these pathways to determine whether CFTR activation, or alternatively blocking detrimental effects on ion transport, confers clinically meaningful benefits.

FUNDING

This research is sponsored by the NIH (R01 HL105487 to S.M. Rowe, P30 DK072482 to S.M. Rowe, and 5UL1 RR025777) and the Cystic Fibrosis Foundation (CLANCY09Y0 to S.M. Rowe and R464-CF to S.M. Rowe). S.V. Raju is supported by American Lung Association (RG-305752) and the Flight Attendants Medical Research Association (YFA130008).

CONFLICTS OF INTEREST

G.M. Solomon has served on CF-related advisory boards for Bayer and Gilead. He has served as site principal investigator (PI) for contracted CF clinical trials sponsored by Nivalis Therapeutics. M.T. Dransfield has served on COPD-related advisory boards for Forest, GlaxoSmithKline, and Boehringer Ingelheim. He has served as site PI for contracted COPD clinical trials sponsored by GlaxoSmithKline and Boehringer Ingelheim. He has received COPD-related grant funding from National Heart, Lung and Blood Institute (NHLBI R01HL105487). The University of Alabama at Birmingham (UAB) received compensation for S.M. Rowe's role as a consultant for Vertex Pharmaceuticals, Novartis, and Galapagos for the design of CF clinical trials and sponsored research agreements. S.M. Rowe also served as PI for CF clinical trials sponsored by Vertex Pharmaceuticals and Novartis conducted at UAB. He has received COPD-related grant funding from NHLBI. The funders had no role in study design, data collection and analysis, decision to publish, or preparation of the article.

REFERENCES

1. Ford ES, Murphy LB, Khavjou O, et al. Total and state-specific medical and absenteeism costs of COPD among adults aged ≥ 18 years in the United States for 2010 and projections through 2020. Chest 2015;147(1):31–45.
2. Hoyert DL, Xu JQ. Deaths: preliminary data for 2011. Natl Vital Stat Rep 2012;61(6):1–65.
3. Vestbo J, Prescott E, Lange P. Association of chronic mucus hypersecretion with FEV1 decline and chronic obstructive pulmonary disease

morbidity. Copenhagen City Heart Study Group. Am J Respir Crit Care Med 1996;153:1530–5.

4. Vestbo J. Epidemiological studies in mucus hypersecretion. Novartis Found Symp 2002;248:3–12 [discussion: 12–9, 277–82].

5. Hogg JC, Chu F, Utokaparch S, et al. The nature of small-airway obstruction in chronic obstructive pulmonary disease. N Engl J Med 2004;350:2645–53.

6. Sloane PA, Shastry S, Wilhelm A, et al. A pharmacologic approach to acquired cystic fibrosis transmembrane conductance regulator dysfunction in smoking related lung disease. PLoS One 2012;7:e39809.

7. Cantin AM, Hanrahan JW, Bilodeau G, et al. Cystic fibrosis transmembrane conductance regulator function is suppressed in cigarette smokers. Am J Respir Crit Care Med 2006;173:1139–44.

8. Kreindler JL, Jackson AD, Kemp PA, et al. Inhibition of chloride secretion in human bronchial epithelial cells by cigarette smoke extract. Am J Physiol Lung Cell Mol Physiol 2005;288:L894–902.

9. Clunes LA, Davies CM, Coakley RD, et al. Cigarette smoke exposure induces CFTR internalization and insolubility, leading to airway surface liquid dehydration. FASEB J 2012;26(2):533–45.

10. Savitski AN, Mesaros C, Blair IA, et al. Secondhand smoke inhibits both Cl− and K+ conductances in normal human bronchial epithelial cells. Respir Res 2009;10:120.

11. Raju SV, Jackson PL, Courville CA, et al. Cigarette smoke induces systemic defects in cystic fibrosis transmembrane conductance regulator (CFTR) function. Am J Respir Crit Care Med 2013; 188(11):1321–30.

12. Dransfield MT, Wilhelm AM, Flanagan B, et al. Acquired cystic fibrosis transmembrane conductance regulator dysfunction in the lower airways in COPD. Chest 2013;144:498–506.

13. Rab A, Rowe SM, Raju SV, et al. Cigarette smoke and CFTR: implications in the pathogenesis of COPD. Am J Physiol Lung Cell Mol Physiol 2013; 305(8):L530–41.

14. Crystal RG. Are the smoking-induced diseases an acquired form of cystic fibrosis? Am J Respir Crit Care Med 2013;188:1277–8.

15. Jain M, Goss CH. Update in cystic fibrosis 2013. Am J Respir Crit Care Med 2014;189:1181–6.

16. Dolgin E. Orphan cystic fibrosis drugs find sister diseases. Nat Med 2011;17:397.

17. Cohn JA, Friedman KJ, Noone PG, et al. Relation between mutations of the cystic fibrosis gene and idiopathic pancreatitis. N Engl J Med 1998;339:653–8.

18. Sharer N, Schwarz M, Malone G, et al. Mutations of the cystic fibrosis gene in patients with chronic pancreatitis. N Engl J Med 1998;339:645–52.

19. Kerem E, Hirawat S, Armoni S, et al. Effectiveness of PTC124 treatment of cystic fibrosis caused by nonsense mutations: a prospective phase II trial. Lancet 2008;372:719–27.

20. Howard MT, Anderson CB, Fass U, et al. Readthrough of dystrophin stop codon mutations induced by aminoglycosides. Ann Neurol 2004;55:422–6.

21. Howard MT, Shirts BH, Petros LM, et al. Sequence specificity of aminoglycoside-induced stop codon readthrough: potential implications for treatment of Duchenne muscular dystrophy. Ann Neurol 2000;48:164–9.

22. Pignatti PF, Bombieri C, Benetazzo M, et al. CFTR gene variant IVS8-5T in disseminated bronchiectasis. Am J Hum Genet 1996;58:889–92.

23. Girodon E, Cazeneuve C, Lebargy F, et al. CFTR gene mutations in adults with disseminated bronchiectasis. Eur J Hum Genet 1997;5:149–55.

24. Knowles MR, Durie PR. What is cystic fibrosis? N Engl J Med 2002;347:439–42.

25. Mall MA, Hartl D. CFTR: cystic fibrosis and beyond. Eur Respir J 2014;44(4):1042–54.

26. Ratjen F, Doring G. Cystic fibrosis. Lancet 2003; 361:681–9.

27. Kellermayer R, Szigeti R, Keeling KM, et al. Aminoglycosides as potential pharmacogenetic agents in the treatment of Hailey-Hailey disease. J Invest Dermatol 2006;126:229–31.

28. Varga K, Goldstein RF, Jurkuvenaite A, et al. Enhanced cell-surface stability of rescued DeltaF508 cystic fibrosis transmembrane conductance regulator (CFTR) by pharmacological chaperones. Biochem J 2008;410:555–64.

29. Rowe SM, Miller S, Sorscher EJ. Cystic fibrosis. N Engl J Med 2005;352:1992–2001.

30. Rabe KF, Hurd S, Anzueto A, et al. Global strategy for the diagnosis, management, and prevention of chronic obstructive pulmonary disease: GOLD executive summary. Am J Respir Crit Care Med 2007;176:532–55.

31. Houghton AM, Quintero PA, Perkins DL, et al. Elastin fragments drive disease progression in a murine model of emphysema. J Clin Invest 2006; 116:753–9.

32. Bartoszewski R, Rab A, Jurkuvenaite A, et al. Activation of the unfolded protein response by deltaF508 CFTR. Am J Respir Cell Mol Biol 2008;39:448–57.

33. Saetta M, Turato G, Baraldo S, et al. Goblet cell hyperplasia and epithelial inflammation in peripheral airways of smokers with both symptoms of chronic bronchitis and chronic airflow limitation. Am J Respir Crit Care Med 2000;161:1016–21.

34. Martinez-Garcia MA, Soler-Cataluna JJ, Donat Sanz Y, et al. Factors associated with bronchiectasis in patients with COPD. Chest 2011;140: 1130–7.

35. Dransfield MT, Washko GR, Foreman MG, et al. Gender differences in the severity of CT emphysema in COPD. Chest 2007;132:464–70.

36. Hautamaki RD, Kobayashi DK, Senior RM, et al. Requirement for macrophage elastase for cigarette smoke-induced emphysema in mice. Science 1997;277:2002–4.

37. Lim S, Roche N, Oliver BG, et al. Balance of matrix metalloprotease-9 and tissue inhibitor of metalloprotease-1 from alveolar macrophages in cigarette smokers. Regulation by interleukin-10. Am J Respir Crit Care Med 2000;162:1355–60.

38. Turino GM. Proteases in COPD: a critical pathway to injury. Chest 2007;132:1724–5.

39. Shifren A, Mecham RP. The stumbling block in lung repair of emphysema: elastic fiber assembly. Proc Am Thorac Soc 2006;3:428–33.

40. Morgan L, Pearson M, de Iongh R, et al. Scintigraphic measurement of tracheal mucus velocity in vivo. Eur Respir J 2004;23:518–22.

41. Brown JS, Zeman KL, Bennett WD. Ultrafine particle deposition and clearance in the healthy and obstructed lung. Am J Respir Crit Care Med 2002;166:1240–7.

42. Moller W, Felten K, Sommerer K, et al. Deposition, retention, and translocation of ultrafine particles from the central airways and lung periphery. Am J Respir Crit Care Med 2008;177:426–32.

43. Hogg JC, Chu FS, Tan WC, et al. Survival after lung volume reduction in chronic obstructive pulmonary disease: insights from small airway pathology. Am J Respir Crit Care Med 2007;176:454–9.

44. Le Gars M, Descamps D, Roussel D, et al. Neutrophil elastase degrades cystic fibrosis transmembrane conductance regulator via calpains and disables channel function in vitro and in vivo. Am J Respir Crit Care Med 2012;187(2):170–9.

45. Bernard K, Rowe SM, Fan L, et al. Inhibition of CFTR-mediated Cl- current by neutrophil elastase. Pediatr Pulmonol 2008;(Suppl):31.

46. Guimbellot JS, Fortenberry JA, Siegal GP, et al. Role of oxygen availability in CFTR expression and function. Am J Respir Cell Mol Biol 2008;39:514–21.

47. Raju SV, Jackson PL, Courville CA, et al. Cigarette smoke induces systemic defects in cystic fibrosis transmembrane conductance regulator function. Am J Respir Crit Care Med 2013;188:1321–30.

48. Lambert JA, Raju SV, Tang LP, et al. CFTR activation by roflumilast contributes to therapeutic benefit in chronic bronchitis. Am J Respir Cell Mol Biol 2013;50(3):549–58.

49. Courville CA, Tidwell S, Liu B, et al. Acquired defects in CFTR-dependent β-adrenergic sweat secretion in chronic obstructive pulmonary disease. Respir Res 2014;15:25.

50. Friedlander AL, Lynch D, Dyar LA, et al. Phenotypes of chronic obstructive pulmonary disease. COPD 2007;4:355–84.

51. Prescott E, Almdal T, Mikkelsen KL, et al. Prognostic value of weight change in chronic obstructive pulmonary disease: results from the Copenhagen City Heart Study. Eur Respir J 2002;20:539–44.

52. Schols AM, Broekhuizen R, Weling-Scheepers CA, et al. Body composition and mortality in chronic obstructive pulmonary disease. Am J Clin Nutr 2005;82:53–9.

53. Tashkin DP, Altose MD, Connett JE, et al. Methacholine reactivity predicts changes in lung function over time in smokers with early chronic obstructive pulmonary disease. The Lung Health Study Research Group. Am J Respir Crit Care Med 1996;153:1802–11.

54. Han MK, Bartholmai B, Liu LX, et al. Clinical significance of radiologic characterizations in COPD. COPD 2009;6:459–67.

55. Welsh MJ. Cigarette smoke inhibition of ion transport in canine tracheal epithelium. J Clin Invest 1983;71:1614–23.

56. Cohen NA, Zhang S, Sharp DB, et al. Cigarette smoke condensate inhibits transepithelial chloride transport and ciliary beat frequency. Laryngoscope 2009;119:2269–74.

57. Moran AR, Norimatsu Y, Dawson DC, et al. Aqueous cigarette smoke extract induces a voltage-dependent inhibition of CFTR expressed in Xenopus oocytes. Am J Physiol Lung Cell Mol Physiol 2014;306:L284–91.

58. Rasmussen JE, Sheridan JT, Polk W, et al. Cigarette smoke-induced Ca2+ release leads to cystic fibrosis transmembrane conductance regulator (CFTR) dysfunction. J Biol Chem 2014;289:7671–81.

59. Maouche K, Medjber K, Zahm JM, et al. Contribution of alpha7 nicotinic receptor to airway epithelium dysfunction under nicotine exposure. Proc Natl Acad Sci U S A 2013;110:4099–104.

60. Wilschanski M, Dupuis A, Ellis L, et al. Mutations in the cystic fibrosis transmembrane regulator gene and in vivo transepithelial potentials. Am J Respir Crit Care Med 2006;174:787–94.

61. Innes AL, Woodruff PG, Ferrando RE, et al. Epithelial mucin stores are increased in the large airways of smokers with airflow obstruction. Chest 2006;130:1102–8.

62. Tamashiro E, Xiong G, Anselmo-Lima WT, et al. Cigarette smoke exposure impairs respiratory epithelial ciliogenesis. Am J Rhinol Allergy 2009;23:117–22.

63. Leopold PL, O'Mahony MJ, Lian XJ, et al. Smoking is associated with shortened airway cilia. PLoS One 2009;4:e8157.

64. Barnes PJ, Celli BR. Systemic manifestations and comorbidities of COPD. Eur Respir J 2009;33:1165–85.

65. Nussbaumer-Ochsner Y, Rabe KF. Systemic manifestations of COPD. Chest 2011;139:165–73.

66. Quinton P, Molyneux L, Ip W, et al. Beta-adrenergic sweat secretion as a diagnostic test for cystic fibrosis. Am J Respir Crit Care Med 2012;186(8):732–9.

67. Cote GA, Yadav D, Slivka A, et al. Alcohol and smoking as risk factors in an epidemiology study of patients with chronic pancreatitis. Clin Gastroenterol Hepatol 2010;9(3):266–73 [quiz: e27].

68. Xie XT, Liu Q, Wu J, et al. Impact of cigarette smoking in type 2 diabetes development. Acta Pharmacol Sin 2009;30:784–7.

69. Yeh HC, Duncan BB, Schmidt MI, et al. Smoking, smoking cessation, and risk for type 2 diabetes mellitus: a cohort study. Ann Intern Med 2010;152:10–7.

70. Gerber PA, Locher R, Schmid B, et al. Smoking is associated with impaired long-term glucose metabolism in patients with type 1 diabetes mellitus. Nutr Metab Cardiovasc Dis 2011;23(2):102–8.

71. Chia SE, Lim ST, Tay SK. Factors associated with male infertility: a case-control study of 218 infertile and 240 fertile men. BJOG 2000;107:55–61.

72. Uchida K, Kanematsu M, Morimitsu Y, et al. Acrolein is a product of lipid peroxidation reaction. Formation of free acrolein and its conjugate with lysine residues in oxidized low density lipoproteins. J Biol Chem 1998;273:16058–66.

73. Grafstrom RC, Dypbukt JM, Willey JC, et al. Pathobiological effects of acrolein in cultured human bronchial epithelial cells. Cancer Res 1988;48:1717–21.

74. Jia L, Liu Z, Sun L, et al. Acrolein, a toxicant in cigarette smoke, causes oxidative damage and mitochondrial dysfunction in RPE cells: protection by (R)-alpha-lipoic acid. Invest Ophthalmol Vis Sci 2007;48:339–48.

75. Kitaguchi Y, Taraseviciene-Stewart L, Hanaoka M, et al. Acrolein induces endoplasmic reticulum stress and causes airspace enlargement. PLoS One 2012;7:e38038.

76. Caruso RV, O'Connor RJ, Stephens WE, et al. Toxic metal concentrations in cigarettes obtained from U.S. smokers in 2009: results from the International Tobacco Control (ITC) United States survey cohort. Int J Environ Res Public Health 2014;11:202–17.

77. Rennolds J, Butler S, Maloney K, et al. Cadmium regulates the expression of the CFTR chloride channel in human airway epithelial cells. Toxicol Sci 2010;116:349–58.

78. Hassan F, Nuovo GJ, Crawford M, et al. MiR-101 and miR-144 regulate the expression of the CFTR chloride channel in the lung. PLoS One 2012;7:e50837.

79. Bomberger JM, Coutermarsh BA, Barnaby RL, et al. Arsenic promotes ubiquitinylation and lysosomal degradation of cystic fibrosis transmembrane conductance regulator (CFTR) chloride channels in human airway epithelial cells. J Biol Chem 2012;287:17130–9.

80. Mazumdar M, Christiani DC, Biswas SK, et al. Elevated sweat chloride levels due to arsenic toxicity. N Engl J Med 2015;372:582–4.

81. Cantin AM, Bilodeau G, Ouellet C, et al. Oxidant stress suppresses CFTR expression. Am J Physiol Cell Physiol 2006;290:C262–70.

82. Bartoszewski R, Rab A, Fu L, et al. CFTR expression regulation by the unfolded protein response. Methods Enzymol 2011;491:3–24.

83. Ebbert JO, Croghan IT, Schroeder DR, et al. Association between respiratory tract diseases and secondhand smoke exposure among never smoking flight attendants: a cross-sectional survey. Environ Health 2007;6:28.

84. Habesoglu M, Demir K, Yumusakhuylu AC, et al. Does passive smoking have an effect on nasal mucociliary clearance? Otolaryngol Head Neck Surg 2012;147:152–6.

85. Wu CF, Feng NH, Chong IW, et al. Second-hand smoke and chronic bronchitis in Taiwanese women: a health-care based study. BMC Public Health 2010;10:44.

86. Ni I, Ji C, Vij N. Second-hand cigarette smoke impairs bacterial phagocytosis in macrophages by modulating CFTR dependent lipid-rafts. PLoS One 2015;10:e0121200.

87. Lee PN, Chamberlain J, Alderson MR. Relationship of passive smoking to risk of lung cancer and other smoking-associated diseases. Br J Cancer 1986;54:97–105.

88. Lebowitz MD. Influence of passive smoking on pulmonary function: a survey. Prev Med 1984;13:645–55.

89. Olin JT, Wechsler ME. Asthma: pathogenesis and novel drugs for treatment. BMJ 2014;349:g5517.

90. Carolan BJ, Sutherland ER. Clinical phenotypes of chronic obstructive pulmonary disease and asthma: recent advances. J Allergy Clin Immunol 2013;131:627–34 [quiz: 35].

91. Wenzel SE. Asthma phenotypes: the evolution from clinical to molecular approaches. Nat Med 2012;18:716–25.

92. Robinson DS, Hamid Q, Ying S, et al. Predominant TH2-like bronchoalveolar T-lymphocyte population in atopic asthma. N Engl J Med 1992;326:298–304.

93. Jeffery PK. Remodeling in asthma and chronic obstructive lung disease. Am J Respir Crit Care Med 2001;164:S28–38.

94. Fahy JV, Dickey BF. Airway mucus function and dysfunction. N Engl J Med 2010;363:2233–47.

95. Sheehan JK, Richardson PS, Fung DC, et al. Analysis of respiratory mucus glycoproteins in asthma: a detailed study from a patient who died in status

asthmaticus. Am J Respir Cell Mol Biol 1995;13: 748–56.

96. Nakagome K, Matsushita S, Nagata M. Neutrophilic inflammation in severe asthma. Int Arch Allergy Immunol 2012;158(Suppl 1):96–102.

97. Evans CM, Kim K, Tuvim MJ, et al. Mucus hypersecretion in asthma: causes and effects. Curr Opin Pulm Med 2009;15:4–11.

98. Del Donno M, Bittesnich D, Chetta A, et al. The effect of inflammation on mucociliary clearance in asthma: an overview. Chest 2000;118:1142–9.

99. Pavia D, Bateman JR, Sheahan NF, et al. Tracheobronchial mucociliary clearance in asthma: impairment during remission. Thorax 1985;40:171–5.

100. Thomas B, Rutman A, Hirst RA, et al. Ciliary dysfunction and ultrastructural abnormalities are features of severe asthma. J Allergy Clin Immunol 2010;126:722–9.e2.

101. Oguzulgen IK, Kervan F, Ozis T, et al. The impact of bronchiectasis in clinical presentation of asthma. South Med J 2007;100:468–71.

102. Sandford A. The role of CFTR mutations in asthma. Can Respir J 2012;19:44–5.

103. Schroeder SA, Gaughan DM, Swift M. Protection against bronchial asthma by CFTR delta F508 mutation: a heterozygote advantage in cystic fibrosis. Nat Med 1995;1:703–5.

104. Dahl M, Tybjaerg-Hansen A, Lange P, et al. DeltaF508 heterozygosity in cystic fibrosis and susceptibility to asthma. Lancet 1998;351:1911–3.

105. Dahl M, Nordestgaard BG, Lange P, et al. Fifteen-year follow-up of pulmonary function in individuals heterozygous for the cystic fibrosis phenylalanine-508 deletion. J Allergy Clin Immunol 2001;107: 818–23.

106. Maurya N, Awasthi S, Dixit P. Association of CFTR gene mutation with bronchial asthma. Indian J Med Res 2012;135:469–78.

107. Noone PG, Knowles MR. 'CFTR-opathies': disease phenotypes associated with cystic fibrosis transmembrane regulator gene mutations. Respir Res 2001;2:328–32.

108. Goodwin J, Spitale N, Yaghi A, et al. Cystic fibrosis transmembrane conductance regulator gene abnormalities in patients with asthma and recurrent neutrophilic bronchitis. Can Respir J 2012;19:46–8.

109. Anagnostopoulou P, Riederer B, Duerr J, et al. SLC26A9-mediated chloride secretion prevents mucus obstruction in airway inflammation. J Clin Invest 2012;122:3629–34.

110. Huang F, Zhang H, Wu M, et al. Calcium-activated chloride channel TMEM16A modulates mucin secretion and airway smooth muscle contraction. Proc Natl Acad Sci U S A 2012;109:16354–9.

111. Skowron-zwarg M, Boland S, Caruso N, et al. Interleukin-13 interferes with CFTR and AQP5 expression and localization during human airway epithelial cell differentiation. Exp Cell Res 2007; 313:2695–702.

112. Danahay H, Atherton H, Jones G, et al. Interleukin-13 induces a hypersecretory ion transport phenotype in human bronchial epithelial cells. Am J Physiol Lung Cell Mol Physiol 2002;282: L226–36.

113. Galietta LJ, Pagesy P, Folli C, et al. IL-4 is a potent modulator of ion transport in the human bronchial epithelium in vitro. J Immunol 2002;168:839–45.

114. Anagnostopoulou P, Dai L, Schatterny J, et al. Allergic airway inflammation induces a prosecretory epithelial ion transport phenotype in mice. Eur Respir J 2010;36:1436–47.

115. Decramer M, Rutten-van Molken M, Dekhuijzen PN, et al. Effects of N-acetylcysteine on outcomes in chronic obstructive pulmonary disease (Bronchitis Randomized on NAC Cost-Utility Study, BRONCUS): a randomised placebo-controlled trial. Lancet 2005;365:1552–60.

116. Zheng JP, Kang J, Huang SG, et al. Effect of carbocisteine on acute exacerbation of chronic obstructive pulmonary disease (PEACE Study): a randomised placebo-controlled study. Lancet 2008;371:2013–8.

117. Poole PJ, Black PN. Mucolytic agents for chronic bronchitis or chronic obstructive pulmonary disease. Cochrane Database Syst Rev 2006;(3):CD001287.

118. O'Donnell AE, Barker AF, Ilowite JS, et al. Treatment of idiopathic bronchiectasis with aerosolized recombinant human DNase I. rhDNase Study Group. Chest 1998;113:1329–34.

119. Valderramas SR, Atallah AN. Effectiveness and safety of hypertonic saline inhalation combined with exercise training in patients with chronic obstructive pulmonary disease: a randomized trial. Respir Care 2009;54:327–33.

120. Clinical Trial. NCT02135432.

121. Astrand AB, Hemmerling M, Root J, et al. Linking increased airway hydration, ciliary beating, and mucociliary clearance through ENaC inhibition. Am J Physiol Lung Cell Mol Physiol 2015;308: L22–32.

Index

Note: Page numbers of article titles are in **boldface** type.

Clin Chest Med 37 (2016) 159–164
http://dx.doi.org/10.1016/S0272-5231(15)00166-5
0272-5231/16/$ – see front matter © 2016 Elsevier Inc. All rights reserved.

chestmed.theclinics.com

Moving?

Make sure your subscription moves with you!

To notify us of your new address, find your **Clinics Account Number** (located on your mailing label above your name), and contact customer service at:

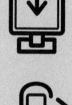

Email: journalscustomerservice-usa@elsevier.com

800-654-2452 (subscribers in the U.S. & Canada)
314-447-8871 (subscribers outside of the U.S. & Canada)

Fax number: 314-447-8029

Elsevier Health Sciences Division
Subscription Customer Service
3251 Riverport Lane
Maryland Heights, MO 63043

*To ensure uninterrupted delivery of your subscription,
please notify us at least 4 weeks in advance of move.

ELSEVIER

Printed and bound by CPI Group (UK) Ltd, Croydon, CR0 4YY

08/05/2025

01864680-0009

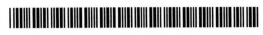